AF556011

Advanced
Extension & Communication Strategies for Sustainable Livelihood Through Animal Husbandry and Allied Farming System

NIPA® GENX ELECTRONIC RESOURCES & SOLUTIONS P. LTD.
New Delhi-110 034

About the Editors

Prof. (Dr). Arunasis Goswami, M.V.Sc, Ph.D., D.Litt., FNAVSc., is presently working as Professor in the Department of Veterinary & A.H. Extension Education, W.B. University of Animal & Fishery Sciences, 68, K.B. Sarani, Belgachia, Kolkata-700037, W.B., India since 2012. He has more than 34 years of vast professional Teaching-Research, Extension & Administrative working experience in various capacities in several reputed higher academic institutions as, University of Kalyani, W.B. State University, Dept. of Animal Resource Development, Govt. of West Bengal. Since 1987 in the state of West Bengal, India.

Dr. Sukanta Biswas, M.V.Sc., Ph.D. PGDAEM, FISRD (UK) Presently working as Associate Professor in the Department of Veterinary & A.H. Extension Education, W.B. University of Animal & Fishery Sciences, Mohanpur, Dist-Nadia, West Bengal-741235, India since 2019. He has more than 16 years of diversified professional Research, Teaching, Extension & Administrative working experience in various capacities in several reputed higher academic institutions, as-Uttar Banga Krishi Viswavidyalaya, and University of Kalyani since 2005 in the state of West Bengal, India.

Advanced Extension & Communication Strategies for Sustainable Livelihood Through Animal Husbandry and Allied Farming System

Chief Editor
Arunasis Goswami
M.V.Sc, Ph.D., D.Litt, FNAVSc.
Professor
Department of Veterinary & A.H. Extension Education
West Bengal University of Animal & Fishery Sciences
68, K.B. Sarani, Belgachia, Kolkata-700037, W.B., India

Editor
Sukanta Biswas
M.V.Sc., Ph.D., PGDAEM, FAVSc.
Associate Professor
Department of Veterinary & A.H. Extension Education
West Bengal University of Animal & Fishery Sciences
Mohanpur, Dist-Nadia, West Bengal-741235, India

NIPA® GENX ELECTRONIC RESOURCES & SOLUTIONS P. LTD.
New Delhi-110 034

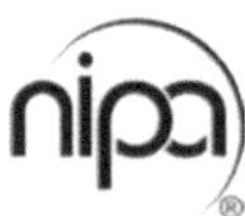

NIPA® GENX ELECTRONIC RESOURCES & SOLUTIONS P. LTD.

101,103, Vikas Surya Plaza, CU Block
L.S.C. Market, Pitam Pura, New Delhi-110 034
Ph : +91 11 27341616, 27341717, 27341718
E-mail: newindiapublishingagency@gmail.com
www: www.nipabooks.com
For customer assistance, please contact
Phone: + 91-11-27 34 17 17
Fax: + 91-11-27 34 16 16
E-Mail: feedbacks@nipabooks.com

ISBN: 978-93-94490-82-6

Composed and Designed by NIPA®.

Preface

The Book on *'Advanced Extension & Communication Strategies for Sustainable Livelihood Through A.H. & Allied Farming System'* is first of its kind is envisaging the importance of extension and communication skills for ushering the growth and development of animal husbandry and allied sectors in India by imbibing the elements of global perspectives and go for the animal Husbandry productivity. Though, the country is highest in milk and second highest producer of cattle and fish, but our contribution to the global market is not up to the desired level. The social ecology of animal husbandry practices are consisted of 536.76 Million no's of livestock distributed amongst 121.0 Million holdings of livestock owners that has invited extreme extension ad communication problems both at farmers and policy maker's level. The brunt of climate change has made the situation further precarious with the reveling truth, that in India alone around 230 million people are going to lose their livelihoods due to migratory impact of climate change.

The extension organization in the country along and across the layers of hierarchy, the decision making level are suffering from lack of professional skills, proper manpower planning and management, insufficient resource management skills and capability to deal with grassroots problems being confronted by the livestock farmers with every picking of times. Although, the KVKs in India have outnumbered 724 and denying the fact, that it is the world's largest number of farm science centers mentoring by any nations, they need to undergo further socialization processes to transform the technology into the voices of 130 million practicing stakeholders. The need of skill development and capacity building of the extension professionals at grass root and higher level of management are well discernible. This book, the first in arrow of this discipline from WBUAFS has accepted the challenge to befit the young scientist and teachers, working at SAU, SVU, KVKs and ICAR institutes with the advanced concept and methodology of communication and management skills having a match with global standards. That's why the aspect of ICT has been attuned to the skills in knowledge management, technology socialization, supply chain management and research prioritization techniques. In addition to that, the basic communication and management skills have been up scaled into problem solving skills, project management skills, social networking, conflict & stress management, emotional intelligence etc. have well been accommodated and supported by advanced research methodology and empirical studies.

The importance of extension & communication methodology has been well accepted by the professional of extension education and allied discipline. Considering the need and importance, this multi-authorship book is compiled to develop competency and efficiency of the extension performers of Pan India. We are confident and hopeful that, the compilation will fulfill its intended purpose for better development role play of the rural stakeholders through advanced as well as applied extension communication strategies in near future.

Prof. Arunasis Goswami
Dr. Sukanta Biswas

Contents

Theme-02: Applied Extension & Communication Strategies for Sustainable Livelihood Through Animal Husbandry and Allied Farming System

Theme-01

Advanced Extension and Communication Strategies for Sustainable Livelihood Through Animal Husbandry and Allied Farming System

1

Training and Capacity Building for Sustainable Entrepreneurship in Animal Husbandry and Allied Sector

Manas Mohan Adhikary
Bidhan Chandra Krishi Viswavidyalaya, Nadia, West Bengal

Training: The Concept

For any kind of development, resource is the basic condition and necessity. Every resource should undergo a process of refinement, up gradation, and integration for being able to contribute to a proper functioning and accomplishment. No exception to human resources, the most splendid and creative resource of the earth. While human resources are unique? The following are the reason:

(a) It can think and create

(b) It can integrate and coordinate

(c) It can ideate and communication

(d) It can support and sustain

Training and capacity building are the two most important component as well as intervention for nurturing, shaping, upgrading human resources to transform an "ordinary man" into an active human entity and there from into an extraordinary personality. This is a continuous and evolving process, its transform imparting cognitive skill and reaches to attend a high end perceptual skill. The other kinds of skills to be imparted and share are motivational skill and motor skill.

What is training?

Training is special and unique skill driven education which focuses on behavioral changes for attaining competency and proficiency for accomplishing a defined goal. While education aims at a comprehensive behavioral change by integrating all the basic component viz. knowledge, skill, attitude and understanding, training is extremely skill cantered and task oriented. These are the following differences or uniqueness between and off training and education.

Training and Education: A comparison

Training	Education
Skill based and task oriented learning	Comprehensive behavioral changes based on understanding and philosophy
It is sectorial	It is totalitarian
Task oriented	Objective oriented
Segmented by time	Arranged over time
Cost dominates in training	Purpose dominate in education
Psychomotor skill with the core feature	Psychosocial performances is the core feature
More applicable in job climate	More applicably in social and institutional climate
It is arranged chronologically and amenable to season and location	It is continuous and amenable to social context and greater ecological set-up..

Training and learning development

Conventional 'training' is required to cover essential work-related skills, techniques and knowledge, and much of this section deals with taking a positive progressive approach to this sort of traditional 'training'.

Lifelong learning and training

The evolution of training and its incessant contribution to personality building is basically a reflection of lifelong learning which results into a capacity building competency and ability to mettle on anything innovative and selective too a problem. (European Commission on Education and Training, 2006).

Improving knowledge through training: In the present knowledge World, collection, collation and integration of information, relevant and relegated to a defined job, is an essential process to be organized through training.

Improving skill in personal perspective: Personality is the combination of all behavioral and situational traits in which an individual expresses himself and get himself related to the surrounding people and institutions.

Improving in skill in civic and social perspective: Learning in improving skill as to socialize one personality in a given framework for social civic structure and in terms of its ethical content and conforming behavior.

Human Resource Management is concerned with the planning, acquisition, training & developing human beings for getting the desired objectives & goals set by the organization. The employees have to be transformed according to the organizations' & global needs. This is done through an organized activity called Training. Training is a process of learning a sequence of programmed behaviour. It is the application of knowledge & gives people an awareness of rules & procedures to guide their behaviour. It helps in bringing about positive change in the knowledge, skills & attitudes of employees. Thus, training is a process that tries to improve skills or add to the existing level of knowledge so that the employee is better equipped to do his present job or to mould him to be fit for a higher job involving higher responsibilities. It bridges the gap between what the employee has & what the job demands. Training is a continuous or never ending process. Even the existing employees need to be trained to refresh them & enable them to keep up with the new methods & techniques of work. This type of training is known as Refresher Training & the training given to new employees is known as Induction Training. Training plays a significant role in human resource development. Human resources are the lifeblood of any organization. Only through trained & efficient employees, can an organization achieve its objectives.

- To impart to the new entrants the basic knowledge & skills they need for an intelligent performance of definite tasks.
- To prepare employees for more responsible positions.
- To bring about change in attitudes of employees in all directions.
- To reduce supervision time, reduce wastage & produce quality products.
- To reduce defects & minimize accident rate.
- To absorb new skills & technology.
- Helpful for the growth & improvement of employee's skills & knowledge.

Successful training - that which produces the desired result - lies almost entirely in the hands of the trainer. In the trainer's hands lies the heavy responsibility for ensuring that the trainees achieve the maximum possible from the training. A measure of the success of training is the relationship that develops between trainer and trainees. In a sound, productive training situation there is mutual respect and trust between them, with the trainer taking care to ensure that even the weakest trainee performs to the highest possible level, and the trainees feeling a desire within themselves to achieve. In this situation the trainer is the motivator and the trainees are the motivated. It is intended that the modules that follow will be of assistance to those wishing to train and those already training.

It is important to note that all employees require different levels and types of development in order to fulfill their job role in the organization. All employees need some type(s) of training and development on an ongoing basis to maintain effective performance, or to adjust to new ways or work, and to remain motivated and engaged. The instructional systems design approach (often referred to as ADDIE model) is great for designing effective learning programs and used for instructional design. Instructional design is the process of designing, developing and delivering learning content. There are 5 phases in the ADDIE model: (1) needs assessment, (2) program design, (3) program development, (4) training delivery or implementation, and (5) evaluation of training.

- **Analyze** - problem identification, (TNA) training needs analysis, target audience determined, stakeholder's needs identified, identify the resources required.
- **Design** - learning intervention/implementation outline and mapped, mapping evaluation methods.
- **Development** - determine delivery method, production of learning product that is in line with design, determine instructional strategies/media/methods, quality evaluation of the learning product, development of communication strategy, development of required technology, development and evaluation of assessments and evaluation tools.
- **Implement** - participation in side-programs, training delivery, learning participation, implementation of a communication plan, evaluation of business, execution of formal evaluations.
- **Evaluation** - (integral part of each step) formal evaluation, continuous learning evaluation, evaluation of business, potential points of improvement.

There are many different training methods that exist today, including both on and off-the-job methods. On-the-job training methods happen within the organization where employees learn by working alongside co-workers in ways such as coaching, mentorship, apprenticeship, job rotation, job instructional technique (JIT), or by being an understudy. To contrast, off-the-job training methods happen outside the organization where employees attend things such as lectures, seminars, and conferences or they take part in simulation exercises like case studies and role-playing. It could also include vestibule, sensitivity or transactional training activities other training methods include:

- **Apprenticeship training:** system of training in which a worker entering the skilled trades is given thorough instruction and experience, both on and off the job, in the practical and theoretical aspects of the work.
- **Co-operative programs and internship programs:** training programs that combine practical, on-the-job experience with formal education. Typically these programs are offered at colleges and universities.

- **Classroom instruction:** information can be presented in lectures, demonstrations, films, and videotapes or through computer instruction. (This includes vestibule training where trainees are given instruction in the operation of equipment.)
- **Self-Directed Learning:** individuals work at their own pace during programmed instruction. Including books, manuals, or computers to break down subject-matter content into highly organized, logical sequences that demand a continuous response on the trainee's part.
- **Audio-visual:** methods used to teach the skills and procedures required for a number of jobs.
- **Simulation:** used when it is not practical or safe to train people on the actual equipment or within the actual work environment.
- **E-learning:** training that uses computer and/or online resources. Such as CBT (computer-based training), videotapes, satellites and broadcast interactive TV/DVD/CD-ROM.

Principles

When a company puts its employees through training programs, it must ensure that they are efficient and relevant to the employees' tasks in the organization as it is estimated that only 20-30% of training given to employees are used in the month later. To help mitigate this issue, some general principles should be followed to increase employees desire to take part in the program. These include:

1. **Self-efficacy:** These means to increase the learner's belief that they can fully comprehend the teachings.
2. **Attitude:** An uncooperative attitude towards learning could hinder the individual's capability to grasp the knowledge being provided.
3. **Competence:** This is the skill an individual develops that enables them to make good decisions in an efficient manner.
4. **External motivators:** These are the behaviors individuals present when a reward or extrinsic goal is given to them.

Motivation is an internal process that leads to an employee's behavior and willingness to achieve organizational goals. Creating a motivational environment within an organization can help ensure employees achieve their highest level of productivity. Motivation can create an engaged workforce that enhances individual and organizational performance. The model for motivation is represented at the most basic level by motivators separated into two different categories:

Intrinsic factors: These represent the internal factors to an individual, such as the difficulty of the work, achievement recognition, responsibility, opportunity for meaningful work, involvement in decision making, and importance within the organization.

Extrinsic factors: These are external factors to the individual, such as job security, salary, benefits, work conditions, and vacations.

Need for Training Policy

To ensure consistency in training and development function, the HR department of each organization develops a suitable training policy, defining the scope, objective, philosophy, and techniques. Such a training policy serves the following purposes:

- It defines what the organization intends to accomplish through training;
- It indicates the type of persons to be responsible for training functions;
- It identifies the formal and informal nature of training;
- It spells out the duration, time, and place of training;
- It indicates the need for engaging outside institutions for training;
- It embraces and includes training about the labor policies of the organization.

Methods for Determining Training Needs

HRM experts have identified the different methods for the identification of training needs.

These methods are briefly discussed below:

- Observation and analysis of job performance;
- Management recommendations;
- Staff conferences and recommendations;
- Analysis of job requirements;
- Consideration of current and projected changes;
- Surveys, reports, and inventories;
- Once it has been determined that training is necessary, training goals must be established. Management should state what changes or results are sought for each employee.

Features of training

- Increases knowledge and skills for doing a particular job; it bridges the gap between job needs and employee skills, knowledge and behaviour.

- Focuses attention on the current job specific and addresses particular performance deficits or problems.
- Concentrate on individual employees changing what employers know, how they work, attitudes toward their work or their interactions with their co-workers or supervisors.
- Tends to be more narrowly focused and oriented towards short term performance concerns.

Training is needed to serve the following purpose

- Newly recruited employees require training so as to perform their tasks effectively. Instructions guidance and coaching help them to handle jobs competently without any wastage.
- Training is necessary to prepare existing employees for higher level jobs (promotion) Existing employees require refresher training so as to keep abreast of the latest development in job operations. In the face of rapid technological changes, this is an absolute necessity.
- Training is necessary when a person moves from one job to another (transfer). After training the employee can change job quickly, improve his performance levels and achieve career goals comfortably.
- Training is necessary to make employees mobile and versatile. They can be placed on various jobs depending on organizational needs.
- Training is needed to bridge the gap between what the employees have and what the job demands. Training is needed to make employees more productive and useful in the long run.
- Training is needed for employees to again acceptance from peers (learning a job quickly and being able to pull their weight is one of the best ways for them to gain acceptance.

Capacity Building Programme

Training & capacity building is an important step to obtain, improve, retain skill & knowledge required to do job competently. To build capacity & create a sustainable Quality culture various training, workshops & courses are led by Quality Improvement division of NHSRC. It targets the health professionals viz. Hospital Superintendents, Quality Managers, Matrons & Nursing Superintendents, Health Administrators, Hospital Managers, Nodal officers for Quality Assurance in State health departments/ NHM, Members of Quality Assurance Teams, Committees and Units, Quality Assessors, Health programme managers, etc.

Capacity Building can be defined as "activities which strengthen the knowledge, abilities, skills and behavior of individuals and improve institutional structures and processes such that the organization can efficiently meet its mission and goals in a sustainable way. Training is one of the essential components of capacity building.

Employ science-based approaches, and local and indigenous knowledge, while undertaking research and development, to improve plant varieties, livestock and soil. Encourage development and adoption of locally appropriate farming systems and agricultural practices.

- Promote the use of soil conservation and improvement techniques, including integrated.
- Nutrient management and nutrient use efficiency
- Promote sound water management and saving
- Strengthen research, education and extension that advance the practice of sustainable agriculture and rural development. Improve linkages among research, instruction in schools and universities, and diffusion of knowledge by extension services.
- Expand agricultural extension services to help small holders to access and take advantage of modern information and communication technology
- Strengthen multi-stakeholder participation and partnerships.
- Foster expanded scientific and technical cooperation, including North-South and South-South cooperation, . . . Sustainable bio-energy production, arid and semi-arid agriculture, and combating desertification
- Diffuse more widely pre-and post-harvest technologies . . .
- Strengthen the assistance from the UN System and all relevant international organizations . . . To help farmers . . . Increase production and integrate with markets.
- **CRED'** Capacity Building and Training Programme enables people, communities and organizations to strengthen their capabilities to develop, implement and maintain effective health sector services. The programme also provides guidance and support on preventing and responding to disasters, conflicts and other humanitarian emergencies.
- The Centre develops implements and evaluates training materials and courses to help international agencies, national governments, non-governmental organizations, research institutes and schools of public health strengthen their technical capacity in emergency public health management.
- CRED strives to improve disaster management capacities through institutional and community capacity-building, information and data management, and

partnerships. In addition, the Centre provides training in public health, epidemiology, natural disaster management and complex emergency intervention.

Summer Course: Assessing Public Health in Emergency Situations (APHES)

This two-week intensive course is designed to familiarize professionals with the epidemiological techniques to determine the health impacts of disasters and conflicts. The course covers the different uses of quantitative tools for the assessment of the health needs of populations affected by catastrophic events. Participants are also given the chance to put the knowledge acquired during theoretical classes into practice.

The course is taught by an international faculty comprised of reputable professors from a range of prestigious Institutions. Topics covered include malnutrition, infectious diseases, mortality, morbidity, mental health, reproductive health, and population displacement.

Why Entrepreneurial Training Development

Training aimed at developing entrepreneurial competence in potential individuals is called entrepreneurial training. Motivating probable entrepreneurs, assisting. these individuals in endeavor to do the appropriate activities and enterprises, improving their enterprise development skills, and facilitating them to make economically and technically feasible project reports are the main activities of entrepreneurial training programmes. The different types of motivational inputs include the wide array of tests, role plays, psychological games, goal-setting exercise and so on. Helping the individuals to have a better understanding of their entrepreneurial personality, changing self-concept and values with the help of self-study and creating the supportive entrepreneurial behavior arc the main motives of these inputs.

Developing Course Content

For various EDPs which are conducted in the country, normally a uniform course curriculum is adopted by the ED institutes. Total 30-35 participants are taken in a group and the training goes for 4-6 weeks. Throughout the training module, the following inputs are normally covered which can be seen as appropriate for having the basic knowledge related to entrepreneurship and enterprise:

1. **Basics of Entrepreneurship:** In this input, the basics of entrepreneurship like its meaning, history, features, qualities, significance, advantages of being an entrepreneur, role in economic development of the country, etc., are discussed with the potential entrepreneurs.

2. **Motivational Inputs:** Various motivational inputs are included in the training course so as to develop entrepreneurial competencies in the potential entrepreneurs. These inputs are called Achievement Motivation Training (AMT). The main objectives of AMT are to enhance the confidence, self-awareness, innovativeness, achievement need, and other entrepreneurial skills among the entrepreneurs. Behavioral psychology techniques are also used here.
3. **Management Inputs:** For starting a new venture and making it profitable, it is very necessary to inculcate management concepts in potential entrepreneurs. That is why, basic management functions like production, marketing, finance and labour relations are taught to them.
4. **Support System and Procedure:** Different supporting institutions are available to support the entrepreneurs and the entrepreneurial ventures. The participants are introduced to the supporting institutions and their schemes and roles.
5. **Project Feasibility Study:** The information related to prospective business opportunities present in the area where EDP is conducted is provided to the trainees. Once the trainees select some business opportunities, assistance is provided to them for preparing the project feasibility reports to be submitted to the banks and various other financial institutions.
6. **Field Visits/Industrial Exposure:** The course curriculum also includes industrial visits so that the trainees can have a real life exposure to industrial activities. Apart from this, first-hand knowledge and exposure related to the various issues and opportunities in industrial enterprises can be gained with the help of industrial visits.
7. **Technical Knowledge:** It is very important for the entrepreneurs to have the technical knowledge about the selected field of enterprise. Therefore, the trainees are required to have information about the economic aspects of the technology such as costs and benefits associated with a particular technology.
8. **Market Survey:** Since, the entrepreneurs should also have enough knowledge about how a market operates, therefore, EDPs also provide the trainees with opportunities to conduct market surveys for project of their choice.

   Various experienced entrepreneurs who have successfully established their businesses are called in these training programmes to share their life experiences with the upcoming entrepreneurs. They serve as role models for the budding entrepreneurs.

Method of Entrepreneurial Training

The various methods of providing training to the entrepreneurs are as follows:

1. **Lecture Method:** As the name suggests, lecture method involves providing information to the trainees orally. In case of any doubt arising in the minds of trainees, clarification can be given spontaneously by the instructors.
2. **Written Instructional Method:** When the training contents are to be used in the future by the trainees, this method is used and it is most popular in case of standardized production system.
3. **Individual Instruction:** In this method, only one person is chosen for providing entrepreneurial training. When a tough skill is to be imparted in the candidate, this type of training becomes very useful.
4. **Group Instruction:** When the training is to be provided to the group of different individuals, this method is adopted particularly when these persons have to perform the same type of activities and similar instructions are to be given to all the candidates.
5. **Demonstration Method:** This method is mainly useful when the physical exposure is to be imparted by the trainer. In this method, the main focus is on providing practical knowledge rather than theoretical knowledge.
6. **Meetings:** This method of training mainly involves the group of people to discuss the different issues faced by them. They share their views, ideas and different conclusions are drawn on the basis of various alternatives and suggestions.
7. **Conference:** This method is generally used for imparting knowledge regarding new ideas and techniques to the trainees. Here, conferences are organized and experts from different fields are called to share their knowledge and experiences useful for the trainees.

2

Communication Styles for Extension Organizations

V.K. Jayaraghavendra Rao

ICAR-Indian Institute of Horticultural Research Bangaluru, Karnataka

Extension organizations are highly sociable organizations with a definite purpose of using the grass root principle and democratic leadership in bringing transience in the organization and society. In this direction the communication styles most suited for these extension functionaries in bringing these transitions need to be studied and understood and developed for effective functioning of these organizations as nucleus of change in transforming societies for development

Learning to identify the different communication styles - and recognizing which one we use most often in our daily interactions with friends, family and colleagues - is essential if we want to develop effective, assertive communication skills. But how can we tell the difference between the styles, and is there a time and place for each one in certain situations?

Being assertive means respecting yourself and other people. It is the ability to clearly express your thoughts and feelings through open, honest and direct communication.

Becoming more assertive does not mean that you will always get what you want - but, it can help you achieve a compromise. And even if you don't get the outcome you want, you will have the satisfaction of knowing that you handled the situation well, and that there are no ill feelings between you and the other person or people involved in the discussion.

Communicating assertively is not a skill reserved for the very few – anyone can do it - but, it does take time and practice if it is not how you are used to communicating. Fortunately, it is a technique you can practice and master at home in your own time – either by yourself or with a friend you can trust to give you honest feedback. Remember to also think about how the person you are talking to may react and how best you might cope with this.

Personality Differences

All extension professionals recruited do not have the same communication style and variety is a fact of group life. No matter how skilled, prepared, motivated and responsible the individuals involved in a group, personality differences exist. Personality "difference" is not the same as personality conflict. Differences can often *lead* to conflict, however, if they are

1. Not understood,
2. Blamed on ethical or intellectual failure rather than individual or cultural preferences, or
3. Not discussed until emotions get out of hand.

Sometimes people think it is impolite to talk about differences honestly. (Your mother probably taught you not to point at kids who were "different.") In other situations, people just don't have the vocabulary to talk about differences productively. (You never learned any other way to describe "weird" people.) Either way, differences can get in the way of group work. Because they can't be discussed productively, they can easily turn into conflict.

Communication Styles

Although the communication styles of individuals in extension organizations might be unfamiliar and even uncomfortable, your communication and work preferences are something you *need* to be able to talk about with your co-workers, supervisors and colleagues in order to work successfully with them. You need to know what you are good at, and what you will need others on your work team to help you with. You need to be able to describe the things that you can only do for a little while, as well as the things are that you'd be happy to do for the rest of your life. Most important for group work, you need to be comfortable explaining to others on your work team how you work best, what you don't do well, and what you can promise to do better than most other people. Your communication style is the "you" that is on display every day—the outer pattern of behavior that others see. If your style is very different from the other person's, it may be difficult for the two of you to develop rapport.

Communication-style bias is a state of mind experienced when we have contact with another person whose communication style is different from our own.

- The learning objective of this session would be
- Discuss influence of communication style bias on relationship process

- Explain benefits of understanding communication styles
- Identify two key dimensions of communication style model
- List and describe four major communication styles in model
- Learn to identify your preferred style and that of your customer
- Learn to overcome communication style bias with style flexing

Communication-Style Principles

- Communication style is a way of thinking and behaving.
- Individual style differences tend to be stable.
- There is a finite number of communication styles.
- We make judgments about people based on communication style.

Improving Relationship Skills

- First Goal—Understand your own communication preferred style
- Second Goal—Develop greater understanding for different styles
- Third Goal—Manage selling relationships by adapting style "style-flexing"

Communication Styles

Before deciding that you would like to communicate assertively, you need to have an understanding of what your usual style of communication is. There are five communication styles, and while many of us may use different styles in different situations, most will fall back on one particular style, which we use as our 'default' style.

The Five Communication Styles

1. Assertive
2. Aggressive
3. Passive-aggressive
4. Submissive
5. Manipulative

Different sorts of behavior and language are characteristic of each.

The Assertive Style

Assertive communication is born of high self-esteem. It is the healthiest and most effective style of communication - the sweet spot between being too aggressive and too passive. When we are assertive, we have the confidence to communicate without resorting to games or manipulation. We know our limits and don't allow ourselves to be pushed beyond them just because someone else wants or needs something from us. Surprisingly, however, Assertive is the style most people use least.

Behavioral Characteristics

- Achieving goals without hurting others
- Protective of own rights and respectful of others' rights
- Socially and emotionally expressive
- Making your own choices and taking responsibility for them
- Asking directly for needs to be met, while accepting the possibility of rejection
- Accepting compliments

Non-Verbal Behavior

- Voice – medium pitch and speed and volume
- Posture – open posture, symmetrical balance, tall, relaxed, no fidgeting
- Gestures – even, rounded, expansive
- Facial expression – good eye contact
- Spatial position – in control, respectful of others

Language

"Please would you turn the volume down? I am really struggling to concentrate on my studies."

"I am so sorry, but I won't be able to help you with your project this afternoon, as I have a dentist appointment."

People on the Receiving end Feel

They can take the person at their word

They know where they stand with the person

The person can cope with justified criticism and accept compliments

The person can look after themselves

Respect for the person

The Aggressive Style

This style is about winning – often at someone else's expense. An aggressive person behaves as if their needs are the most important, as though they have more rights, and have more to contribute than other people. It is an ineffective communication style as the content of the message may get lost because people are too busy reacting to the way it's delivered.

Behavioral Characteristics

- Frightening, threatening, loud, hostile
- Willing to achieve goals at expense of others
- Out to "win"
- Demanding, abrasive
- Belligerent
- Explosive, unpredictable
- Intimidating
- Bullying

Non-Verbal Behavior

- Voice – volume is loud
- Posture – 'bigger than' others
- Gestures – big, fast, sharp/jerky
- Facial expression – scowl, frown, glare
- Spatial position – Invade others' personal space, try to stand 'over' others

Language

"You are crazy!"

"Do it my way!"

"You make me sick!"

"That is just about enough out of you!"

Sarcasm, name-calling, threatening, blaming, insulting.

People on the Receiving end Feel

Defensive, aggressive (withdraw or fight back)

Uncooperative

Resentful/Vengeful

Humiliated/degraded

Hurt

Afraid

A loss of respect for the aggressive person

Mistakes and problems are not reported to an aggressive person in case they "blow up'. Others are afraid of being railroaded, exploited or humiliated.

The Passive-Aggressive Style

This is a style in which people appear passive on the surface, but are actually acting out their anger in indirect or behind-the-scenes ways. Prisoners of War often act in passive-aggressive ways in order to deal with an overwhelming lack of power. People who behave in this manner usually feel powerless and resentful, and express their feelings by subtly undermining the object (real or imagined) of their resentments – even if this ends up sabotaging themselves. The expression "Cut off your nose to spite your face" is a perfect description of passive-aggressive behaviour.

Behavioral Characteristics

- Indirectly aggressive
- Sarcastic
- Devious
- Unreliable
- Complaining
- Sulky
- Patronizing
- Gossips

Two-faced - Pleasant to people to their faces, but poisonous behind their backs (rumors, sabotage etc.) People do things to actively harm the other party e.g. they sabotage a machine by loosening a bolt or put too much salt in their food.

Non-Verbal Behavior

- Voice – Often speaks with a sugary sweet voice.
- Posture – often asymmetrical – e.g. standing with hand on hip, and hip thrust out (when being sarcastic or patronizing)
- Gestures – Can be jerky, quick
- Facial expression – Often looks sweet and innocent
- Spatial position – often too close, even touching other as pretends to be warm and friendly

Language

Passive-aggressive language is when you say something like "Why don't you go ahead and do it; my ideas aren't very good anyway" but maybe with a little sting of irony or even worse, sarcasm, such as "You always know better in any case."

"Oh don't you worry about me, I can sort myself out – like I usually have to."

People on the Receiving end Feel

Confused

Angry

Hurt

Resentful

The Submissive Style

This style is about pleasing other people and avoiding conflict. A submissive person behaves as if other peoples' needs are more important, and other people have more rights and more to contribute.

Behavioral Characteristics

- Apologetic (feel as if you are imposing when you ask for what you want)
- Avoiding any confrontation
- Finding difficulty in taking responsibility or decisions
- Yielding to someone else's preferences (and discounting own rights and needs)
- Opting out
- Feeling like a victim
- Blaming others for events
- Refusing compliments
- Inexpressive (of feelings and desires)

Non-Verbal Behavior

- Voice – Volume is soft
- Posture – make themselves as small as possible, head down
- Gestures – twist and fidget
- Facial expression – no eye contact
- Spatial position – make themselves smaller/lower than others

Submissive behavior is marked by a martyr-like attitude (victim mentality) and a refusal to try out initiatives, which might improve things.

Language

"Oh, it's nothing, really."

"Oh, that's all right; I didn't want it anymore."

"You choose; anything is fine."

People on the Receiving end Feel

Exasperated

Frustrated

Guilty

You don't know what you want (and so discount you)

They can take advantage of you.

Others resent the low energy surrounding the submissive person and eventually give up trying to help them because their efforts are subtly or overtly rejected.

The Manipulative Style

This style is scheming, calculating and shrewd. Manipulative communicators are skilled at influencing or controlling others to their own advantage. Their spoken words hide an underlying message, of which the other person may be totally unaware.

Behavioral Characteristics

- Cunning
- Controlling of others in an insidious way – for example, by sulking
- Asking indirectly for needs to be met
- Making others feel obliged or sorry for them.
- Uses 'artificial' tears

Non-Verbal Behavior

- Voice – Patronizing, envious, ingratiating, often high pitch
- Facial expression – Can put on the 'hang dog" expression

Language

"You are so lucky to have those chocolates, I wish I had some. I can't afford such expensive chocolates."

"I didn't have time to buy anything, so I had to wear this dress. I just hope I don't look too awful in it." ('Fishing' for a compliment).

People on the Receiving end Feel

Guilty

Frustrated

Angry, irritated or annoyed

Resentful

Others feel they never know where they stand with a manipulative person and are annoyed at constantly having to try to work out what is going on.

The Benefits of Understanding the Different Styles of Communication

A good understanding of the five basic styles of communication will help you learn how to react most effectively when confronted with a difficult person. It will also help you recognize when you are not being assertive or not behaving in the most effective way. Remember, you always have a choice as to which communication style you use. Being assertive is usually the most effective, but other styles are, of course, necessary in certain situations – such as being submissive when under physical threat (a mugging, hijacking etc.).

Good communication skills require a high level of self-awareness. Once you understand your own communication style, it is much easier to identify any shortcomings or areas which can be improved on, if you want to start communicating in a more assertive manner.

If you're serious about strengthening your relationships, reducing stress from conflict and decreasing unnecessary anxiety in your life, practice being more assertive. It will help you diffuse anger, reduce guilt and build better relationships both personally and professionally.

Remember the first rule of effective communication: The success of the communication is the responsibility of the communicator.

Based on the sociable and dominance continuums and ideal extension organization/worker should have a high sociable and least dominance communication style , however it may vary with the situation and one may have to do adapt a style called as "style-flexing". Based on this we have four communicating styles as shown in the figure below:

1. Emotive- characterized by high sociability and high dominance
2. Director-characterized by low sociability and high dominance

3. Reflective-characterized by low sociability and low dominance
4. Supportive- characterized by high sociability and low dominance

Although it appears that the 4th communication style with high sociability and low dominance suits extension organizations other styles need not be discounted for as they are suitable on other situations.

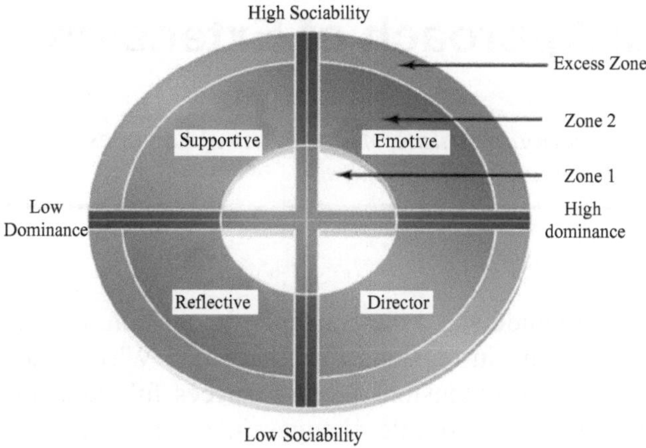

Conclusion

Communication styles of individuals need to be integrated in the organizational and client expectations by way of "style-flexing" and adapting new styles suitable to extension organizations. As far as possible facilitating and less dominating styles are suited for extension organizations however the other styles could be adopted based on situations. Eg., Emotive style to motivate employees, Director style to deal with theory x type individuals, and reflective style in controversial situations and supportive style in situation based extension systems.

Activity – Communication Style Self-Assessment

On each line, read the 4 choices, and select (by placing a checkmark) the word or phrase that is most descriptive of you. There is no such thing as a 'best' style, so do not choose what sounds 'best'. Choose one per line working from left to right, going across.

3

Paradigm Shift in Role of Extension Educationist with Special Reference to Educational Approach of Extension

Basavaprabhu Jirli

Department of Extension Education, Institute of Agricultural Sciences Banaras Hindu University, Varanasi, Uttar Pradesh

Introduction

Enough literature is available to understand the concept of extension. But are there any efforts to understand the in-tensions of ex-tension? Why should we emphasize on inner tensions of extension? to be a successful extension professional for bringing about the desirable changes in the behaviour of stakeholders, we need to understand the inner-tensions of extension in addition to the concept of extension.

Since inception of extension services, the model adopted for transfer of technology was dominated Technology, wherein the core emphasis was on the transfer of technology. The end product was the partial adoption of the technology or non-adoption of the technology. Learning from the experiences, modifications were made in the model and came out with extension mediated technology transfer system, wherein the technology is inseparable component of extension, which was combined with the human element or the societal element. The approaches adopted by different models of extension service delivery were also diverse.

The first model of extension service delivery the Public extension system or the Ministry of Agriculture, which delivers the extension services in the form of a systems approach. The relationship with the farmers or the end users is 'take it or leave it'. Whether the receivers are gaining it or not, whether they do understand it or not, ultimately we are transferring it, and are ending it with the target oriented approach.

The second model was participatory approach of extension service delivery. The relationship with the farmers was 'take it or demand different packages of programs', wherein we can see the approaches of extension that were adopted in the post 1990's have invariably participatory in nature. People started demanding the things, wherein the Ministry of Agriculture and farmers associations came together.

The third model was the private extension efforts, the examples like the contract farming, wherein everything is compulsory. This model emphasizes on profit. The approach and the relationship with the end users is more of a 'compulsion on the receivers'. Many reports till date reveal that, the end users are being exploited to the maximum extent because of the lack of the legal support systems. In all these three models the end user is the most deprived entity. How we can overcome these types of situations? The way out can be by understanding the basic processes of extension, the fundamentals of extension, which include in the definition of the In-Tension of Ex-Tension.

The concept of In-Tension of Ex-Tension has been conceptualized as the degree to which

The philosophy, the content, ideas, objectives, techniques, principles, theory and models of extension have been internalized by extensionist.

Let's understand the concept of In-Tension of Ex-Tension in right perspective. As an extension professional while delivering the extension services, the first and foremost question to be asked to oneself is, whether I am making use of principles of extension in my service approach?, whether I am delivering extension services as per objectives of extension? Whether, I am exploiting the dimensions of extension in my service delivery efforts? Whether, can I visualize implications of the processes of extension and methods of extension? These are the basic questions that extension professionals need to put to oneself before delivering extension services or acting as an extension professional.

The moment we ask such these questions, the emerging answer is leading towards the holistic approach of extension. That is what is the role of an extension educationist, to give due emphasis on the inner-tensions of extension. The extension educationist is providing you the basic inputs that are necessary for the process of transfer of technology. When we go through the evaluation reports of many of the developmental programs, one thing that is mentioned in all the reports in common is, the extension professionals were loaded with the technology, but lack in skills/technology of extension. Means the extension technology is missing, but the "technology" *per se* which is associated with the crop production or the animal production or the issues associated with, are dominating. Lack of extension technology needs to be taken care of, wherein the extension educationist is going to play key role. The role of extension service provider is, in addition to the technology that they are specializing with learn techniques of extension and influence behaviour of the end user. Technology per sec cannot work on its own and do any wonders until and unless it is understood by the end user.

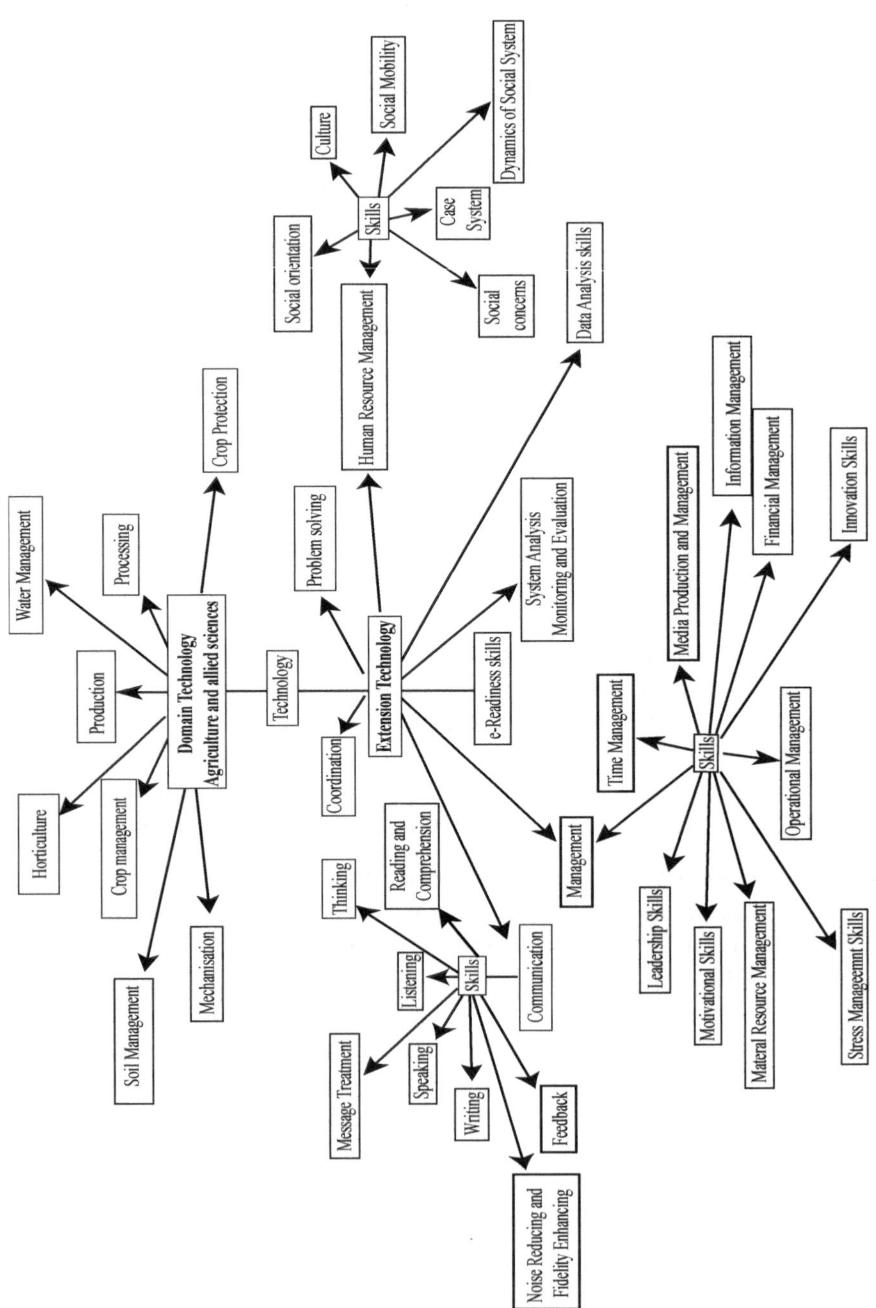
Domain Technology
Agriculture and allied sciences
Water Management
Processing
Crop Protection
Production
Horticulture
Crop management
Soil Management
Mechanisation
Technology
Extension Technology
Problem solving
Human Resource Management
Coordination
Skills
Social orientation
Culture
Social Mobility
Dynamics of Social System
Case System
Social concerns
Data Analysis skills
System Analysis Monitoring and Evaluation
e-Readiness skills
Management
Communication
Thinking
Reading and Comprehension
Listening
Speaking
Message Treatment
Writing
Feedback
Noise Reducing and Fidelity Enhancing
Time Management
Media Production and Management
Information Management
Financial Management
Innovation Skills
Operational Management
Leadership Skills
Motivational Skills
Materal Resource Management
Stress Manageemnt Skills

Extension technology

The emphasis of extension educator is on empowering the stakeholders, which can be understood with the saying, *"If you give a fish to a hungry person, you are satisfying his hunger for a day, but if he is being taught how to catch the fish, it means we are feeding him for the life"*.

The process of extension does not stop there. The inner-tensions of extension go beyond that. What is that? It says that, teach them how to process and package the fish for export, which stimulates the economic development. Bringing in the desirable changes is being emphasized upon with the inner-tensions of extension.

Extension educationist and extension service provider are different entities and have a definite role to play. Apply the techniques of extension while providing the extension services in addition to the technology which is essential for our target community, and make the process of extension more holistic. 'What is extension' is discussed everywhere but what extension is not about is not discussed anywhere. There are many misconceptions regarding the concept of extension. Because of these misconceptions, people don't understand holistically extension as a profession and as a discipline.

What is not Extension?

The perception of people who don't understand the concept of extension say that extension is nothing but a type of gossip, is not a science, not for intellectuals, not academic discipline etc. Since beginning it is being emphasized on that it is the service as well as a profession. Because it is a service, it has developed as profession. Since it is academic discipline, it has its own subject matter, contents, syllabus and offers postgraduate degree programs. Some say that it is nothing but the act of photography, yes; extension makes use of the appropriate photographs, videos and everything for the benefit of the stakeholders for ensuring efficient services.

Extension education is not the process of story writing and it is also said extension education is a type of journalistic process. Developing success story and making use of few aspects of journalism in extension processes and models does not make them the profession of journalist. These misconceptions emerge because of the meaning attached to the concept of extension as the transfer of technology. There is another connotation attached with extension is the postman's job of transferring the information from resource institution to that place of information deficit. In between there are good number of educational events that are part of the extension service efforts, it proves to be not the postman's job because, until and unless there is change in knowledge, attitude and skill, we cannot say that extension has taken place.

Also few people say that it's a vague, hazy, indistinct and a fuzzy subject. People perceive it because they feel it is difficult to understand the processes of extension. It is difficult to understand all the nuances of extension. Hence it is not easy to prove, to be a professional extension educator or service provider. Extension deals with the most dynamic animal on this earth; that is human being, who is having competencies in various specialized areas. Extension Professional makes use of all techniques to convince every stakeholder. If he fails, then he starts feeling that, it's a vague subject, fuzzy subject, an indistinct subject.

Next misconception in the line is extension means crowd pulling or bringing the people to programmes. Obviously we need the people to understand the technology, to understand the information which is appropriate for them. It is not that sole responsibility of extension professional is bringing the crowd of people for some other purposes. The purpose is educational activities, for the purpose of changing their behaviour, making them educated, changing their practices etc.

There is another understanding of extension; it is nothing but a propaganda activity. What do we mean by propaganda? Propaganda is the information especially biased or misleading in nature, used to promote a political cause or a point of view. When this concept 'propaganda' itself is having so many negativities within it how can we equate it with extension which has nothing to do with these negativities.

One more meaning attached with is extension means advertising, basically, advertising is an audio or visual form of marketing communication that employs an openly sponsored non- personal message to promote or sell a product, service or an idea. Extension deals with the information and innovative ideas, but they are not non-personal in nature. Extension does not market or sells ideas or innovations. But efforts are directed towards changing behaviour, practices, living standards and ultimately leading towards enhanced production and productivity of its stakeholders.

Extension is not the process of mass communication. Because mass communication is a study of how people exchange information through mass media to large segments of the population at the same time. The Process of extension deals with a particular target community. The information needs of target communities of extensions service are totally distinct. But in case of mass communication they are dealing the entire community as a whole. On the contrary extension segments the entire population based on their needs and provide information which is relevant to them. If you take a village as a unit, within the village, there are different information needs that the farmers have.

There might be 10-15 groups of people who are in need of different types of information. Accordingly extension provides services to them.

Extension Educator vs Extension Service Provider

What are the difference between the person who is acting as an extension educationist and who acts as an extension service provider? These are the people who are responsible for providing the extension services for the benefit of the people, hence there is need to overcome the misconceptions that we are trying to discuss about.

Extension Educationist is a person with a background of education in agriculture and allied sciences and specialization in extension science and provides the knowledge and skills of extension and communication tools and techniques to the extension service providers at regular intervals to bring the desirable changes in the behaviour of extension service provider. This is the role of an extension educationist who has specialized himself in extension science.

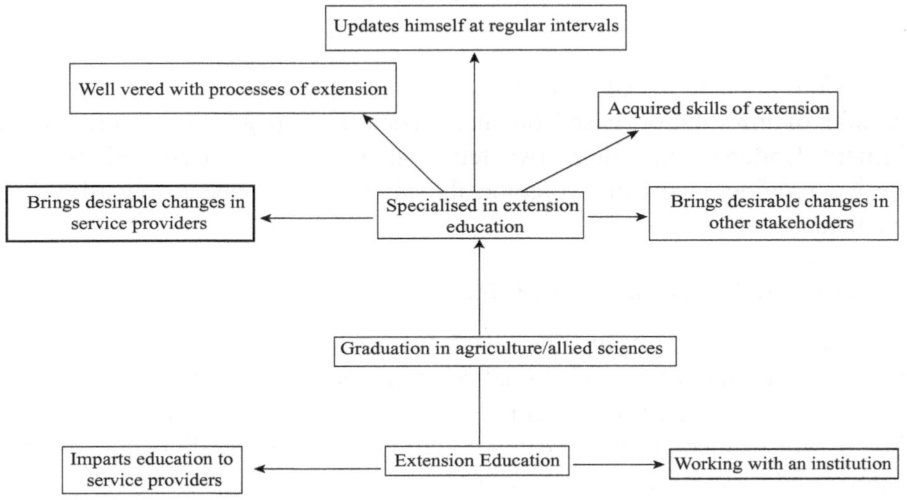

Who are the extension service providers? The service provider is a person with a background of education in agriculture and/or allied sciences and specializations in the discipline of agriculture and allied sciences, who is serving in a public or private institution and meant for dissemination of technological advances to the intended communities and institutions based on the needs, after acquiring the extension and communication tools and techniques from extension educationist.

The extension service provider is an individual with the specialization of his own subject, in addition to that, he is getting the additional information of how to transfer that technology from extension educationist, and then only he becomes service provider. For example entomologist, pathologist, agricultural engineer, agronomist, horticulturist, animal husbandry etc.

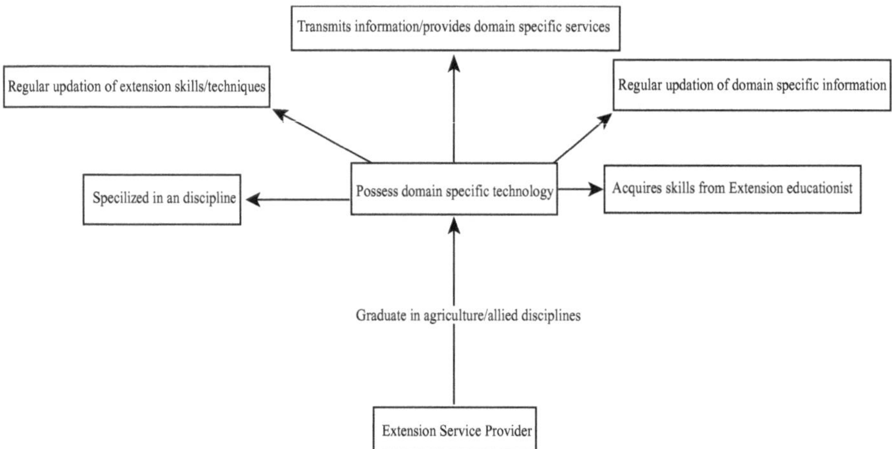

Extension Educators and Extension Service providers are responsible for transfer of information based on their specialization for the benefit of the farmers. Understanding these two terms, that is extension educationist and service provider, we can overcome the misleading concepts regarding the extension.

Pluralism in Agricultural Extension

The term pluralism means the existence of variety of agencies, service providers, models and institutional arrangements; especially including the public institutions, the private institutions, the community based organizations, the non-governmental organizations, catering to the information and advisory support and service needs of the farmers.

The institutional mechanisms are available for satisfying the information needs. When the numbers of such institutions are increasing, the concept of pluralism comes into the picture. It is not one institution but many institutions are providing the similar services. Why such situations are emerging especially in Indian context? Because the population dependent on agriculture is huge. Even today more than 50% of the population is still dependent on agriculture. And the number of service providers to the population needs to be huge, but various players are interested in providing similar services.

According to the statistics available in the State of Andhra Pradesh, one extension worker is catering to the needs of 3,162 farmers, and when you look into input supply agencies, specially the fertilizer, which is one of the critical inputs for agriculture, for 1622 farmers, there is one fertilizer shop. Rest of the follow the suite. What does this mean? It means there is need for multiple institutions (pluralism) catering to the needs of extension services.

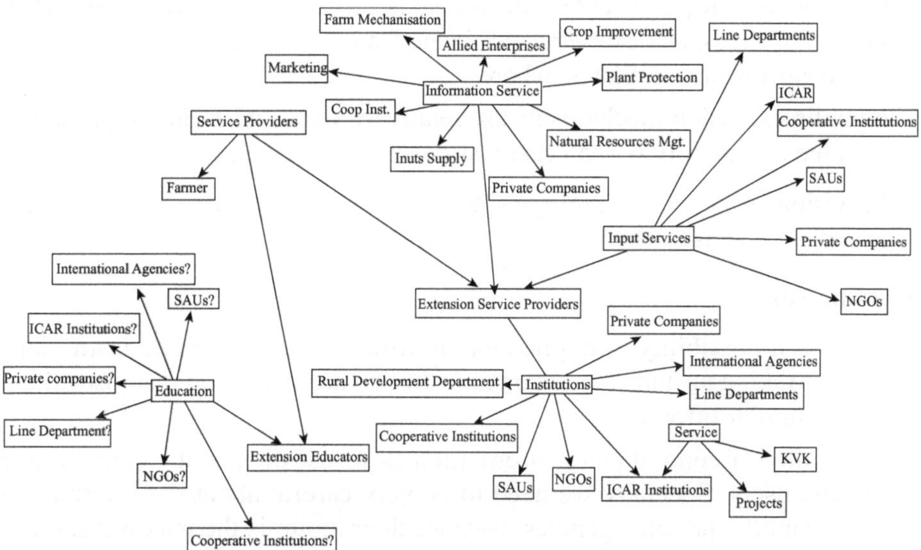

Strengths of Pluralism

- The diversity in approaches and the target groups covered, so that we can easily reach our clients in a comfortable manner and their needs are also satisfied.
- Can complement and supplement the efforts of each other. If the public extension mechanism is lacking in any of the efforts, the private can take care of that and if private is not able to do that, public extension agencies can do that, if both are not able to take up some issues the community based organizations or the non-governmental organizations can take into account.
- The private agencies can cater to the demands of the farmers, prominently observed in case of seed, plant protection chemicals etc.
- Help to overcome the paucity of human resource in the public extension system which is one of the major issues. Once the private players, the non-governmental organizations or the community based organizations is there, the paucity of the extension professionals can be easily taken care of. This is what the strength of pluralism is.

- It can help address varying needs of the farming community. The public extension mechanism (any such institution) may not be having expertise in all the areas as desired by the farming community. But the private institutions are coming out with their own super-specializations and accordingly they are catering to the needs of the farmers.
- Increase in outreach where public extension system is weak. There are many places where the public extension system is very difficult to reach, especially in the hilly areas, in the desert areas, in the States of Jharkhand or Uttarakhand or the North-Eastern States, where

The public extension mechanisms are relatively weak, wherein the private as well as the community based organizations are taking care of such issues.

- Provision of newer technologies and skills to the farmers. So the private agencies can easily cater to these issues.

Weaknesses

- There is a possibility of duplication of effort, which the public institutions are also taking up and at the same time the private institutions are also taking up the similar efforts.
- Possibility of contradictory information flow and the resultant gap among the end-users. Specially we need to be very careful about the information flow from the private agencies, because their motto is the maximization of the profits. Then there are possibilities of creating some hype regarding the products. Such things we cannot expect from the public agencies. The validity and reliability of the information is being checked by various agencies, which is largely absent in case of the private agencies.
- Problem with the quality of the message from the public agencies. Whether we are satisfying the demands of the farmers or our clients is one of the issues, which is largely very weak in case of public extension system.
- Motives and objectives of all agencies may not be aligned with the needs of the farmers. Farmer is in need of something else, but as a private agency or as a community based organization or as a non-governmental organization my priorities are something different. So under such circumstances, there are certain gaps that might be existing between these service providers.
- It makes the extension system more complex, because of number of players that are coming on the same platform and making use of the same concepts of extension. So that is how the concept of pluralistic extension is becoming bit complex

Opportunities

- Harness the synergy of all the actors through convergence. The problems and the weaknesses can be addressed once we come on a common platform. This is an opportunity that we can think of, and address the issues and we can sort out the issues.
- Delineation of the roles of each agency or actor to avoid the duplication of efforts. If various agencies are on a common platform, we can resolve these issues and avoid duplication.
- Offering choice to the farmers among different agencies. So that lets farmer choose whether he wants the services from the public agencies or a private agency or a community based organization or an NGO so that we can provide them services accordingly.
- Enhancing the participation in case of extension programs is one of the opportunities, because as on date the real participation of the farming community in the extension programs is relatively less, but with pluralism we can enhance this participation.
- Public extension can play the role of a leader of pluralistic extension system. Because being part of the government mechanism, they can take the establish coordination among various agencies.
- Potential to create a linkage of the farmers with other actors and across the value chain. So that once the government takes the lead or the public institutions take the lead then automatically things can take a different shape. This is an opportunity.

Threats

- Lack of effective coordination among the agencies. This is currently being experienced and over a period of time it may emerge as a threat also.
- Absence of platform for coordination. Some efforts are being carried out through ATMA. But still lot needs to be done in this sector.
- Efforts of collaboration without imbibing the spirit. Observed with the non-governmental organizations as well as the private sector organizations. The spirit of extension should not be compromised, while providing the services.
- Mismatch between the organizational agenda and the problems due to the hidden agenda. Generally we observe such things in case of the private agencies. Their agenda is profit maximization, while the agenda of the public institutions is the development of the society, enhancing the living standards of the farmers. There are obvious possibilities of mismatch between these agendas, the hidden agendas as well as the declared agenda.

- Lack of leadership and the conflict resolution mechanism may hamper the effective collaboration. Because when these institutions are to come together, even though their target groups are same, their commodities are same, the way of delivering the mechanisms, all are common. But whether these institutions are ready to come together or if there are any conflict that exist, do we have that conflict resolution mechanism? This is the biggest issue which is acting as a threat.
- Political and economic aspects preventing the collaboration. Because the motto of the private agencies and public extension agencies are diagonally opposite, is one of the hindering factors.
- Doubt about the sustainability of the government promoted convergence initiatives is creating another threat in case of pluralism in extension.

If you look into this diagram, the services we are providing to the client *i.e.* farmer. He needs the services. The services can largely be identified as the services to be provided by the extension educators and extension service providers. So when we look into the extension educational efforts, they are being taken up by the State Agricultural Universities, the international agencies, the ICAR institutions, the private agencies, the line departments, the non-governmental organizations, cooperative societies number of institutions which are involved in educating the farming community.

Similarly when it comes to the service, the institutions which are involved in the service may it be the department of rural development, the cooperative institutions, the state agricultural universities, non-governmental organizations, ICAR institutions, KVK's as well as the projects, they are reaching the farmers. The line depts., international agencies and the private agencies are also providing services.

1. The institutions discussed under the extension education as well as extension service are almost same. This is what is leading towards the pluralism. The input services are being provided again by line depts., ICAR institutions, cooperatives, state agriculture universities, private companies, NGO's. They are all involved in the inputs and at the same time the information services, which is again the domain of the public extension agencies. The private players are also coming here, the similar institutions are there. So this is what we are emphasizing on. Similar services are the institutions discussed under the extension education as well as extension service are almost same. This is what is leading towards the pluralism. The input services are being provided again by line depts., ICAR institutions, cooperatives, state agriculture universities, private companies, NGO's. They are all involved in the inputs and at the same

time the information services, which is again the domain of the public extension agencies. The private players are also coming here, the similar institutions are there. So this is what we are emphasizing on. Similar services are

2. **Affective domain:** the approach/way technology is being handled with emotions. This is, inclusive of enthusiasm of source and receiver, motivations, attitudes, value systems and appreciation of technological intervention. These complex issues can better be explained with simple behavioral ephemeron (Bloom1956):

3. **Receiving phenomena:** conscious hearing to others for the purpose of remembering. The key issue is willingness to listen, its responsibility of source to bring the listener to the level, grab his attention, make him aware of, ask questions if doubts exist, follow the contents and understand for application

   a. **Respond to the phenomena**: depicts the dynamic participation of end user. Learning outcomes lead to action/application.

   b. **Valuing phenomena:** reveals the ability to solve the problems. In regular interaction with both upper and lower sections of profession. Propose a plan for social improvement and commitment to implement it.

   c. **Organizational phenomena:** educates to establish balance between systematic ways adopted to solve problem and follow professional ethical standards.

   d. **Characterization (Internalization of values) phenomena:** adopting instructional objectives commensurate with learners patterns adjustment to the learning situation.

4. **Psychomotor domain:** deals with skill aspects of learning. Educational interventions lead to physical movement, coordination and use of acquired skills. The skills range from manual/mechanical tasks to machine operated tasks. These skills are quantified (measured) in terms of speed of performance/execution, precision in implementation, distance covered and methods/procedures used in implementation.

The categories of skill phenomena include (Dave, 1975):

- **Imitation phenomena:** observation leading to following behavioral pattern of somebody. Reproduction of others methods, processes, skills etc. Though it is a method of acquiring skill, in the long run yields low quality and productivity.

- **Manipulation phenomena**: begins with recalling memory of things learnt during educational efforts. Based on memory, individual makes an effort to perform certain actions by following instructions. Indigenous knowledge is largely memory based. The oral tradition played dominant role in keeping indigenous traditions alive even today. Over a period of time we observe certain changes in adoption of indigenous knowledge also.
- **Precision phenomena:** performing a skill with high degree of accuracy. Get rid of any deviation to be more precise.
- **Articulation phenomena**: establishing coordination between a series of skills to produce desirable product. Every operation in agriculture and allied sciences involves a series of activities involving skills. It needs perfect coordination between various sub units of a particular operation.
- **Naturalization phenomena:** running behind a particular skill until mastery is achieved in performing. Regular and continuous practice leads to naturalization of skill. The ultimate output is achieving high level of skill performance.

Why social media platforms for agricultural extension?

- Easy access to the electronic gadgets and the Internet facilities including the rural population. We have already observed the statistics that almost equal numbers of people in urban as well as rural area are having access to the Internet as well as the modern information-communication technology tools and techniques. So that is how the social media has a huge potential specially for providing the extension services.
- For delivering information to the target communities at anytime, anyplace and from any place to any place, from any place. At any point of time we can provide the extension services or the information services to the farmer.

Challenges before Social Media

- The institutional awareness about the social media as potential is one of the important challenge. The institutions should recognize the potential of the social media, so that they can make use of the potential of social media as an instrument for delivering extension services.
- Encouraging the stakeholders to access the social media links. So the figures what we have seen, so they are all for using the social media for the purpose of entertainment. But whether they are making use of this for educational purpose, for getting extension service purpose. That is what the challenge before the professionals is.
- The skilled human resource to maintain the social media interactions. We need the people who can manage these platforms, so wherein the skills are essential, that is another challenge.

- Internet and information technology infrastructure is another issue. So that needs to be maintained and that needs to be promoted.
- Then satisfying the heterogeneous users is another challenge for the professionals. Because as we have number of people on these platforms, their demands are also diverse in nature. So whether we are able to cater to all the needs. So that's what an issue is.
- Measuring impact is another challenge. So because of the social media, what are the changes that occurred into the technological scenario or the adoption scenario that is another issue.
- Continuous engagement of the population is one of the challenges.

Opportunities for Social Media in Extension Services

- Formation of global/national interest groups is possible. So right now we are thinking of formation of the groups at the local and regional level. But that can be extended to national as well as global level. Then can act as a catalyst for resource mobilization that resource maybe technology, organization, finances etc.
- Integration of wide range of stakeholders. All the stakeholders can come on a common platform. Maybe it is the technology users, technology providers, the input suppliers, the processors, the marketers. All the stakeholders can come on a common platform is an opportunity.
- Then reaching one to many. One institution is there but it has an access to each and every individual.

(Adopted from Jirli Basavaprabhu (2021) "Use of Social Media in Agricultural Extension with special reference to Facebook, Youtube, Whatsapp and Instagram" Lecture delivered in BAU- MANAGE Collaborative Training Programme on ICT and Mass Media in Agricultural Extension, May 05, 2021)

Conclusion

The results of the effort indicate that there is growing inclination towards user friendly platforms. Given an opportunity stakeholders are participating and getting the benefits, but how many such programs are being offered? How to ensure the quality aspects of content? How to treat the message as per the needs to stakeholders? How to document and interpret the needs of stakeholders? Who and how to decide the appropriate platforms for various stakeholders? And so on. The list of questions to be answered is growing, its only the extension educationist. This is the opportune time to extension educationist to recognize his role and begin with the educational activities of extension service providers and other stakeholders.

There is a need to create awareness among the extension professionals and build the capacities to share more information on the social media platforms. Institutionalizing the use of social media for sustained momentum and for better sharing as well as networking for the purpose of delivering extension services. Then encouraging self-publication and collective collaboration, so that each and every professional can add the content on his own and he can develop the content for the social media. Extension organizations need to encourage the stakeholders to use the social media for interaction and obtaining the feedback. Research on social media is one of the important issue that need to be taken care of in the days to come.

4

ICT Tools & Application for Effective Dissemination & Development of Extension System

R.K. Sohane

Extension Education, Bihar Agricultural University
Sabour, Bhagalpur - 813210

Abstract

Information and communications technology (ICT) is an extended term for information technology (IT) which stresses the role of unified communications and the integration of telecommunications (telephone lines and wireless signals), computers as well as necessary enterprise software, middleware, storage, and audio-visual systems, *which enable users to access, store, transmit, and manipulate information.*

The term *ICT* is also used to refer to the convergence of audio-visual and telephone networks with computer networks through a single cabling or link system. There are large CoymeBoang incentives (huge cost savings due to elimination of the telephone network) to merge the telephone network with the computer network system using a single unified system of cabling, signal distribution and management.

However, ICT has no universal definition, as "the concepts, methods and applications involved in ICT are constantly evolving on an almost daily basis." The broadness of ICT covers any product that will store, retrieve, manipulate, transmit or receive information electronically in a digital form, e.g. personal computers, digital television, email, robots. For clarity, Zuppo provided an ICT hierarchy where all levels of the hierarchy "contain some degree of commonality in that they are related to technologies that facilitate the transfer of information and various types of electronically mediated communications." Skills Framework for the Information Age is one of many models for describing and managing competencies for ICT professionals for the 21st century.

Keywords*: *ICT Tools, Gadgets, Software, Apps, Networking Technologies.

Introduction

In the recent years, Information and Communication Technology (ICT) have been widely used to improve productivity and reduce costs for the enhancement of agricultural and rural development. The increase in internet penetration with the wide use of smart phones, internet connectivity and broadband coverage has enabled the widening coverage of ICT in agriculture. Over the years, it has led to accurate and timely information on markets, production processes, crops and livestock disease, as well as access to services such as land registration databases, permits, and information on government regulations. The magnitude of impact varies with the region under implementation. Agriculture in developing countries is facing challenges of enhancing production in a situation of decreasing natural resources for efficient productivity. The growing demand for agricultural products to feed a growing and increasingly requires compliance with more stringent quality standards and regulations for the production and handling of agricultural produce. The ICT project for agriculture undertaken by the alliance of private and public-sector stakeholders is useful for effective collaboration which is at large serving the needs of the involved beneficiaries on a wider scale. It is widely accepted that increased information flow is having a positive effect on the agricultural sector and individual firms. The collection and dissemination of information has enabled use of IT in a faster and more convenient form than others.

Role of ICT in Agriculture

ICT is playing a major role in the agricultural sector to bridge the communications divide created by geographical barriers. ICT has enabled the provision of better education, capacity building and training to rural people all over the world. The individuals having access to new technologies are also prone to better adoption and use of innovations. A popular phrase "information and communications technology for development (ICT4D)" is changing the landscape for a favorable working relationship with the farmers on the ground, with district and national government bodies. The social and policy context must be well understood when designing and implementing ICT solutions for the farming community. Farmers and extension agents must also be provided better capacity building for achieving the desired agricultural transformation and rural prosperity.

Opportunities of ICT in agriculture:

The sustainable rural livelihoods to improve the efficiency and effectiveness of the agricultural sector for the contribution to poverty alleviation should be directed to achieve the following condition which is largely possible using Information and Communication Technologies. The improvements in the scenario due to the implementation of ICTs are as follows:

- increased farm family income (which is spent on agricultural livelihood improvements, investments in smaller operations, shelter, and improvements in access to basic rural infrastructure such as electricity, potable water, telecommunications and waste management),
- increased farm family savings (which can be invested in livelihood strategies that directly or indirectly improve the efficiency and effectiveness of agricultural production)
- improved family health (related to improvements in income and food security, and relevant knowledge), greater access to education and training, reduced vulnerability to unexpected losses and the effects of natural disasters, reduced rural out-migration, sustainable use of natural resources evidenced by the implementation of land ownership policies and procedures.

The important roles which can be played by ICTs in enhancing agricultural production are discussed below:

Enhancement in Agricultural Production

Farmers are often facing threats like poor soils, drought, erosion and pests. The key areas where ICT can help in improvement is by providing up-to-date information about pest and disease control, early warning systems, new varieties, new ways to optimize production and regulations for quality control.

Improvement in access to Markets

With up-to-date information on the market prices of commodities, the farmers can make better decisions about future crops and commodities, and know the best time and place to sell and buy goods.

Capacity-building and empowerment

ICT technologies is also helping to strengthen communities and farmer organizations with better options for negotiating on input and output prices along with land claims, resource rights and infrastructure projects. The rural communities can interact with others with the use of ICT sources helping to strengthen and facilitate the processes like law-making and land-title approvals more transparent.

Challenges for ICT

There are several challenges involved in effective agricultural technology dissemination because of limited access to the market information, low literacy level among the farmers, inadequate channels of distribution involving adoption, access to IT, demographic, IT training/ education, perception, trust, and time. Other factors that lead to the challenges in this sector are as follows: **Poor substitute for face-to-face communication:** Sometimes, less time to talk to each other and know each other better leads to inefficient utilization of the recommendations. This further leads to inefficient utilization of the advisories provided.

Expensive: It can be very expensive to install a new communication technology system in a very big setting. The creation of strong data base which will handle all the queries made by the farmers is still not evident in the agricultural setting.

Not Safe: Since information has been centralized under one database, the information can be attacked by a hacker or a virus and all data will be lost in a minute. There is a need to pay an extra cost to keep this information safe which makes the services costlier.

Conclusion

Adoption of ICT enabled information systems for agricultural development and rural viability is a strategic issue which requires the overcoming of barriers for effective ICT uptake for agriculture, agricultural development and rural viability. ICTs are enablers for economic growth in a better way. With the adoption and proper utilization of ICTs, it will lead to increased yields and quality production of goods and services. The use of ICT's will also help farmers to develop local content through engaging in various projects for mutual benefits and increased agricultural productivity.

5

Gender Mainstreaming in Animal Husbandry: Needs and Prospects

S. S. Dana*, Animesh Maity
Department of Fisheries Extension, Faculty of Fishery Sciences WBUAFS, Kolkata – 700094, India

Amitava Ghosh, Pranab Rudra Paul
College of Fisheries, CAU (Imphal), Tripura, India

Abstract

Livestock remain a lifeline for many of the world's poorest people. Cattle, goats, sheep, pigs, chickens and other farm animals form part of the livelihood portfolios of an estimated 70 per cent of the world's rural poor women and men. For many smallholder farmers, livestock are essentially four-legged bank accounts, allowing hundreds of millions of unbanked poor to build assets and to insure themselves against shocks such crop failures, accidents and illnesses. Such assets and insurance are particularly important to women, who remain the backbone of global smallholder agriculture and who are one of the best hopes for ensuring future global food security. Across the world's varied livestock production systems, women are main actors in poultry, small ruminant and micro livestock production as well as in dairying including the processing and marketing of milk and milk products. But women are often still excluded from household decision-making processes, especially regarding the disposal of animals and animal products. This lack of female control over livestock assets and income impinges on family welfare as well as economic growth.

Key words: Economic growth, Livestock assets, Insurance, Women.

Livestock sector is an important sub-sector of Indian agricultural economy. It is an integral part of livelihood activity for most of the farmers and help sustaining farm activity. Besides, it is supplementary and complementary to agriculture in the form of critical inputs, contributing to health and nutrition of the household, supplementing incomes, offering employment opportunities, and finally being dependable "banks on hooves" in times of need. About 97 per cent of world's total livestock population is in Asia. India has the world's largest livestock population accounting for over 37.28 per cent of cattle, 21.23 per cent of buffalo, 26.40 per cent of goats and 12.17 per cent of sheep (Sonavale *et al.*, 2020).India is blessed with vast livestock resources in the form of varieties of livestock breeds which include 43 indigenous cattle, 16 buffaloes, 34 goat and 43 sheep breeds (DARE, 2019). Livestock sector contributes 4.11per cent in Gross Domestic Product (GDP) and 25.6per cent of total agricultural GDP (DAHDF, 2019).Livestock production is an essential part of rural livelihood for many poor. It is more popular among the marginal and small farmers as more than 62 per cent of marginal household directly associated with livestock sector (Das *et al.*, 2020). It has the potentiality to overcome poverty and household which are associated with livestock has less chance to fall into poverty. It provides employment to about 8.8 % of the population in India. Livestock provide nutrient rich food products, draught power, dung as organic manure and domestic fuel, hides and skin and are a regular source of cash income for rural livelihood.

Gender identifies the social relations between men and women, boys and girls, and how this is socially constructed. So, gender refers to the socially constructed roles and responsibilities of men and women in a given culture or location. These roles are influenced by perception and expectations arising from cultural, political, environmental, economic, social and religious factors as well as customs, law, class, ethnicity and individuals or institutional bias (WHO, 2003).

Gender issues focus not only on women, but on the relationship between men and women, their roles, access to and control over resources, and division of labour and needs. Gender relations determine household security, well-being of the family, planning, production and many other aspects of life. Livestock is generally considered as a key asset for rural livelihoods. It offers advantages over other agricultural sectors and is an entry point for promoting gender balance in rural areas. In particular, because (a) in most societies, all household members have access to livestock and are involved in production; (b) livestock activities are a daily occupation: animal products such as eggs and milk are produced, processed and marketed throughout the year, without seasonal restrictions, in all livestock-keeping communities, with women responsible for the bulk of the work; (c) livestock production systems offer the potential for introducing a wide range of project activities relating to gender mainstreaming, including improved production methods, and redistribution of intra-household tasks and responsibilities.

Women play an important role in livestock management, processing and marketing, acting as care providers, feed gatherers, and birth attendants.

They are major contributors in the agricultural economy, but face various constraints that limit them from achieving optimal livestock production and agricultural development. These constraints include: (i) Limited access to productive resources, including land, water and credit. (ii) Limited access to market information and market prices. (iii) Limited decision-making powers because of unequal power relations within the household and the community. A report by FAO argues that if women were to have access to the same level of resources as men, agricultural productivity would increase by up to 30 percent, agricultural output by up to 4percent, and the number of poor people would reduce by up to 17percent(Njuki and Sanginga, 2013).

Livestock are an asset that women can more easily own. It is generally easier for women in developing countries to acquire livestock assets, whether through inheritance, markets or collective action processes, than it is for them to purchase land or other physical or financial assets for the family. Putting assets in the hands of women increases their bargaining power, their role in household decision-making and household spending on children's education and health (Njuki and Sanginga, 2013). Women's ability to manage their income is vital to the survival of many households. Studies have shown that women spend close to 90 percent of their income on their family while men spend 30-40 percent, even when the overall income is not sufficient to meet family needs. Income under the management of women can increase their bargaining power, reduce domestic violence and improve the nutritional status of their children.

Gender mainstreaming is the process of assessing the implications for women and men of any planned action, including legislation, policies or programs in any area and at all levels. It is the strategy for making the concern and experiences of women as well as men, an integral part of the design implementation, monitoring and evaluation of policies and programs in all political economic and societal spheres so that women and men benefit equally (United Nations, 1997). So, it can be said that the ultimate goal of gender mainstreaming is to achieve gender equality. There are different principles of gender mainstreaming. They are i) identification of issues and problems across all areas of activity should be such that gender differences and disparities can be diagnosed ii) gender analysis should always be carried out iii) political will and allocation of adequate resources for mainstreaming, including additional financial and human resources, if necessary, are important for transformation of the concept into practice and iv) women and men are equally involved in decision making process.

Rural women's contribution to livestock development remains concealed because they are invisible in plans and programmes of livestock development.

They have poor access to resources and information regarding livestock development programmes. So, there is a need for gender mainstreaming by which equal treatment is integrated into steering process. Rural poverty is deeply rooted in imbalances between what women do and what they have(FAO,2007). Different studies show that almost 70percent of economically active women in low-income group are employed in animal husbandry sector and therefore they play a vital role in production of milk, meat, eggs and wools. It is well established fact that animal husbandry involves both self-employment and wage employment. In fact, livestock holdings of 80percent of rural community being small as a situation demands an understanding of activity performance of men, women and children, girls and boys, whose life are fundamentally structured in different ways. Their living pattern, working pattern, interaction style and sharing of scientific information differs from community to community and culture to culture. So, during formulation of livestock projects, more attention is needed to incorporate women livestock farmer into project design to guarantee women's active participation and involvement in the different phases and activities. Achieving equality between women and men is a pre-condition for sustainable livestock production.

Agricultural extension programmes ensure that information on new technologies, plant varieties and cultural practices reaches farmers. However, in the developing world it is common practice to direct extension and training services primarily towards men. A recent FAO survey showed that female farmers receive only five percent of all agricultural extension services worldwide and that only 15 percent of the world's extension agents are women. As rural women are a vital in livestock farming, it is essential that they take their place alongside men as full participants in and beneficiaries of extension programmes to develop new skills and to get hand on experience of livestock farming from the extension agent.

Livestock farming in India is a female-dominated enterprise (Fulzule and Meena,1995). About 75 million women as against 15 million men engaged in dairying in India (Thakur and Chandra, 2006). So, gender mainstreaming approach does not look at women in isolation but looks at women and men both as actors in the developmental process and as its beneficiaries. Women make an essential contribution in small ruminant management particularly goat and pig rearing and backyard poultry rearing in tribal areas.

In India, women face disproportionate challenges compared to men in accessing livestock services and information. Women account for 55 percent of livestock farming labour, whereas, their participation in works related to the care of animals is above 77 percent. Rural women make up for 93 percent of overall employment in dairying and their average contribution to the entire farm production is estimated around 45 percent to 56 percent of the total labour. Given the strong informal association of rural women with livestock, it is essential to create matching programs with sufficient funds so that their participation gets institutionalized. Several studies have shown that most of the conventional training and extension program are oriented at men. It would be effective if women farmers are reached through women extension workers. Appreciably few dairy co-operatives have done some good work in this regard, but such initiatives need more encouragement and policy support (Chander, 2013).

Credit and capital are basic requisites to increase livestock production. Women and men farmers need short term credit to buy livestock, chicks, feeds, equipment, medicines, vaccines etc. Although, both women and men, small livestock farmers have problems getting credit. The situation facing women is more serious because they lack collateral security. Different studies reveal that when women succeed in obtaining credit, they are more reliable than men in their debt repayments. Although women own only 2 percent of the land and receive only 1 percent of all agricultural credit and 5 percent of all agricultural extension resources, which are directed towards them but their contribution in livestock development is immense. So, it can be said that gender mainstreaming is a long and slow process which requires many inputs on many fronts over a long period of time including advice, support, competence, development of methods and tools for evaluating progress.

The focus of any extension service needs to be on building the capabilities of the women farmers to take care of their animal and crop apart from transfer of technology and strengthening of various infrastructure and support services. The veterinarians are supposed to educate the women farmers on scientific management practices, sustainability of livestock farming, ways to meet scarcity of animal feed and fodder, marketing of livestock, livestock products processing, environmental issues due to livestock, social entrepreneurship development.

6

Farmer Outreach Through Innovative Extension Methodology

Mahesh Chander

Division of Extension Education
ICAR-Indian Veterinary Research Institute, Izatnagar-243122
Uttar Pradesh, India

Abstract

Extension and Advisory Services (EAS) are delivered by millions of extension professionals representing the public, private and civil society located across the globe and have been helping in addressing farmers' needs over the years. However, public sector has been a major agency dealing with EAS in India and is facing several challenges and constraints to fulfill the demands of farmers on timely basis. The challenge today is to change the organizational culture to incorporate innovation as a core value and to institutionalize the emerging paradigms. Further, different strategies and measures need to be taken to ensure timely and quality EAS by reorienting extension priorities. This paper has highlighted on strengthening extension and feedback mechanism, improving research-extension linkages, capacity building, public-private partnership (PPP), developing infrastructure, mass media support and use of Information and Communication Technologies (ICTs) etc. to improve the efficiency as the time demands. The paper concludes that reorienting extension priorities is very essential with a vast network of various stakeholders by adapting effective approaches like utilization of social media, human resource development, PPP, farmer groups etc. during and post pandemic scenario. Further, empirical efforts are also needed to develop reliable, location-specific, participatory, gender-sensitive and inexpensive extension methodologies and materials to meet the emerging demands. Further, developing countries like India have to invest in terms of various resources like financial, human resource etc. for promoting higher productivity and sustainability through EAS.

Introduction

Extension and Advisory Services (EAS) across the world have been helping in addressing farmers' needs over the years. However, as the world struggles to fight the pandemic, farmers across the globe face the dual burden of inadequate health services coupled with timely extension services for sustaining their livelihoods (FAO, 2020). Further, it also reported that about 3–6% increase in total production value could be achieved if only EAS services are provided the way farmers want on real time basis (World Economic Forum, 2018). Although EAS are delivered by millions of extension professionals representing the public, private and civil society located across the globe, public sector has been a major agency dealing with EAS in India. However, Swanson and Mathur (2003) have also depicted narrow focus of extension, lack of farmers involvement in extension programme planning, supply rather than market driven extension, lack of transparency and accountability, inadequate technical capacity, lack of local capacity to validate and refine technologies, inadequate communication capacity and inadequate operating resources and financial sustainability as other major challenges for Indian extension system. Further, a study conducted by Babu *et al.* (2012) has indicated that quality and reliability of public extension system is still a constraint while, Rivera and Sulaiman (2009) have indicated that public-sector extension agencies and extension workers are finding it difficult to translate their roles from the classical model of agricultural extension to the innovation system perspective.

Owing to static and inflexible nature of the organizations, where a top-down hierarchical approach continues (Raabe 2008), farmers' see the quality of the information provided by the public extension staff as a major shortcoming (GOI 2005) and information flow is considered to be supply driven and not need-based or area-specific (Raabe 2008). Also, in a developing country like India, extension models are usually top–down structures, often located within the ministry of agriculture, not usually formally associated with universities (Boone 1989) and therefore, have poor linkages with research and extension. In this context, there must be innovations in EAS delivery that embrace different methods and offer flexible adaptations to cater to the needs of users across states, regions, and communities (Glendenning *et al.* 2010). The challenge is to change the organizational culture to incorporate innovation as a core value and to institutionalize the emerging paradigms into research for development processes. Further, different strategies and measures need to be taken to ensure timely and quality EAS by reorienting extension priorities in such emergency situations and later too.

Need and Importance for Reorienting Priorities

EAS in the past have helped countries move towards meeting food needs, conserving natural resources and developing human and social capital. However, the need for new extension functionalities and job charts are echoed all over the world. Especially, the small holder farmers need real time solutions and become connected to the service providers (even at affordable costs). Over last few months, many organizations have realized that there's need for innovation and functional transformation to mitigate the crisis. Suddenly, there is a demand for shift in the approach of EAS from traditional face-to-face farm advisory to supporting farmers with marketing and use of ICTs in supply chain management. In this context, EAS organizations need to innovate continuously with the better functionalities like data driven personalized services in credit, insurance, markets, inputs supplies, aggregation models, traceability etc. (Meera, 2020) and improve the efficiency as the time demands.

There are other aspects of transformation that should be simultaneously taken care such as building appropriate infrastructure with proper scales of economy, building relevant capacities of extension professionals, integrating the complex digital processes into the basic agricultural workflows etc. (Meera, 2020). In this context, different strategies and measures are necessary to reorient extension priorities and ensure food security. Also, as large numbers of migrants are returning to their respective villages, active support of the agriculture and an allied department in the states needs to be emphasized at all levels. Hence, reorienting extension priorities is very essential with a vast network of various stakeholders involved in research, extension, education, marketing, agro-processing etc.

Changing Priorities of Extension and Advisory Services

An effort has been made to identify the extension mechanism followed across India including reorienting extension priorities. Some of the important components have been discussed.

- **Strengthening Extension and feedback mechanism:** The extension wing at different levels is looking after activities and ensures effective coordination with all agencies like ATMA, KVK, programmes and schemes of Extension. These agencies shall liaison and encourage participation of private organizations and NGOs for their active involvement in delivery of extension services. Problems which need new technology to confront crisis have to be addressed and communicated as feedback to researchers. Such feedback in general is often missing due to poor linkage and feedback mechanism among research, extension and farmers leading to poor dissemination of agricultural technologies from researchers to farmers. Based on the farmers' feedback, the research can be field tested by various interdisciplinary teams on location and resource specific scientific recommendations. The feedback from multi-stakeholders in generation, development and transfer of technologies is highly necessary in the present scenario.

- **Improving Research-Extension linkages:** The public system heavily suffers from failures of various issues like infrastructure, weak linkages and market structure failures. Hence, to improve the relevance, effectiveness, and efficiency of research outputs, stronger linkages are also needed between the performers of research and its end users in the region. Developing a social network involving all the stakeholders of EAS for timely information dissemination to all agricultural subsectors is very essential at this point of time. An interaction between different multi-stakeholders should be organized at the grass root levels to establish policy dialogues and programme plans for the future (Rathore *et al.* 2008).
    - ***Promotion of direct interface between farmers and scientists:*** There are relatively high costs attached to this direct mode of technology transfer and the outreach of scientists is limited. State and region level meetings between line departments and universities must be activated in the existing interface mechanisms. In this changing time, online media may be emphasized for organizing such meetings and activities.
    - ***Research priority setting based on SREP.*** Micro-level extension strategies reflected in the Strategic Research and Extension Plans (SREPs) based on PRA and developed jointly by the district technology teams including the marketing department officials and scientists of the KVKs/ ZRS or SAUs should formally feedback into the research systems. Participatory Technology Development is another way of connecting farmers with the scientists thus leading to need based researches.
- **Capacity Building in Extension:** An optimal requirement of human resource to support various programmes must be worked out and steps can be taken to generate the same through involvement of Government Agencies, reputed NGOs and private sector. Many young people and women need to be empowered to lead farming as heads of their households.
    - ***Diploma Courses***: The Diploma holders can supplement the efforts of extension officers at the grassroots level by providing practical production guidelines to both, commercial and small-scale farmers helping them towards developing a sustainable agriculture and allied sector enterprise.
    - ***Training of Para-professionals:*** The training programmes for Para-professionals and similarly placed personnel must be undertaken on regular basis.

- ***Entrepreneurship and Vocational Training:*** Vocational training of rural youths and farm women in the areas of agriculture and allied sector needs to be augmented. There are various enterprises, which can be practiced on commercial scale and can be started with small investment on scientific lines by the rural youth.
- ***Farmers' training and Farmer led approach:*** Farmers' training and demonstration needs may be assessed in participatory mode so that area specific tailor-made training programmes are designed by effective linkages of organizations depending on socio-economic background of the farmers. Progressive farmers after various scientific orientations can be encouraged to act as extension agents by giving them due recognition.
- ***Merging of Extension with other activities***: It is very pertinent to note that any programme can be successful when it is merged with extension activities. A carefully designed extension education campaign initiated before and after by the professional extension personnel would be highly beneficial.
- **Gender and Extension:** Since there is a strong informal association of rural women with agriculture and livestock, it is necessary to create matching programmes and budgeting for women. The conventional training and extension programmes must be oriented to suit women also. It would be more effective, if women Extension workers disseminate the technologies to the women farmers both in formal and informal mode. Further, with a group mobilization approach few leading women farmers may be trained for transfer of technologies and deployed as link women extension functionaries between farmers and Department/NGO personnel.
- **Developing infrastructure in Extension:** The single-discipline, single-commodity based approach gradually must be replaced by an integrated systems-oriented research which demands high extension infrastructure at all the levels from village to central government and universities. The training infrastructure, by and large, is very poor in terms of facilities like hostel, classrooms, laboratories, audio-visuals, farms etc. There is a need to have equipment's for print, photostat, content development and validation mechanism and printing of extension literature at state and central headquarters and universities. Further, equipment's like display boards, Audio-visual aids and mobile extension vehicles may also be needed at the institution or college level to reach the farmers. In this era of pandemic, the globe has realized the importance of online tools and media in transferring and sharing information apart from networking.
- **Role of public-private partnership in Extension:** The public-private partnerships which do not exist effectively (Singh *et al.* 2013) can be one of the best modes of strengthening linkages among various stakeholders

for effective research and extension activities. In this context, Public-private partnerships should be the thought pattern and 'method of choice' underpinning the government's stance in extension. The ICAR draft policy of November 2012 recommends evolving appropriate models of public private partnership (ICAR 2012). As per NASSCOM's 2019 report, India is home to more than 450 Agri-tech start-ups, growing at 25% annually and hence, new digital partnership may evolve among different agencies or start-ups for improving the impact of EAS (Meera, 2020).

- **Extensionist's competency development:** Though the extension system has taken many pro-active measures to help farmers, there is a need for more involvement and formulation of innovative practices to enable them to address different challenges. EAS providers need to be properly equipped so as to address changes in the development scenario, as well as to meet the emerging demands and needs of farmers and FPOs, especially on agribusiness, value addition, and marketing (Wadkar, 2020).

  Extensionist's need to be trained on next generation extension tools and media. COVID-19 like situations demands more knowledge and skills in social media and its uses, including the current tools, methods and models for crisis communication. Extensionist's need to be equipped to use Facebook, WhatsApp, Twitter, YouTube, etc. They need to learn and master skills to disseminate information and monitor, track, measure, and analyse social media traffic (Chander, 2020a). Besides, skills in mobilizing farmers and facilitating interaction are very much needed to secure coordination of different agencies to broker gains for farmers.

- **Mass Media Support & Use of Information and Communication Technologies (ICTs):** ICTs have created positive impact on income growth in developing and developed countries (Waverman *et al.* 2005). In rural areas, ICTs can raise incomes by increasing agricultural productivity (Lio and Liu 2006) and introducing income channels other than traditional farm jobs. Studies depicted that ICTs can improve incomes and quality of life among the rural poor (Goyal 2010, Jensen 2007). In this context, an effort to deliver information to rural masses through ICT, free or at nominal cost, can increase the timely and transparent flow of information to build or strengthen the innovation networks among different stakeholders (Chander and Rathod, 2015). Further, ICTs can also revolutionize the interaction through Information Kiosks, Tele-centres, toll-free Call Centers, websites, mobile phones software applications etc. New advanced instruments like Personal Digital Assistants may be provided to the Extension agents for technical information, communicating, field recording, database maintenance and scheduling. It is important to use ICT in combination with the more traditional extension methods such as mass media, group meetings, field days, demonstrations and exchange visits with the objective to make the information available to all the stakeholders very effectively, efficiently and quickly. Community radio is also doing tremendous service during the lockdown by organizing pertinent programmes in local dialects, which makes them effective in conveying the desired information (Chander, 2020b). Partnering with community radio stations to broadcast information to farmers would be beneficial to their production.

The scope of social media in offering EAS is tremendous. Social media such as Whats app, Telegram, Facebook and YouTube are successfully used by extensionist's to offer EAS. Plethora of studies have already indicated the benefits of using social media like whatsapp, youtube, telegram etc. (Thakur and Chander, 2018; Dileep Kumar, 2020 and Tamizhkumaran and Saravanan Raj, 2020) but needs to emphasized on priority basis. Webpages of official websites of EAS offering institutes, containing advisory information on different relevant topics is being made directly accessible at free or very nominal cost. Hence, there is a need to synthesize learning's from different success stories and case studies and translate them into digital extension frameworks to formulate better extension strategies and policies. Extensive adoption of digital technology in EAS has been very successful during this pandemic and needs to continue in future too.

- **Market driven approach:** Production and marketing of agricultural and allied sector products through creation of basic market facilities and market information for the farmers is very essential. As Swanson (2009) has pointed out that market-oriented extension is relevant in economies that are experiencing growth and changes in consumer preferences that create markets for high-value products, India can be effective in making some of their extension market-driven. Although creation of market or linkage with markets has been emphasized long before, but linking producers and small farm businesses to market and input agencies was very poor over the years. However, with an online marketing platform, the agricultural produce can also be traded at a location or with a buyer of choice. Farmers are being encouraged to use e-NAM facilities and hedge through futures and increased use of warehouse receipts (Prasad, 2020). In the same way, market is also created through various social media tools like Facebook, Whats App etc. and needs to continue post pandemic situation.
- **Role of Farmer producer Organizations (FPO) and Farmers Groups/ associations:** The extension approach needs to be changed from individual to group or association approach to have effective decision making. The Interest Groups, SHGs or Cooperatives have been very successful models

for effective production or marketing. In the similar way, farm women or youth may also be promoted in the form of Joint Liability Groups for effective production and marketing. Very recently, FPOs have become an integral part of coordination and convergence of EAS along with ATMA and KVK in the district during this crisis. The Indian government directed state governments to make efforts to connect FPOs to the processing industry, exporters, bulk buyers and big retailers to maintain the supply line. This will help FPOs get remunerative prices for their produce and help track transportation online. Various state governments allowed FPOs to sell their produce by facilitating packaging, transport and marketing of their produce by relaxing limitations and providing certificates to them.

Farmers' organizations and agro-dealers (small-scale operations that stock farming inputs) also play a key role in bridging extension services to farmers, especially when they are already equipped with ICT tools. In Maharashtra, for example, 265,000 farmers' organization members are using Whatsapp for exchange and learning purposes (Even and Nyathi, 2020).Further, this is also the time for strengthening and gearing up farmers groups and cooperatives to play a major role in aggregation and distribution of agriculture and allied farm produce. Some of the examples in different states of India (Nikam and Kale, 2020; Kanatt and Jos, 2020; Patil. *et al.*, 2020 and Shabong, 2020) depict the fact that multi-stakeholder linkages and ICT can successfully benefit the farmers. The potential of FPOs and cooperatives needs to be effectively utilized by EAS to help farmers sell their products and share information and updates on farming post pandemic scenario also.

- **Farmers as Extension Agents:** The extension systems must promote innovative farmers to play local "farmer professor" roles to scale up the enterprises among different groups of farmers which can lead to effective market-driven extension system (Davis *et al.* 2010). The experienced farmer in Indian context needs to be encouraged to act as EAS providers with very nominal incentives. These farmers who stay in their own villages act as resource persons in villages and need not depend on the external extension agents regularly. In some situations, if the movement of project staff and government extension agents is restricted, the services of these farmers may be utilized for EAS by preparing pre-recorded videos and picture-based materials to provide quality training to their peers in the villages. Further, these farmers can also conduct trainings and field visits of their peers in smaller groups.
- **Role of Institutions and Organizations:** Since the extension efforts by ICAR institutes have very limited reach (Chander *et al.* 2010), efforts for effective university curricula involving farmers, private sector and other organizations can be planned. In this context, different universities or institutions and

their associated KVKs are issuing location specific advisories on crop, livestock, fisheries and related matters using information and communication technologies (ICTs). Also, several information related to markets, availability of critical inputs, maintaining social distance, facilitating the installation of Aarogya Setu app, immunity enhancing protocol, etc. are being shared by these institutions. Interestingly, extension organizations in last few months have tried to solve immediate problems of farmers through online mode. The pandemic has compelled extension organizations and personnel to explore different online channels to remain connected with the farmers and other stakeholders. EAS is increasingly depending on these online resources indicating the fact that digital extension efforts have been emphasized during this pandemic. However, the organizations and institutions need to continue these transformational changes in EAS post the pandemic.

These universities and institutions may establish internship and exchange programmes for under-graduate and post graduate student with a task to develop different extension models and improve their performance to bring them on par with private organizations. Further, these institutions need to have package of practices including "Do's &Don'ts" which farmers can follow to confront the crisis and also should have provision to update them regularly.

- **Investment in EAS:** The economic studies from developing and developed countries have indicated that high monetary returns to extension activity (Gill 1991, Chand et al. 2011) provide solid evidence as investment with high returns. However, in recent years, the GOI has spent only about 0.14% of Agricultural Gross Domestic Product (GDP) on extension services (Chand et *al.* 2011). Further, I case of animal husbandry, Chander and Rathod and (2013) have recommended that each State should create an extension and training wing at state headquarters with regional/local wings, staffed and equipped with trained livestock extension specialists, audio-visual (AV) equipment and mobile publicity vans along with budgetary allocations of at least 10% of the departmental budget for extension activities. Hence, in the present situation, the Govt. has to invest considerable budget for EAS in the years to come.
- **Strengthening Government Schemes and programmes:** The demand for agricultural products is expected to increase with a major focus on health-conscious population. It is also good time to bring primary processing and marketing facilities closer to the farm gates and help producers gather market intelligence and manage the value chain better with digital agriculture tools. Further, EAS agencies also needs to educate the farmers about machineries for smooth procurement and marketing operations apart from information about different inputs and their role in farm production.

Conclusion

An effort has been made to review the extension mechanism followed across India and also have focused on reorienting extension priorities post COVID-19 scenario. The strengthening extension and feedback mechanism, improving research-extension linkages, capacity building, public-private partnership (PPP), developing infrastructure, mass media support and use of Information and Communication Technologies (ICTs) etc. to improve the efficiency as the time demands has been highlighted. The innovative extension practices to be followed is very essential with a vast network of various stakeholders by adapting effective approaches like utilization of social media, human resource development, PPP, farmer groups etc. during and post pandemic scenario. Further, empirical efforts are also needed to develop reliable, location-specific, participatory, gender-sensitive and inexpensive extension methodologies and materials to meet the demands during such crisis. Further, developing countries like India have to invest in terms of various resources like financial, human resource etc. for promoting higher productivity and sustainability through EAS.

Finally, the Committee constituted to work out modalities for Doubling the Farmers' Income has redefined, Agricultural extension as given below:

"Agricultural Extension is an empowering system of sharing information, knowledge, technology, skills, risk & farm management practices, across agricultural sub-sectors and along all aspects of the agricultural supply chain, so as to enable the farmers to realize higher net income from their enterprise on a sustainable basis (Committee on Doubling the Farmers' Income (DFI), 2017)."

We should keep note of this fresh definition of Agricultural Extension, which emphasizes on supply chain, market oriented/led value chain extension. References: References will be provided on request.

7

Managing Extension Projects Instruments and Application

Siddhartha D. Mukhopadhyay

Department of Agricultural Extension Palli Siksha Bhavana (Institute of Agriculture), Visva-Bharati, Sriniketan

Abstract

Extension education as a subject field as well as extending services to clients is found to be associated with the bio-production system and some service areas where the actual stakeholders are not a part of the specified field of knowledge and technology. Taking the example of a bio-production system like agriculture, horticulture, fishery, animal and veterinary science, sericulture, forestry, etc. – paradoxically contrasting to an industrial production system, in which actual practitioners (farmers) do not come to respective institutions where the S & T inputs in the respective fields are generated and disseminated. There lies the necessity and importance of extension in order to reach them with appropriate S & T inputs which can boost up the production and productivity of crops and lands. This is particularly necessary for meeting the food, feed, fiber requirement of the ever-increasing human and animal population as well as to maintain seed reserve. Improvement of bio-production systems in terms of their production and productivity is largely dependent on public (government) funds and efforts are being made to improve these sectors through a different extension program. Since independence through different projects and programme, like, IAAP, IADP, HYVP, IRDP, Training & Visit, IVLP, NAIP, NATP, and many others have been launched. But there was criticism that these projects were not managed efficiently to yield the expected outcome.

Managing Extension Projects: A great task indeed as well as involving lots of S & T of project management. In this article, different instruments of project management and their application will be discussed. Let that be started with a definition of the project and the key elements of project management.

Definition of Project / Programme

According to Price Gittinger (1984), "a project is an activity on which money will be spent in expectation of returns and which logically seems to lend itself to planning, financing, and implementation as a unit".

According to Project Management Institute, USA, "a project is a one-shot, time-limited, goal-directed, major undertaking, requiring the commitment of varied skills and resources.

In the context of rural development, "A development project may be defined as an investment of resources on a package of inter-related, time-bound activities.

The simplest possible definition of the project can be "a set of inter-related activities undertaken to achieve some objectives or goals within a given period of time through consumption of some resources".

Basic Elements of a Project

- Objective
- Activities
- Time
- Resources
- Client

Characteristic Feature of a Project

- Objectives – Should have fixed set of objectives
- Life Span – Having a fixed life span, cannot continue endlessly.
- Single Entity – Usually one entity with responsibility entrusted to one center.
- Life Cycle – Is having a life-cycle reflected by growth, maturity, and decay.
- Uniqueness – All projects are unique in nature.
- Successive Principle – Final results of any project are not known at any stage of the life-cycle and the details get finalized with the passage of time.
- Change – A project is supposed to bring about change.
- Unity in Diversity – Diverse technology, process, and manpower are untidily directed towards the achievement of project goals.
- Risk and Uncertainty – Every project has a certain amount of risk and uncertainty.

Why Project Management

Project Management is necessary for addressing the following issues:

- Time Factor – Timely completion of any project is necessary
- Availability of resources required for the completion of any project is limited.
- Project must be completed as early as possible.
- Element of risks and uncertainties must be considered.
- Continuous planning is necessary.
- Unity of objectives to be ensured.
- A project is executed once only.
- Project should be kept within budget and schedule.

Project management with the proper application of different tools helps in addressing the above-stated issues.

Steps in Project Management

- Project Planning
    - Provides a basis for organization of work and assignment of responsibilities
    - Provides coordination
    - Includes time consciousness
    - Provide a basis for monitoring and evaluation
- Project Scheduling
    - Activates are decided
    - Arranged in time scale in chronological order
    - Resource requirements for each activity are decided
    - Starting and completion times as well as the duration of each activity are determined.
- Project Controlling
    - It provides a basis for a continuous check on the performance of the project.
    - Variance Analysis Control
    - Variance is determined by comparing the actual cost with the budgeted cost. It tells us what has happened in the past but did not tell us what will happen in the future.
    - Performance Analysis Control
    - Systematically analyses the performance of the project.

Step I – Find whether the entire project is within the schedule or not. If any departure following question arises:

Where did it occur?

What would be its implication?

How can it be corrected?

Step II – Find whether the cost of the project is within or out of budget estimates. In the case of departure, the same questions arise.

Step III – Check the trend of performance, that is estimate (a) the expected cost of the project, (b) the expected duration of the project.

The instruments for Project Schedule /Activities Management

1. **Bar Chart** – Developed by Gantt in connection with Military requirements of World War I. In the Bar Chart activities of the project are depicted by a horizontal bar with their scheduled start and finish time and their current status.

   Advantages of Bar Chart

   - Plan, schedule and progress of the project are represented graphically.
   - Gives an estimate of the progress of each activity.

   Disadvantages of Bar Chart

   - Does not show the relationships between activities.
   - Difficult for a large project.
   - Becomes outdated.

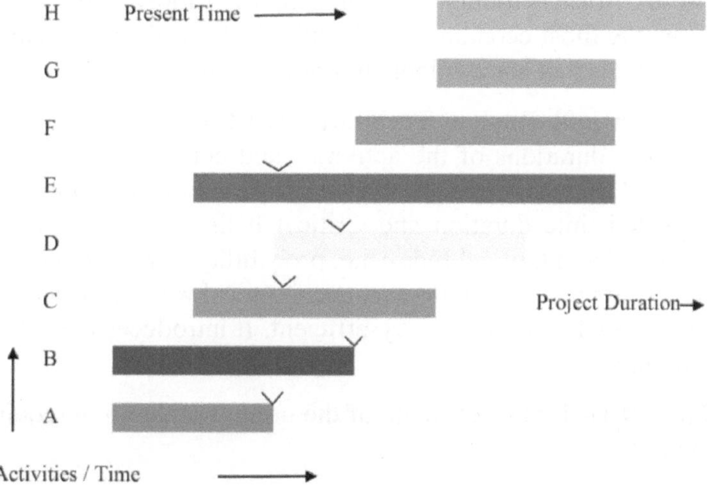

2. **Network Method** – Powerful tools for the management of all types of projects. Represents the project plan by a schematic diagram called a network that clearly depicts the sequence and inter-relation between activities. There are three basic network methods, namely, Critical Path Method (CPM), Project Evaluation and Review Technique (PERT), and Graphical Evaluation Technique (GERT).

Network Representation of a Project

- Each activity must be represented by one and only one arrow.
- The Letter above each arrow represents the Activity Code.
- The number over each arrow represents the duration of each activity.
  - The specific time at which each activity begin or end is called a Node & represented by a circle
  - The number inside the circle is the Node Number.
- No two activities should have the same initial and same terminal nodes.
- The arrowheads should not form a closed loop.
- The starting and terminal nodes must be unique.
- Dummy Activity may be inserted in the network (represented by dotted lines) for establishing a relationship between activities which doesn't consume any time/resource.

Critical Path Method (CPM) – This is the logical-mathematical model based upon the optimal duration required for each activity and optimal use of available resources. In CPM the durations of different activities are deterministic (fixed). It ascertains Critical activities whose completion determines the completion of the project. These Critical activities together form the Critical Path. For a fixed duration, it gives the most economical schedule. It determines the pattern of allocation of resources that are available in limited quantity.

Project Evaluation and Review Technique (PERT) – PERT introduces uncertainties on the durations of the activities and consequently on project duration. It is well suited where the duration of activities is uncertain. It determines expected time duration and Critical Path as well Semi Critical Path. Every activity has a Critical Index, i.e. probability of becoming Critical. It allocates the limited resource in the most economical way. If the simulation technique is introduced it becomes very efficient. It introduces the following time duration of an activity.

Optimistic Time (t_o) – It is an estimate of the minimum duration required to complete an activity.

Most Likely Time (t_m) – It is duration if the activity is repeated several times under unchanged conditions.

Pessimistic Time (t_p) – It is an estimate of the maximum duration required to complete the

$$t_o < t_m < t_p.$$

Expected Time Duration for an Activity:

$$E(Tij) = (t_o + 4t_m + t_p) / 6 \quad (1)$$

The measure of variability, the standard deviation V_{ij} of the activity (i,j) is introduced by assuming that 90% of data falls within $[t_o, t_p]$. This leads to –

$$V_{ij}^2 = \{(t_p - t_o) / 2\}^2 \quad (2)$$

Graphical Evaluation and Review Technique (GERT) – In GERT looping is allowed in contrast to CPM and PERT. This is very suitable for R & D Projects where the process is repeated until the desired result is not obtained. In GERT probabilistic events are allowed. For example, if activities A and B are completed then either activity C, D or E starts with probability p_1, p_2, p_3 $(p_1 + p_2 + p_3 = 1)$ Which cannot be considered under CPM and PERT. In GERT network only simulation can be used.

Comparison between CPM, PERT and GERT

S. No	CPM	PERT	GERT
1	Time duration are deterministic	Time duration are probabilistic	Time duration are probabilistic
2	Time duration of the project is fixed	Expected duration of the project	Expected duration of the project
3	Looping and probabilistic events are not allowed	Looping and probabilistic events are not allowed	Includes looping and probabilistic events.
4		Simulation can be used	Simulation is the only technique

Network Example

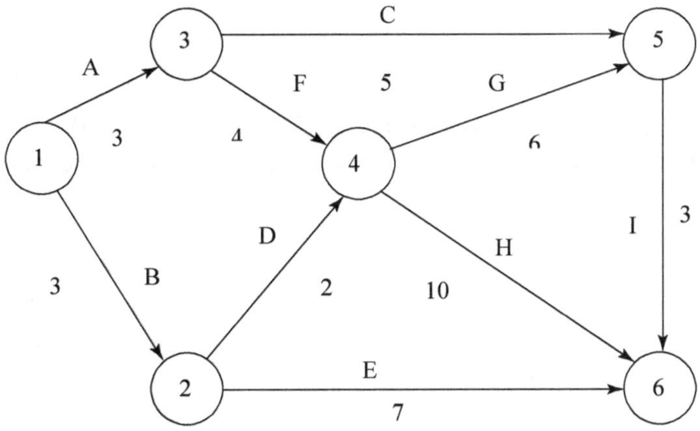

Critical Path under CPM

T_{ij} denote the duration of activity between node i,j.
Let ES_k denote the earliest start time of activities emanating from node k. Then: $ES_1 = 0$
ES_k = Max of ($ES_j + t_{ij}$) for all incoming activities.
For the above network (**Forward Phase**)– $ES_1 = 0$
ES_2 = Max of (ES_1 + 3) = (0 + 3) = **3**
ES_3 = Max of (ES_1 + 3) = (0 + 3) = **3**
ES_4 = Max of (ES_2 + 2), (ES_3 + 4) = 5, **7**
ES_5 = Max of (ES_3 + 5), (ES_4 + 6) = **8, 13**
ES_6 = Max of (ES_2 + 7), (ES_4 + 10), (ES_5 + 3) = 9, **17**, 16
ES_ks are entered into a rectangle at each node.

Backward Phase

Let, LCi denote the latest completion time activities coming into node i. Then,

LCi = ESi for the last node.
LCi = Min (LCj –tij) for all outgoing activities (i,j)
In the above example: LC6 = ES6 = 17
LC5 = Min (LC6 – 3) = 14
LC4 = Min (LC6-10), (LC5 – 6) = **7**
LC3 = Min (LC5 – 5), (LC4 – 4) = 3
LC2 = Min (LC6 – 7), (LC4 – 2) = 5
LC1 = Min (LC3 – 3), (LC2 – 3) = 0

LCi for every node is entered into a triangle over the rectangle. This completes the backward phase of calculation.

Critical Activity: An activity is called Critical activity if,

$ES_i = LC_i$
$ES_j = LC_j$
$ES_j - ES_i = LC_j - LC_i = t_{ij}$

In the above example, Critical Activities are (1,3), (3,4) and (4,6). The summation of duration of Critical Activities is the duration of the project and in this case, it is 17.

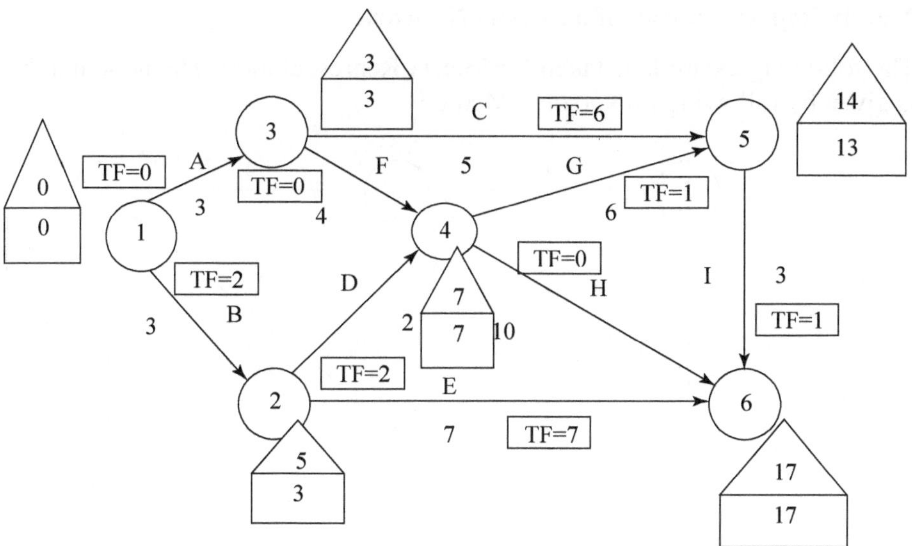

Float – Total Float of an activity (i,j) is denoted by TF_{ij} is the largest time available to complete the activity minus the time required to complete the activity. Thus,

$$\begin{aligned} TF_{ij} &= (LC_j - ES_i) - t_{ij} \\ &= LC_j - EC_{ij} \\ &= LS_{ij} - ES_i \end{aligned}$$

Free Float of an activity (i,j), denoted by FFij, is the excess of available time over the time required to complete the activity. Thus,

$$\begin{aligned} FF_{ij} &= (ES_j - ES_i) - t_{ij} \\ &= ES_j - EC_{ij} \end{aligned}$$

In the above example, we have,

$TF_{12} = 2$ $FF_{12} = 0$

$TF_{13} = 0$ $FF_{13} = 0$

$TF_{24} = 2$ $FF_{24} = 2$

$TF_{26} = 7$ $FF_{26} = 7$

$TF_{34} = 0$ $FF_{34} = 0$

$TF_{35} = 6$ $FF_{35} = 5$

$TF_{45} = 1$ $FF_{45} = 0$

$TF_{46} = 0$ $FF_{46} = 0$

$TF_{56} = 1$ $FF_{56} = 1$

It is observed from the definition of Total Float and Free Float for an activity (i,j),

$TF_{ij} = 0$ implies $FF_{ij} = 0$

$FF_{ij} = 0$ need not imply $TF_{ij} = 0$

Activity (i.j) is critical if and only if $TF_{ij} = 0$

Matrix Representation of a Project Network

The following example is taken for Matrix Representation. The node number is given by following Fulkerson's Method

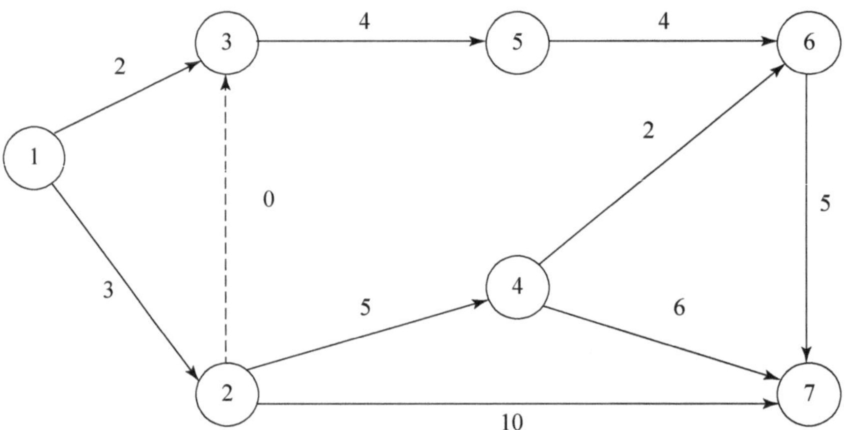

Matrix Representation

Initial Event	Terminal Events j							
i	**1**	**2**	**3**	**4**	**5**	**6**	**7**	**ES_i**
1		3	2					$ES_1 = 0$
2			0	5			10	$ES_2 = 3$
3					4			$ES_3 = 3$
4						2	6	$ES_4 = 8$
5						4		$ES_5 = 7$
6							5	$ES_6 = 11$
7								$ES_7 = 16$
LC_i	$LC_1 = 0$	$LC_2 = 3$	$LC_3 = 3$	$LC_4 = 9$	$LC_5 = 7$	$LC_6 = 11$	$LC_7 = 16$	

Critical Path under PERT

In this case, a Critical Path is ascertained by following the same method followed in the case of CPM. The only difference is in the case of CPM we talk about Time (as it is deterministic) but in the case of PERT we talk about Expected Time and that is calculated by the formula --

$E(Tij) = (t_o + 4t_m + t_p) / 6$ for each activity and thus,

$T = \text{Sum}\ (T_{ij})$

The Expected project duration (taking all critical activities together) E(T) is given by

$$E(T) = \text{Sum }(E(T_{ij}))$$

As T_{ij} are independent random variables, the variance V_T^2 of T is given by

$$V_T^2 = \text{Sum } V_{ij}^2$$

Optimal Scheduling by CPM

In a project two types of costs are involved – **Direct Costs** – associated with individual activity and these are resources required for an activity. And **Indirect Costs** – is the overhead expenditure associated with the project in terms of supervision costs etc. **The Direct Cost increases with decrease in duration of an activity whereas, Indirect Costs of a project decrease with reduction of time of the project**. The Cost of the project is the sum of its Direct and Indirect costs. There is something called Cost-Duration relationship of the project.

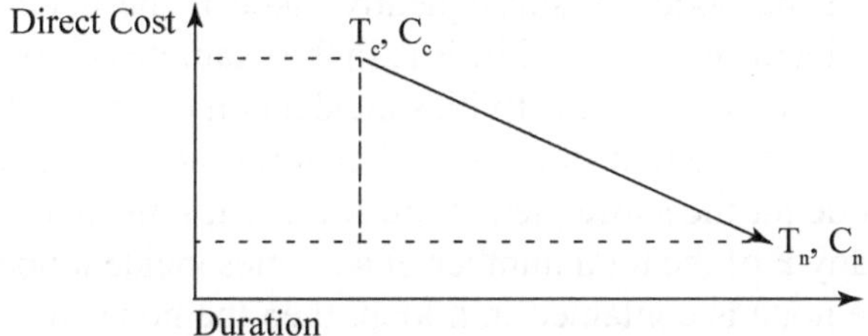

Here, T_n, C_n represents the duration and direct costs of an activity under normal condition. The Crash Point is denoted by T_c, C_c beyond which the duration of an activity cannot be reduced any more.

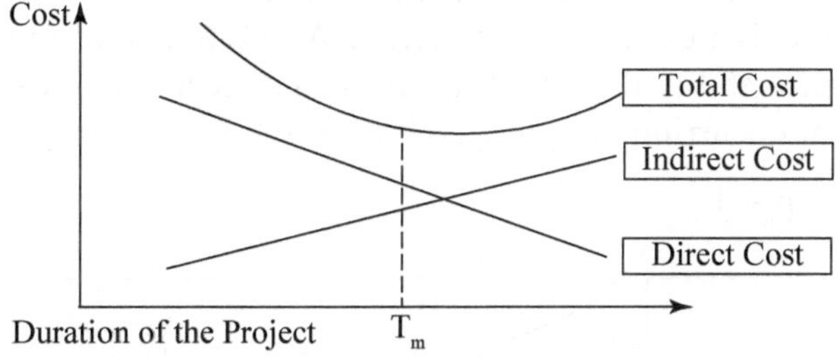

The Direct Cost of the project increase and Indirect Costs decrease if the duration of the project is reduced. Here duration Tm of the project is ascertained which minimizes the total cost of the project.

Graphical Evaluation and Review Technique (GERT)

In CPM and PERT, it is demanded that all preceding activities be completed before a node is reached or realized. But in a situation where the realization of a node depends on the completion of not all but one or more incoming activities then GERT is useful. It allows a loop that may start from any node and may incident upon any previous node. For GERT network simulation is needed. It differs from the PERT network in following aspects:

- It includes probabilistic nodes.
- It includes loop in the network.
- The realization of a node for the first time and subsequent times depends on not all incident activities.
- The terminal node need not be unique.

Deterministic Node

All activities emanating from the node are subsequently taken if the node is realized, this is somewhat similar as in CPM and PERT. In the example below N is the node number, F denotes the number of activities incident on the node that must be completed for the first realization of a node. S denotes the number of activities, incidents on the node for the subsequent realization. Thus, the node is realized the first time when any F of the total number of activities incident upon the node is completed. If the node is contained in a loop, then the node can be realized in the second and subsequent times when any S of the total number of activities incident upon the node are completed. In general F > S.

Probabilistic Node

Only one activity emanating from the node is taken if the node is realized. In the example the outgoing activities are A_1, A_2 .... A_n. Only one of these will occur at a time. The probability that the Activity Ai will occur is p_i (i=1). The sum of probabilities of occurring outgoing activities is 1.

Thus, $p_1 + p_2 + \dots\dots\dots + p_n = 1$

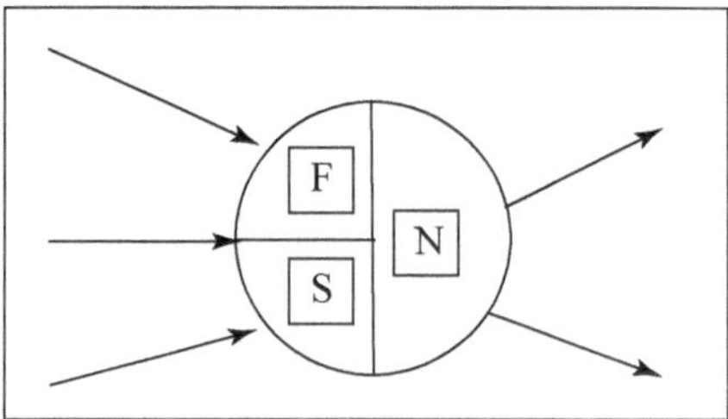

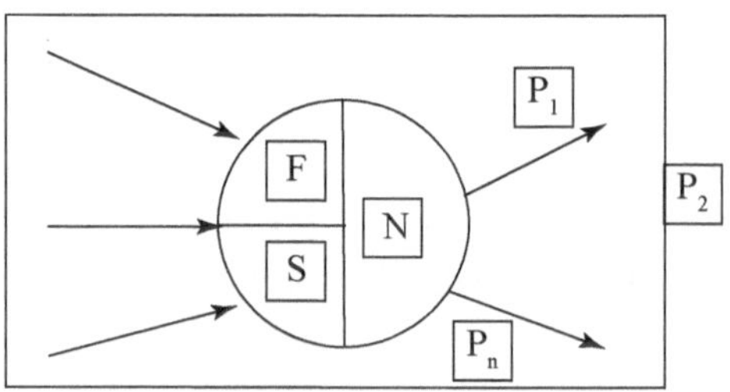

Logical Framework Approach (LFA)

LFA is result based and not activity driven approach used for systematic planning, implementation, monitoring and evaluating project. It envisages stakeholder involvement and need-based approach. It is based on logical intervention approach involving vertical and horizontal logic. It logically sets the objectives and their causal relationships. It shows whether objectives have been achieved in terms of indicators. Also analyses the external factors. Thus, it provides the framework for assessing relevance, feasibility and sustainability.

LFA is the main tool used for project design during identification and formulation phases. It is divided into two phases:

Phase I – The Analysis Phase to develop a vision of the "future desired situation" and strategies thereof.

Phase II – The Planning Phase.

Phase I: Analysis Phase

Includes:

- Problem Analysis
- Stakeholder analysis
- Gender consideration
- Planning workshop
- Objective analysis
- Strategy analysis

Problem Tree

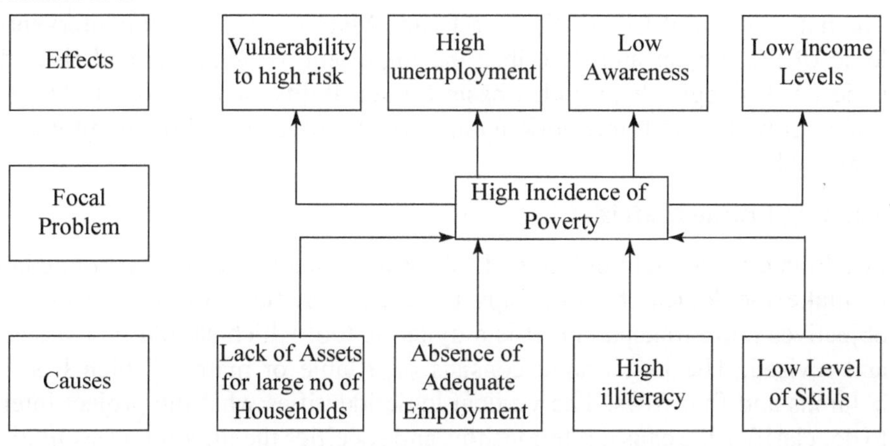

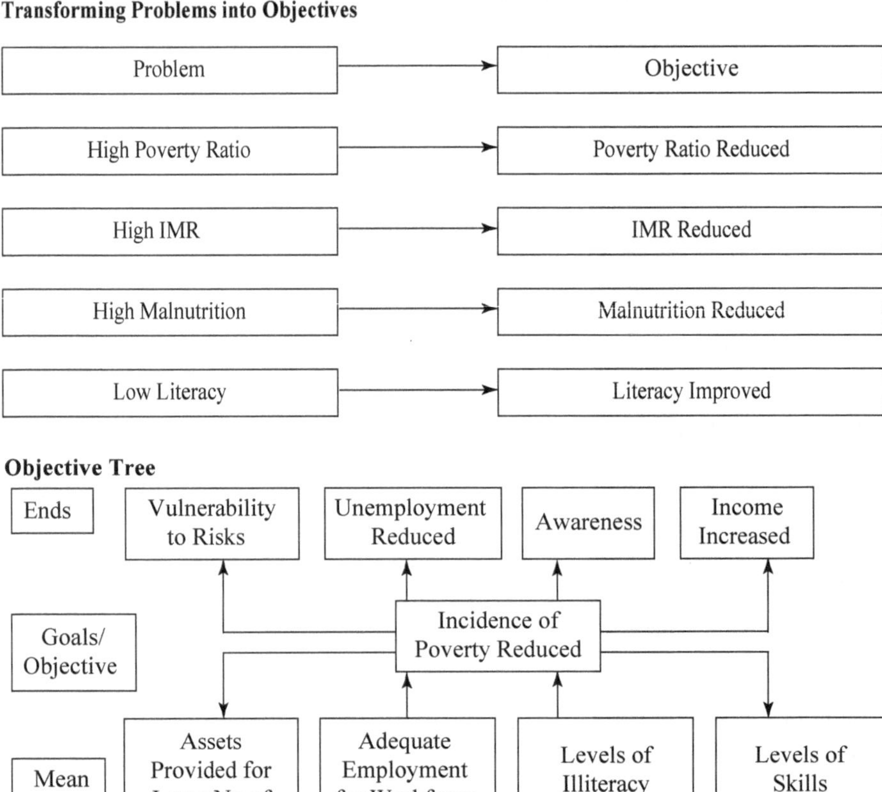

Phase II: The Planning Phase

The main output of LFA is the Log Frame Matrix. It sets out the intervention logic of the project and describes the important assumptions and risks that underlie this logic. It provides basis for feasibility of the project. The Log Frame provides the framework against which progress will be monitored and evaluated.

The Log Frame Matrix

Log Frame is the main output of LFA. When used properly Log Frame helps to make the logical relationships between activities, results, purpose and objectives more transparent. It is a dynamic tool which should be reassessed and revised. The Log Frame consists of a table or matrix, which has four columns and four rows. The vertical logic identifies what the project intends to do, clarifies the causal relationships and specifies the important assumptions and uncertainties. The horizontal logic relates to the measurement of the effects of, and resources used by, the project through the specification of key indicators of measurement, and the means by which the measurement will be verified The Logical Framework is shown below.

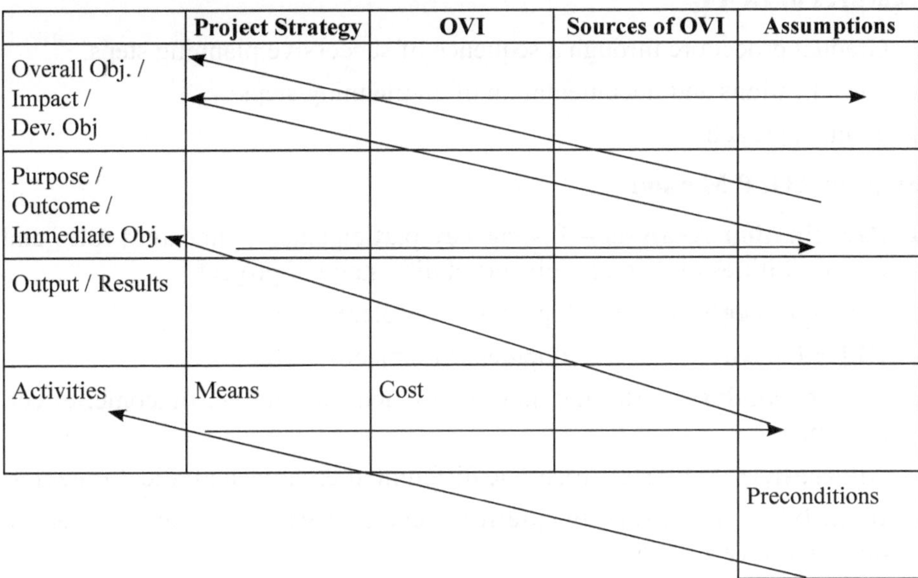

	Project Strategy	OVI	Sources of OVI	Assumptions
Overall Obj. / Impact / Dev. Obj				
Purpose / Outcome / Immediate Obj.				
Output / Results				
Activities	Means	Cost		
				Preconditions

ZOPP Method (Objective Oriented Planning)

The German Development Cooperation (GTZ) developed ZOPP methods, to bring about an improvement in the quality of project design and management and to ensure effectiveness. These methods can be considered as alternatives to LFA.

ZOPP (Ziel orientierte Projekt planung) meaning "Objectives-oriented Project Planning" incorporated LFA into its model. Through ZOPP Method **Project Planning / Design Matrix** is developed which is shown below.

Summary of Objectives / Activities	**OVI**	**Sources of OVI**	**Assumptions**
Project Goal			
Project Purpose			
Results			
Activities			

Objectives of ZOPP

- To identify realistic and specific objectives;
- To improve communication and cooperation;

- To clarify the scope of responsibility of project teams; and
- To provide indicators for monitoring and evaluation.

Features of ZOPP

- Gradual procedure through a sequence of successive planning steps.
- Visualizations and documentation of all planning steps
- Team approach

Steps in ZOPP Method

- **Participation Analysis** – Listing key participants; Delineating roles and responsibilities of diff. participants at diff. stage of project
- **Problem Analysis** – Development of Problem Tree.
- **Objective Analysis** – Development of Objective Tree.
- **Results Analysis** – Results may be divided into output, outcome, effect, and impact.
- **Alternatives Analysis** – Examine different alternative activities/strategies.
- **Identifying Indicators to quantify levels of achievements** – Must be objectively verifiable.
- **Risk and assumptions involved**-Analyzing the risks & assumptions surrounding the project
- **Action Plan** – Action Plan is prepared based on the results of the analyses to execute the project in a given time including resources required.

Between 1992 and 1995 GTZ tackled different criticism related with the ZOPP system. GTZ defined what it understands by quality in Project management and introduced flexibility in the procedure for project preparation and developed its "**Project Cycle management**" procedure.

Project Cycle Management Method (PCM)

The European Commission introduced PCM in the early 1990s to improve the quality of project design and management and thereby to improve effectiveness. It incorporates the application of project planning and appraisal tools like ZOPP, PRA, gender analysis, and others. The core of the philosophy of PCM is based on the principle that the initiative for a technical cooperation project must be born from a self-help development process in which only the genuine actors are involved.

PCM is based on six principles, these are:

- **Project Cycle analysis** – Distinguishes phases in project Cycle; stating roles of stakeholders at different phases; decisions, etc.

- **Beneficiary Focus and Ownership orientation** – Beneficiary oriented problem analyses; type of interventions required.
- **Logical Framework Planning based on thorough Analysis**–Produces LFA-based transparent Project Design.
- **Sustainability** – Results and activities are tested for sustainability.
- **Transparent, Standardized Documentation** – Introduces Transparent, Standardized Documentation.
- **Framework for Learning and Decision Making** – Provides systematic framework for learning from experience based on improved monitoring and evaluation practices; ensures:
- Projects are relevant to the agreed strategy and needs of stakeholders.
- Project is feasible and objectives can be realistically achieved
- Projects are sustainable.

Participatory Project Cycle Management (PPCM)

This variant of PCM enables a structured, cyclic, bottom-up planning process throughout different stages of identification, conception, and implementation with the following advantages.

- Problem-solutions can be tried out at the planning phase; experience can be used as feedback for progressive planning.
- Appreciation of stakeholders' problems, cultural context, possibilities (Ownership – People's Project).
- People's motivation to participate actively.
- Visions, problems, potentials, and solutions are clarified and analyzed systematically.

Concept of PPCM

- Project is perceived as an organized social process with phases of identification, conceptualization, and implementation with the active involvement of stakeholders.
- Everybody involved in Project must perform to reach the milestones.
- Interrelations between objectives and activities on a priority basis must be outlined before taking a decision.
- In PPCM, planning is conducted as a rolling plan in a cyclic process with many feedback loops.
- All decisions must be regularly reviewed and modified. The provisional nature of the decisions and plans is regarded as the strength of a process that evolves as a cyclic communication and learning process.

Steps in PCM

1. Idea Generation

- Based on vision/mission and the overall goal of the organization
- Discussion with organization
- Comparing with sectoral and developmental goals of donor partners.

2. Objective Setting

- Situation / Problem / Project Environment analysis through PRA.
- Participatory development of action plan.
- Participatory development of objectives, purpose, results, activities, indicators, risks and assumptions.
- Discuss the responsibilities.
- Specifying accountability.
- Practice transparency.
- Practice monitoring (self and external).
- Incorporation of lessons in the next phase of project.

3. Implementation

- Participation of people in implantation, identification of indicators, monitoring etc.
- Periodic monitoring of effects.
- Yearly monitoring and evaluation.
- Study the implications monitoring is having on project purpose, goal, results etc.

Annexure I: Activity Scheduling (Dummy)

Project Title: Promotion of Entrepreneurship among Rural Women of Bolpur-Sriniketan C D Block

S. No	Objective	Activity	Activity Code	EST	LST	Dura tion (Days)	ECT	LCT	Assumption about type and amount / no of resources required
1	Selection of willing rural women	Preparing List of interested Women	A	01/06	10/06	15	15/06	25/06	Remuneration for data collector (10 nos.). Stationery
		Organizing Workshop on entre-preneurship (in groups)	B	20/06	25/06	20	10/07	15/07	Rem for trainer. Tiffin / Lunch/Organizing Cost
		Selection of first group of women (100 No's)	C	10/07	12/07	05	15/07	17/07	Office Expenditure
2	Selection ofenterprises (10 no)	Organizing workshop							
3	Selection of site	Conducting field survey							
4	Imparting entrepreneurial training	Holding no. of training for each enterprise							

Annexure-II: Log Frame Matrix (Dummy)

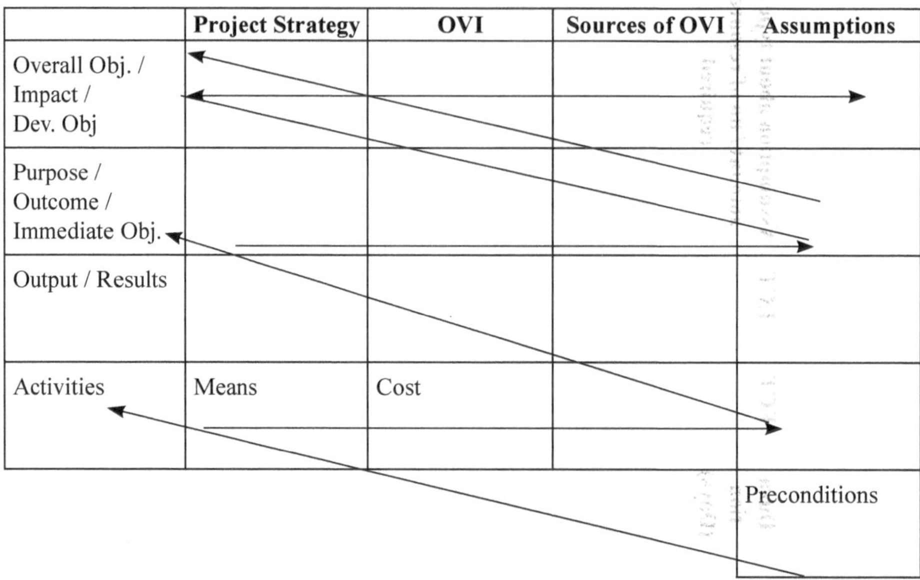

	Project Strategy	OVI	Sources of OVI	Assumptions
Overall Obj. / Impact / Dev. Obj				
Purpose / Outcome / Immediate Obj.				
Output / Results				
Activities	Means	Cost		
				Preconditions

Annexure-III: Effect of River Water Pollution in Fishery (Dummy) Problem Tree

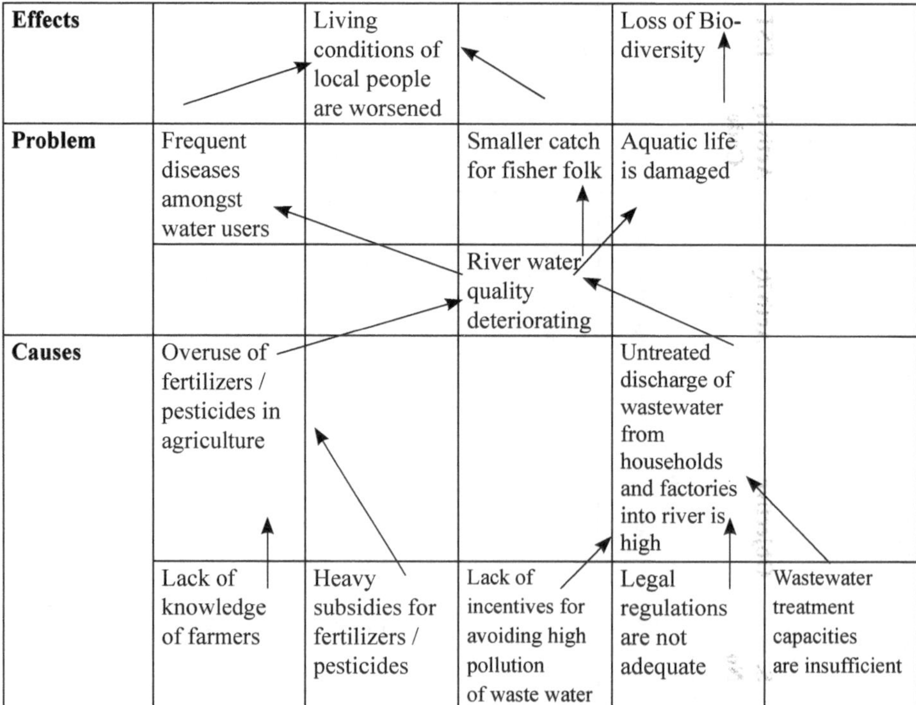

Effects		Living conditions of local people are worsened		Loss of Bio-diversity	
Problem	Frequent diseases amongst water users		Smaller catch for fisher folk	Aquatic life is damaged	
			River water quality deteriorating		
Causes	Overuse of fertilizers / pesticides in agriculture			Untreated discharge of wastewater from households and factories into river is high	
	Lack of knowledge of farmers	Heavy subsidies for fertilizers / pesticides	Lack of incentives for avoiding high pollution of waste water	Legal regulations are not adequate	Wastewater treatment capacities are insufficient

8

Good Governance Concept and Issues

Debabrata Basu

Department of Agricultural Extension, BCKV, Nadia, West Bengal

Introduction

Recently the terms "governance" and "good governance" are being increasingly used in development literature. Bad governance is being increasingly regarded as one of the root causes of all evil within our societies. Major donors and international financial institutions are increasingly basing their aid and loans on the condition that reforms that ensure "good governance" are undertaken.

Good governance is an essential complement to sound economic policies. Efficient and accountable management by the public sector and a predictable and transparent policy framework are critical to the efficiency of markets and governments, and hence to economic development. Good governance, for the World Bank, is synonymous with sound development management The Bank's experience has shown that the programs and projects it helps finance may be technically sound, but fail to deliver anticipated results for reasons connected to the quality of government action. Legal reforms, however urgent, may come to naught if the new laws are not enforced consistently or there are severe delays in implementation. Efforts to develop privatized production and encourage market-led growth may not succeed unless investors face dear rules and institutions that reduce uncertainty about future government action.

Vital reforms of public expenditure may flounder if accounting systems are so weak that budgetary policies cannot be implemented or monitored or if poor procurement systems encourage corruption and distort public investment priorities. Failure to involve beneficiaries and others affected in the design and implementation of projects can substantially erode their sustainability.

These examples illustrate a broader point: good governance is central to creating and sustaining an environment which fosters strong and equitable development, and it is an essential complement to sound economic policies. Governments play a key role in the provision of public goods. They establish the rules that make markets work efficiently and, more problematically, they correct for market failure. In order to play this role, they need revenues, and agents to collect revenues and produce the public goods. This in turn requires systems of accountability, adequate and reliable information, and efficiency in resource management and the delivery of public services. Yet there is no certainty that institutional frameworks conducive to growth and poverty alleviation will evolve on their own. The emergence of such frameworks needs incentives, and adequate institutional capacity to create and sustain them.

The World Bank, along with other external aid and finance agencies, is involved in assisting developing countries build these incentives and develops such capacity. Thus, for example, in public sector management, the Bank's work has broadened from assisting in improving the management of project-related agencies to addressing such systematic constraints on sound management as weaknesses in the civil service, in wage structures, and in the central economic agencies that are responsible for policy formulation. This broader approach is also under way in other areas of governance, such as action to clarify accountability and strengthen the legal framework.

Governance

The concept of "governance" is not new. It is as old as human civilization. Simply put "governance" means: **the process of decision-making and the process by which decisions are implemented (or not implemented)**. Governance can be used in several contexts such as corporate governance, international governance, national governance and local governance. Since governance is the process of decision making and the process by which decisions are implemented, an analysis of governance focuses on the formal and informal actors involved in decision-making and implementing the decisions made and the formal and informal structures that have been set in place to arrive at and implement the decision.

Government is one of the actors in governance. Other actors involved in governance vary depending on the level of government that is under discussion. In rural areas, for example, other actors may include influential land lords, associations of peasant farmers, cooperatives, NGOs, research institutes, religious leaders, finance institutions political parties, the military etc. The situation in urban areas is much more complex. Figure 1 provides the interconnections between actors involved in urban governance. At the national level, in addition to the above actors, media, lobbyists, international donors, multi-national corporations, etc. may play a role in decision making or in influencing the decision-making process.

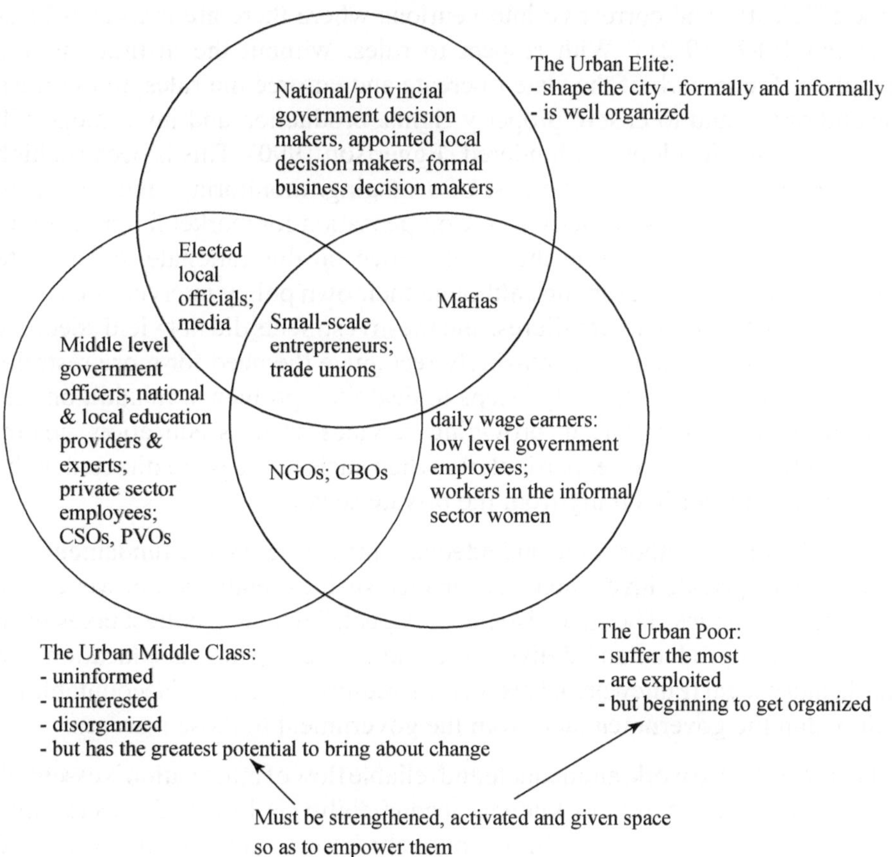

Fig 1. Urban Actors

All actors other than government and the military are grouped together as part of the "civil society." In some countries in addition to the civil society, organized crime syndicates also influence decision-making, particularly in urban areas and at the national level. Similarly formal government structures are one means by which decisions are arrived at and implemented. At the national level, informal decision-making structures, such as "kitchen cabinets" or informal advisors may exist. In urban areas, organized crime syndicates such as the "land Mafia" may influence decision-making. In some rural areas locally powerful families may make or influence decision-making. Such, informal decision-making is often the result of corrupt practices or leads to corrupt practices.

The Nature of the Problem

The Role of Governments even in societies that are highly market-oriented, only governments can provide two sorts of public goods: rules to make markets work efficiently and corrective interventions where there are market failures (McLean 1987: 19-21). With respect to rules, without the institutions and supportive framework of the state to create and enforce the rules, to establish law and order, and to ensure property rights, production and investment will be deterred and development hindered (Eggertson 1990). This is because high "transaction costs" (that is, the cost of arranging, monitoring, and enforcing contracts) will inhibit such activities. Compensation for market failure is more problematic. Governments in the 1970s relied on this rationale to rush into unwise policies and investments, although their own policy interventions often were responsible for market failures, and the investments did not yield adequate returns. Governments now increasingly recognize the need for more restraint and for taking "market-friendly" steps to deal with problems. In addition, the state must play a key role in providing services such as education, health, and essential infrastructure, particularly when such services are directed at the poor and are not forthcoming from the private sector.

A well-educated labor force and adequate infrastructure are fundamental to the quality of private investment. To finance such expenditures, however, the state needs revenues. The state also needs "agents" who will collect taxes from the public and produce and deliver essential services (such as education and health, and a legal framework).This, in turn, requires systems of accountability-both within the government and from the government to those it serves.

For the system to work, an adequate and reliable flow of information is essential. Without it, the rules are not known, accountability is low, and uncertainties are excessive. Thus, accountability, publicly known rules, information, and transparency are all elements of sound development management. Moreover, the institutional framework needed to provide these public goods must be managed efficiently. Productive institutional arrangements will vary between countries on the basis of their cultural traditions and historic relationships. And they will continue to evolve as the economy grows and becomes more complex and more integrated with international markets. Mature institutional frameworks take a great deal of time to develop, but there is no guarantee that arrangements which are supportive of economic growth and poverty alleviation will, in fact, emerge.

When Governance Fails

The institutional characteristics for managing development thus vary widely among countries and do not permit easy generalization. Nor is it practical to attempt taxonomy, classifying states, say, by different characteristics of governance. This complexity arises from the unique imprint of history, geography, and culture on each country's institutions and rules, and the multi-dimensional nature of governance as a concept. Thus each country is at a different level of political, economic, and social development reflecting a wide array of historical, geographic, and cultural factors. A number of the World Bank's borrowers have been relatively successful in creating the institutions and rules that promote broadly based economic development. Some others are on their way to doing so, whereas yet others still labor under severe political, institutional, and economic constraints on better government performance.

But poor governance is readily recognizable. Some of its main symptoms are:

- Failure to make a clear separation between what is public and what is private, hence, a tendency to divert public resources for private gain.
- Failure to establish a predictable framework of law and government behavior conducive to development, or arbitrariness in the application of rules and laws.
- Excessive rules, regulations, licensing requirements, and so forth, which impede the functioning of markets and encourage rent-seeking
- Priorities inconsistent with development, resulting in a misallocation of resources
- Excessively narrowly based or nontransparent decision making.

Such "problems" may be due to lack of capacity or to volition, or both, and may be of varying severity. It is when they are sufficiently severe and occur together, however, that they create an environment hostile to development. In such circumstances, the authority of governments over their peoples tends to be progressively eroded. This reduces compliance with decisions and regulations. Governments then tend to respond through populist measures or, as in some authoritarian regimes, they resort to coercion. Either way, the economic cost can be high, including a diversion of resources to internal security and escalating corruption. Poor development performance can in turn contribute to poor governance by further eroding the confidence of citizens in their governments and causing governments to behave insecurely.

The absence of good governance has proved to be particularly damaging to the "corrective intervention" role of government. Programs for poverty alleviation and environmental protection, for example, can be totally undermined by a lack of public accountability, corruption, and the "capture" of public services by elites. Funds intended for the poor may be directed to the benefit of special interest groups, and the poor may have inadequate access to legal remedies. Similarly, the enforcement of environmental standards, which benefit the population as a whole but which may be costly to powerful industrial and commercial groups, can be emasculated by poor governance. Industrial emissions standards, forest protection policies, and guidelines for the incorporation of environmental concerns into public expenditure decisions may be worth little more than the paper they are written on unless rules are dear, information is available to the public, and government officials are accountable.

In the case of the environment, problems are magnified by difficulties of monitoring and enforcement, which enable official government policies to be ignored. Among the underlying causes of poor development management is the level of economic, human, and institutional development. Lack of an educated and trained work force and weak institutions can substantially reduce the capacity of countries to provide sound development management. Poverty and illiteracy make poor governance more likely. This is not, though, to suggest that development automatically brings good governance; nor to imply that sound economic management is not possible in poor countries. There are a number of Asian counter-examples, both authoritarian and democratic. It is simply that poverty, illiteracy, and weak institutions make the task of good development management much more complicated and problematic. Pervasive corruption is particularly damaging to development. Corruption occurs in all countries and in many different forms. It tends to thrive when resources are scarce, and governments, rather than markets, allocate them; when civil servants are underpaid; when rules are unreasonable or unclear; when controls are pervasive and regulations are excessive; and when disclosure and punishment are unlikely.

Although there have been isolated instances of governments being both corrupt and successful at promoting development, in general, corruption weakens the ability of governments to carry out their functions efficiently. "Bribery, nepotism, and venality," notes World Development Report 1991, "can cripple administration and dilute equity from the provision of government services-and thus also undermine social cohesiveness" (World Bank 1991d: 131). Graft on a large scale is not possible without collusion with private companies or foreign suppliers, with officials of foreign governments sometimes turning a blind eye-a problem of international governance. Other causes of poor development management are a high degree of concentration of political power and the colonial inheritance. On the positive side, many former colonies inherited systems of financial accountability, an independent civil service, and a legal framework. Because these were imported from outside, however, they have not always taken root. Colonial rule implied accountability to the colonial power, rather than to citizens; it thus sometimes destroyed indigenous systems of accountability.

These symptoms and causes of poor governance are not unique to any particular form of government. World Development Report 1991 examined the evidence on the relative performance records of democracies and authoritarian regimes and noted that the democratic-authoritarian distinction itself "fails to explain adequately whether or not countries initiate reform, implement it effectively, or survive its political fallout" (World Bank 1991d: 134). Authoritarian regimes were just as likely to yield to the interests of narrow constituencies.

Good governance

Good governance has 8 major characteristics. It is participatory, consensus oriented, accountable, transparent, responsive, effective and efficient, equitable and inclusive and follows the rule of law. It assures that corruption is minimized, the views of minorities are taken into account and that the voices of the most vulnerable in society are heard in decision-making. It is also responsive to the present and future needs of society.

Participation

Participation by both men and women is a key cornerstone of good governance. Participation could be either direct or through legitimate intermediate institutions or representatives. It is important to point out that representative democracy does not necessarily mean that the concerns of the most vulnerable in society would be taken into consideration in decision making.

Participation needs to be informed and organized. This means freedom of association and expression on the one hand and an organized civil society on the other hand.

Rule of law

Good governance requires fair legal frameworks that are enforced impartially. It also requires full protection of human rights, particularly those of minorities. Impartial enforcement of laws requires an independent judiciary and an impartial and incorruptible police force.

Transparency

Transparency means that decisions taken and their enforcement are done in a manner that follows rules and regulations. It also means that information is freely available and directly accessible to those who will be affected by such decisions and their enforcement. It also means that enough information is provided and that it is provided in easily understandable forms and media.

Responsiveness

Good governance requires that institutions and processes try to serve all stakeholders within a reasonable time frame.

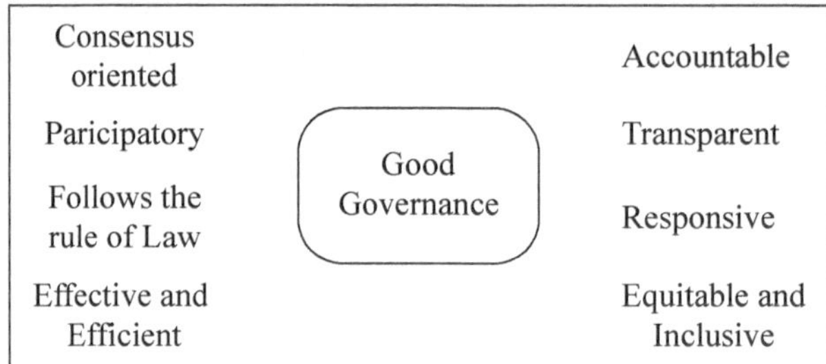

Fig 2. Characteristics of Good Governance

Consensus oriented

There are several actors and as many viewpoints in a given society. Good governance requires mediation of the different interests in society to reach a broad consensus in society on what is in the best interest of the whole community and how this can be achieved. It also requires a broad and long-term perspective on what is needed for sustainable human development and how to achieve the goals of such development. This can only result from an understanding of the historical, cultural and social contexts of a given society or community.

Equity and inclusiveness

A society's well-being depends on ensuring that all its members feel that they have a stake in it and do not feel excluded from the mainstream of society. This requires all groups, but particularly the most vulnerable, have opportunities to improve or maintain their well-being.

Effectiveness and efficiency

Good governance means that processes and institutions produce results that meet the needs of society while making the best use of resources at their disposal. The concept of efficiency in the context of good governance also covers the sustainable use of natural resources and the protection of the environment.

Accountability

Accountability is a key requirement of good governance. Not only governmental institutions but also the private sector and civil society organizations must be accountable to the public and to their institutional stakeholders. Who is accountable to whom varies depending on whether decisions or actions taken are internal or external to an organization or institution. In general an organization or an institution is accountable to those who will be affected by its decisions or actions. Accountability cannot be enforced without transparency and the rule of law.

Conclusion

From the above discussion it should be clear that good governance is an ideal which is difficult to achieve in its totality. Very few countries and societies have come close to achieving good governance in its totality. However, to ensure sustainable human development, actions must be taken to work towards this ideal with the aim of making it a reality. In sum, governance is a continuum, and not necessarily unidirectional: it does not automatically improve over time. It is a plant that needs constant tending. Citizens need to demand good governance. Their ability to do so is enhanced by literacy, education, and employment opportunities. Governments need to prove responsive to those demands. Neither of these can be taken for granted. Change occurs sometimes in response to external or internal threats. It also occurs through pressures from different interest groups, some of which may be in the form of populist demands.

9

Interpersonal Behaviour & Relationship in Extension

Atul Borgohain

Department of Extension Education
Assam Agricultural University, Khanapara, Guwahati-22

Interpersonal Behavior is the study of one's own perception, knowledge, attitude & motivation and how these affect one's behavior to the self & with others. It is characterized mainly by 3 factors. A. Communication skill (Knowledge / literacy / intelligence, Listening skill, Verbal skill and Active listening/feedback). B. Emotional intelligence (Self-awareness and Emotional maturity) C. Social skill (Good eye contact, Body language and Empathy/ understanding & assimilating ability). For Understanding Interpersonal Behaviors, Behavioral scientists recommend the use of Johari Window & Transactional Analysis (TA).

Johari Window is a psychological too created by Joseph Luft& Harry Ingham in 1955 in USA.. It helps people to understand their better interpersonal relations & communication. The Johari Window model is also referred to as a 'disclosure/feedback model of self-awareness', and by some people an 'information processing tool'. The Johari Window actually represents information - feelings, experience, views, attitudes, skills, intentions, motivation, etc - within or about a person - in relation to their group, from four perspectives. Johari window four quadrants: 1. what is known by the person about him/herself and is also known by others - open area, open self, free area, free self, or 'the arena'. 2. what is unknown by the person about him/herself but which others know - blind area, blind self, or 'blind spot'. 3. what the person knows about him/herself that others do not know - hidden area, hidden self, avoided area, avoided self or 'facade'. 4. What is unknown by the person about him/herself and is also unknown by others - unknown area or unknown self.

Transactional Analysis: When two people interact with each other, they engage in social transactions, in which one person responds to the other. Study of such "Social Transactions" is called 'Transactional Analysis'. What is a

Transaction? A Transaction is an exchange of two strokes between two people. The first stroke is called 'Stimulus'; the second is called the 'Response'.

Type of Transactions

1. Complementary
2. Non-Complementary.

To understand Transactional Analysis we must first understand EGO STATES:

Ego States: Within each human being, several human beings are existing at the same time, depending upon how the person is behaving at any given time. Advantages of T.A it improves Interpersonal Communication, Simple to learn, Applicable to Motivation, Helps in Organizational Development, Can be used at home as well as in office. One of the most distinctive aspects of human beings is that we are social beings & Nursing is therapeutic processes have been the core of our social system since the dawn of civilization. & demands an association between the nurse & the patient. Interpersonal relationships refer to reciprocal social & Interpersonal relationship is defined as a close association between individuals who share common interests, emotional interactions between two or more individuals in an environment & goals. One person relays a message It is the simplest of the three interpersonal dynamics. It is also one of the most intimate interpersonal dynamic as the focus of listening.

The johari window model is a simple}& useful tool for illustrating & improving self-awareness & the johari window terminology refers to self} mutual understanding between individuals within a group. & self refers to the person subject to the Johari window analysis}others. & others refer to other people in the person's group or tea. The johari window model was devised by American psychologist; Joseph Luft & the Johari window model represents self- awareness of an individual towards himself or herself. The upper left quadrant of the window represents the part of the self that is public; that is, aspect of the self about which both the individual & others are aware. The upper right (blind) quadrant of the window represents the part of the self that is known to others but remains hidden from the awareness of the individual. The lower left quadrant of the window represents the part of the self that is known to the individual, but which the individual deliberately & consciously conceals from others. The lower right quadrant of the window represents the part of the self that is unknown to both the individual & to others. The model is a simple & useful tool for illustrating & improving self-awareness & mutual understanding between individuals in a group.

- The Johari model can also be used to assess & improving self-awareness & mutual understanding between individuals in a group.
- The johari window actually represents information – feelings, experiences, views attitudes, skills, intentions, motivation, etc. - within or about a person in relation to their group from four perspectives. The Johari window provides a useful way to graphically visualize the process of self-disclosure.

10

Performance Appraisal & Logical Framework Analysis Application in Extension

Asif Mohammad

ICAR-National Dairy Research Institute, Kalynai-741235, West Bengal

Abstract

In any extension organization, performance appraisal is critical for human resource management. Extension professionals or employees will have a better grasp of their roles and obligations, as well as recommendations on how to improve their performance, if the performance appraisal process is formal and well-structured. The Logical Framework Analysis (LFA) is also described as the project-planning matrix, is a planning, monitoring and evaluation technique for extension projects. The steps in the performance appraisal process are as follows: setting performance benchmarks, communicating standards to employees, evaluating actual performance, comparing actual to desired performance, discussing the results and making a conclusion. Critical Incidence Technique, confidential report, weighted checklists, visual rating scales, behaviorally anchored rating scales, forced choice approach, Management by Objectives (MBO) etc. are commonly used performance appraisal methods. The essential components of Logical Framework Analysis, on the other hand, comprise of hierarchy of objectives, objectively verifiable indicators, verification means and critical assumptions and risks. The logical framework isn't a universal remedy for all development project problems, but it can help policymakers and financial agencies/donors to understand what a project is trying to achieve. Not only that, LFA may also describe in simple terms how the project will achieve its goal.

Introduction

Performance assessment is required to assess employee including extension functionaries and organizational performance in order to track progress toward desired goals and objectives that are aligned with the organization's mission.

Performance appraisal plays pivotal role in managing human resources in any organization (Judge and Ferris, 1993; Boswell and Boudreau, 2002). Employees are now being paid based on their contribution to the system, which is becoming increasingly popular around the world. Individual innovation emerges as a key competence required from workers, in turn crucially affecting the way managers make employees contribute to organizational goals and assess their performance (Curzi *et al.,* 2019). As a result, the companies' primary focus has turned to performance management, specifically individual performance. Employee performance is rated and their contribution to the organization's goals is evaluated through performance appraisal. If the performance appraisal process is formal and well-structured, employees will have a better understanding of their duties and responsibilities, as well as guidance on how to improve their performance. On the other hand, the logical framework, commonly known as the project-planning matrix, is a technique used to plan, monitor, and evaluate extension projects. The Logical Framework was initially developed for the U.S. Agency for International Development (USAID) in 1970 as an evaluation tool to help increase accountability to Congress (Sartorius,1991). It's a type of matrix in which a descriptive impression of the hierarchy of objectives is presented alongside components of key management activities for evaluation, performance measurement, external conditions etc. Evaluation of a project at any stage of its life cycle, especially at its planning stage, is necessary for its successful execution and completion. The Logical Framework Analysis or the Logical Framework Approach (LFA) is an essential tool in designing such evaluation because it is a process that serves as a reference guide in carrying out the evaluation (Barau and Olukosi, 2011). It also provides a prospect to make reasoning from the standpoint of criticism, monitoring, and evolution. The logical framework is a tool for management by objective (MBO). It is depicted as a pair wise matrix of project component and their explanations.

Performance Appraisal Process

The following is a simplified description of the performance appraisal process:

Creating performance benchmarks

The first step in the performance appraisal process is to establish the criteria that will be used as a yardstick to compare the actual performance of the employees. This phase entails determining the criteria for determining whether an employee's performance was successful or unsuccessful, as well as the extent to which they contributed to the organization's goals and objectives. The standards established should be explicit, intelligible, and measurable.

Communicating standards to the employee

It is the obligation of management to convey the standards to all of the organization's personnel once they have been established. Employees should be informed and the standards should be explained to them in detail. This will assist them in understanding their roles and what is expected from them. The standards should also be presented to the appraisers or evaluators and the set standards can be amended at this stage based on the relevant input from the workers or evaluators if necessary.

Actual performance evaluation

The most challenging component of the performance assessment process is measuring actual performance, which refers to the work done by employees over the given period of time during which the performance will be evaluated. It's an ongoing procedure that entails tracking performance throughout the year. This stage necessitates the careful selection of acceptable measurement methodologies, ensuring that personal bias does not influence the process' outcome and assisting rather than interfering with the job.

Comparison of actual vs. desired performance

The actual performance is compared to what is desired or expected. The comparison shows how far the employees' performance deviates from the established benchmarks. The actual performance can either be higher than the anticipated performance or lower than the expected performance, indicating a negative variance in organizational performance. It entails recollecting, evaluating and analyzing data about the performance of employees.

Discussion on the Result

The appraisal results are communicated and discussed with staff on a one-on-one basis. This discussion focuses on communication and listening. The findings, issues and potential solutions are addressed in order to solve difficulties and to reach an agreement. Because feedback might affect an employee's future performance, it should be offered with a constructive attitude. The meeting's goal should be to resolve issues and motivate staff to improve their performance.

Making a Decision

The final phase in the process is to make decisions, which can be used to improve employee performance, implement necessary corrective actions or make relevant decisions such as incentives, promotions, demotions, transfers and so on.

Performance evaluation methods

Several methods are used for performance evaluation. They are discussed in the subsequent paragraphs by following Mohammad and Singh (2010):

(a) Confidential report: This type of report is commonly utilized in government agencies including extension organization. It is a descriptive report written by the employee's immediate superior at the completion of each year. The report outlines the subordinate's strengths and flaws. It usually does not provide any feedback to the employee. The employee is unsure why his ratings have dropped despite his best efforts, why others are rated higher when compared to him,

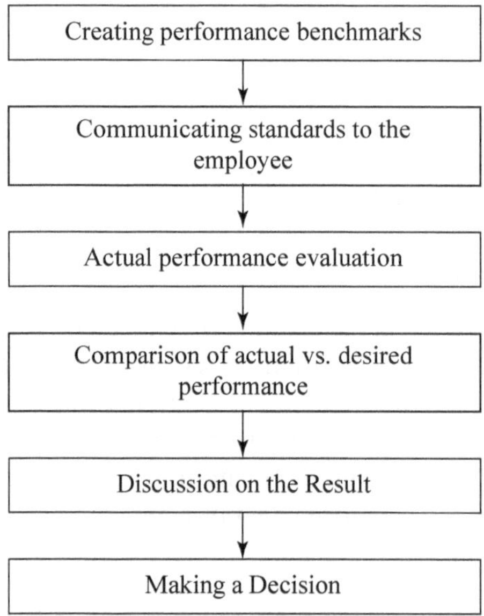

Figure 1: Performance appraisal process

how to correct any mistakes he may have made and on what basis he will be evaluated next year, among other things.

(b) Essay evaluation: In this method, the rate is required to convey both the positive and negative aspects of the employee's performance. Because the rater can elaborately portray the scale by substantiating an explanation for his rating, this technique is typically employed in conjunction with a visual rating scale. The rater considers the following aspects when writing the employee essay: (i) The employee's job knowledge and potential; (ii) The employee's understanding of the organization's programmes, policies and objectives; (iii) The employee's relationships with coworkers and superiors;

(iv)The employee's general planning, organizing and controlling ability; (v) The employee's general attitudes and perceptions. Essay assessment is a non-quantitative method. This method is beneficial in at least one way: the essay provides a wealth of information about the employee while also revealing more about the evaluator. The essay evaluation approach, on the other hand, has the following drawbacks:

- It is extremely subjective; the supervisor's essay may be biased. Employees who serve as acolytes will be rated higher than other employees.
- Some evaluators may struggle to write effective essays on employee performance. Others may be superficial in their explanations and use flowery language, which may not accurately reflect the employee's actual performance.
- The appraiser must allocate enough time to write the essay. A hurried appraiser may compose the essay without thoroughly assessing the worker's actual performance. The appraiser, on the other hand, takes a long time; this becomes uneconomical from the perspective of the organization because the evaluator's (supervisor's) time is expensive.

(c) Critical incident technique: The supervisor compiles a collection of remarks describing an employee's very effective and ineffective actions. These critical incidents or events illustrate the remarkable or poor performance of service workers. The manager keeps a log for each employee in which he captures key instances of the employee's behaviour on a regular basis. These key incidences are used in the evaluation of the workers' performance at the end of the rating period. This strategy provides an objective foundation for discussing an employee's performance in depth. This approach avoids focusing on the most recent instances.

However, this strategy has the following drawbacks:

- Negative incidents may be more visible than positive incidents.
- During an annual performance review session, supervisors have a tendency to unleash a series of complaints regarding incidents.
- It leads to intense supervision, which the employee may not appreciate. The critical events technique of appraisal is most commonly used to assess superiors' performance rather than that of subordinates' peers.

(d) Weighted checklists and checklists: The checklist is another basic approach of evaluating an individual. A checklist is a series of objective or descriptive statements concerning an employee's performance. If the rate is confident that the employee possesses one of the mentioned characteristics, he checks the box; otherwise, he leaves the box blank. The weighted list is a more contemporary variant of the checklist method. Each question's value may be equally weighted or select questions may be weighted more highly than others. The following are some of the checklist's sample questions.

Is the individual genuinely enthusiastic about the task at hand?	Yes/No
Is he well-liked by his co-workers?	Yes/No
Is he respectful of his superiors?	Yes/No
Is he a good follower of instructions?	Yes/No
Is he prone to making mistakes?	Yes/No

The management can use the rating score from the checklist to evaluate the employee's performance. The checklist technique has a significant flaw. The rater's ability to discern between positive and negative questions may be skewed. He might give the questions skewed weights. Another drawback is that this procedure is costly and time-consuming. Identifying, assembling, analyzing and weighing a multitude of assertions about an employee's characteristics, contributions and actions is extremely tough. Despite these drawbacks, the checklist approach is the most commonly utilized way for evaluating an employee's performance.

(e) Graphic rating scale: This is one of the most often used methods for evaluating performance. It is, of course, one of the oldest methods of appraisal now in use. A printed form, such as the one shown below, is used to evaluate an employee's performance in this approach. These types of grading systems can use a range of attributes, the most frequent of which are the quantity and quality of work. The rating scales can also be customized to include characteristics that the organization thinks vital for work performance. A graphic rating scale model is shown below.

Example of one 'Graphic Rating Scale'

Name.................. Department......................Rate .... Date.............

Table 1: Tabular representation of 'Graphic Rating Scale'

Parameters	**Rating**				
	Unsatisfactory	**Fair**	**Satisfactory**	**Good**	**Outstanding**
Work quantity: The amount of work completed under regular working conditions					
Work quality includes neatness, thoroughness and accuracy of Job-related knowledge					
A thorough awareness of the issues affecting the job					
On-the-job attitude: Exhibits excitement and cooperation.					
Dependability					
Cooperation: The willingness and ability to collaborate with others in order to achieve a common goal.					

Today's most prevalent technique of evaluating an employee's performance is the rating scale. One advantage of the rating scale is that it is simple to comprehend and utilize & allows for statistical tabulation of employee scores. When ratings are objective, they can be utilized as evaluators effectively. The graphic rating scale, on the other hand, may have a long-standing flaw: it may be arbitrary and the rating may be subjective. Another issue is that in evaluating an employee's performance, each feature is weighted equally.

(f) Behaviorally anchored rating scales: Also known as the behavioral expectations scale, this method is the most recent advancement in performance evaluation. It's a hybrid of the rating scale and critical incident procedures for evaluating employee performance. The key occurrences serve as anchor statements on a scale and the rating form typically includes six to eight performance characteristics that are clearly specified.

(g) Forced choice technique: This method was created to remove bias and the overabundance of positive ratings that can occur in some institutes. The major goal of the forced choice method is to correct a rater's inclination to consistently give all employees high or bad evaluations. This method employs a series of pair phrases, two of which may be positive and two of which may be negative; with the rater being asked to determine which of the four phrases is the most and least descriptive of a certain worker. In fact, the statement items are structured in such a way that the rater has difficulty in determining which statements applies to the most effective employee.

The following is an example of items that are used as forced choice items in an institute

1. Least	Most
1. Does not foresee problems	A
2. Easily and swiftly grasps explanations	B
3. Does not squander time	C
4. A very easy person to chat to	D
2. Least	Most
1. Can act as a leader	A
2. Spends time on items that aren't productive	B
3. Keep a cool and collected demeanor at all times	C
4. Smart worker	D

A plus credit is awarded for positive attributes, and a minus credit is provided for negative qualities. When the positive aspects outweigh the negative ones or when one of the negative words is marked as insignificantly scored, the worker advances to the next level.

(h) Management by Objectives (MBO): MBO is a modern approach of assessing employee performance. Traditional performance evaluation systems are characterized by relatively adversarial judgments on the part of the rater, as thoughtful managers have grown increasingly conscious. Nowadays, there is a rising belief that it is preferable for superiors to collaborate with subordinates in achieving objectives. Subordinates would be able to exercise self-control over their performance behaviors as a result of this. The concept of management by objectives is the result of Peter Drucker's, McGregor's, and Odiorne's pioneering work in management science.

Logical Framework Analysis (LFA)

It is practically impossible to plan, operate, analyze and monitor an extension project in isolation. It must always be contextualized in relation to other circumstances. For example, it is impractical to undertake or design a project that is not in the line of national development goals and as a result of that no donor will support such a project; if the project objectives are vague or the project outcomes are insignificant then the project will be unsustainable. There is also slender chance of a project to be successful if the project environment is not conducive and full of risk. As a result, while planning the project, a thorough awareness of the context is a must. Logical Framework Analysis (LFA) facilitates in this aspect by helping in analyzing the situation thoroughly by creating premise for development of sound project which are scientific and whose output are measureable and attainable.

Basic elements of logical framework

There are several elements in logical framework and those are discussed in subsequent paragraphs by following Soam (2009):

a. Hierarchy of objectives

Goal, purpose, outputs, activities and inputs are included in the hierarchy of objectives. The cause-and-effect relationship is the foundation of hierarchy. Disconnecting the cause from the impact while writing this column is very much important and use of short, brief words with strong action verbs are required while writing the hierarchy of objectives. The extension project's objective is defined in terms of purpose of the project as the project's goals. The Projects' deliverables are referred to as outputs. The actions that must be taken in order to achieve outcomes are referred to as activities. Inputs include personnel, money, services, equipment, information and databases, as well as other soft and hard requirements for completing tasks.

b. Objectively Verifiable indicators (OVI)

Objectively Verifiable indicators (OVIs) are performance measurement indicators that are used to confirm that a hierarchy of objectives has been met. The indicator at the purpose level measures the end of the project impact and must be targeted in terms of quantity, quality, and time. The indicator should be quantitative, sensitive to project activity, critical to project success and readily available for decision-making. Project reports frequently provide information on inputs.

c. Means of Verification (MOV)

Indicators can be evaluated for performance measurement, but where do users access the information? For this, researchers need some tools, such as sources of data (MOV) that can be used to verify the progress of objectives at various levels. Typically, project reports and baseline reports are MOVs that can be used to track down the information we require.

d. Critical Assumptions & Risks

Many extension project/ programme do not get success not only due to external factors beyond the project's control but also due to unreasonable structure of the project. National policies, environmental variables, access to resources, political, social and religious issues etc. are some examples of these conditions. Analyze the importance and probability of these assumptions while describing them because this will help to manage more actively during project design and implementation. Documentation of any external circumstances that are required to achieve specific objectives is very important. In some circumstances, project managers become more creative and smart by creating a contingency plan to achieve the objectives of the projects.

Benefits of using Logical Framework Analysis (LFA) in extension programme planning

- LFA reveals the project's major elements in a way that allows the link between them to be easily understood, exposing the project's logic to evaluate and monitor.
- Ensure that the hierarchy of objectives is clear
- Assist in monitoring on time to time basis
- Clearly identifies the critical assumptions that are required for project completion
- Project managers are clear about the goals right in the beginning
- Responsibility and accountability standards can be established. The Logical Framework Approach (LFA) has proved to be a valuable tool for project approval, design, and evaluation (Couillard *et al.,*2009).
- The sustainability of the project can be understood by using the LFA which aids in determining the project's long run effectiveness.

Table 2: Simplified tabulation of components in Logical Framework analysis

Hierarchy of objectives	Objectively Verifiable indicators(OVI)	Means of Verification(MOV)	Critical Assumptions & Risks
Goal	Measures used to determine whether or not a goal has been met	Data sources required to confirm the status of goal level indicators	External elements required to achieve the long-term objective
Purpose	Measures to ensure that the Purpose level has been met	Data sources required to confirm the status of Purpose level indicators	External variables required to achieve the goal
Output	Measures taken to ensure that the output level is met	Data sources required to confirm the status of output level indicators	External variables required to achieve the output
Activities	Measures to ensure that activities level are completed	Data sources required to confirm the condition of activity level indicators	External influences required in order to complete activities
Inputs or resources	Measures to ensure that the Input level is met	Data sources required to confirm the status of input level indicators	External factors affecting input availability

Conclusion

The systematic examination of employee performance and understanding of a person's talents/ capabilities for future growth and development of an extension organization is the basic aim of performance appraisal. Supervisors can use performance appraisal to plan promotion programmes for productive staff. Performance appraisal determines compensation packages, which include bonuses, high salary rates, additional benefits, allowances etc. This effectively inspires a worker to do a better job and aids in future performance improvement. Performance appraisal aids in the analysis of employees' strengths and limitations so that new positions can be tailored for efficient workers and helps in the formulation of future development programmes. On the other hand, it can be said that the logical framework isn't a panacea for all development issues, but it does help policy makers and funding agency/ donors to grasp what a project is trying to accomplish. Not only that, LFA can also explain that how the project is going to achieve its objective in simple terms. Major criteria and factors for success of the project are also understood by the LFA. Extension project's long-term sustainability after the project completion is also understood by this methodology.

11

Problem Solving Skills: Essential to Perform in Extension Organization

Biswarup Saha

Department of Fishery Extension
Faculty of Fishery Sciences, WBUAFS, Chakgaria, Kolkata

"Most people spend more time and energy going around problems than in trying to solve them."

— Henry Ford

A problem can be defined as a situation that prevents us from achieving the goals we have set for ourselves. It can be anything from financial, personal to work-related. Problems can arise anywhere, and any activity that helps to end our problem results in problem-solving. Being a part of an extension organization we have to come across different kinds of problems. Every job role has its problems. But how well do we cope up with the everyday problems that we often face? Some people are good at problem-solving. Others may think they are not. Most are somewhere in between.

Good problem solving skills empower managers in their professional and personal lives. Good problem solving skills seldom come naturally; they are consciously learnt and nurtured. The selection of good problem solving skills includes:

- developing creative and innovative solutions;
- developing practical solutions;
- showing independence and initiative in identifying problems and solving them;
- applying a range of strategies to problem-solving;
- applying problem-solving strategies across a range of areas;

What is a Problem?

1. **A problem is an opportunity for improvement**. "Every problem has a gift for you in its hands," says Richard Bach (1936). Someone coined the word "probortunity" – an acronym combining the words "problem" and

"opportunity". A probortunity is a reminder to look at problems as possible opportunities. An optimist looks at challenging or problematic events as potential opportunities for improvement. He is seen always seeking answers for the questions such as:

- Is there more than one probortunity?
- Is it my personal probortunity? Is it the organization's probortunity?
- Is it an actual probortunity or just an annoyance?
- Is this the real probortunity, or merely a symptom of a larger one?

2. A problem is the difference between the actual state and desired state. A problem could also be the result of the knowledge that there is a gap between the actual and desired or ideal state of objectives. Clarity of the problem is determined by the clarity of the knowledge of what precisely one wants and what one has. Greater clarity of the problem helps in finding a better and effective solution.

3. A problem results from the recognition of a present imperfect and the belief in the possibility of a better future. The belief that one's hopes can be achieved will give one the will to aim towards a better future. Hopes challenge one's potential, and challenge is another definition of a problem. When confronted with a problem, according to Robert (1995), people are likely to adopt either of the two approaches – spot it or mop it.

1. Stop It

A stop-it approach seeks to solve a problem, so that the problem no longer exists. Its three forms are prevention, elimination, and reduction.

- Prevent It. Preventing a problem from occurring or recurring is the most ideal solution. The prevention approach is often a difficult one to apply because it requires predictive foresight ("this might be a problem someday if we don't act now"). For example, by preventing a cold, or an automobile accident, one can avoid the need to deal any further with a problem or its effects.
- Eliminate It. Eliminating a problem once and for all is also an ideal way of attacking a problem. If a tank were leaking, an elimination solution would be to plug/seal or otherwise repair the leak, the cause of the problem. To solve by eliminating should be considered in nearly every problem situation.
- Reduce It. The magnitude of any problem can be lessened by reducing its size. Suppose the tank is leaking and a repair (an elimination-solution) is not possible until a day or two later. The problem could be reduced by turning off the incoming water. Without line pressure on the tank, the leak would slow down; that would be better than a full force leak.

2. Mop It

A mop-it approach focuses on the effects of a problem. Instead of treating the leak itself, the water on the floor is mopped up - the effects of the problem.

- Treat It. Here the damage caused by the problem is repaired or treated. The water on the floor is mopped up and the damaged floor is fixed. But, it should be noted that: (1) by itself a treat-it solution is not going to be nearly as effective as some form of stop-it solution and (2) treat-it solutions are often needed in addition to an elimination or reduction form of solution.
- Tolerate It. In this form of mop-it approach, the effects of the problem are put up with. In the leaky water example, one might install a drain in the floor, or waterproof the floor. The effects are taken for granted and measures are taken to endure them.
- Redirect It. Here the problem is deflected. Sometimes the problem will simply be redefined as not a problem. It is hard to think of a legitimate redirection for the leaking water problem, but suppose that the leak is small and the floor is not being damaged. One might say, "Well, I need the humidity; the leak is actually a good thing." It should be remembered that a problem is a problem only when someone defines it as such.

Managers must take cognizance of the fact that problem solving is an ongoing activity. Prof. Jeff Malpas ("Problem solving for Managers") says: "No problem is ever totally solved. Every problem has a solution, but every solution with it brings a new problem. Some well-known management techniques emphasize the idea of continuous improvement and successful problem-solving is seen as part of such continuous improvement."

Managers should know that problem-solving is less a matter of continuous improvement as of continuous adjustment. Every solution will have unintended consequences. Every effective system gives rise to friction and failure. Good management and effective problem-solving depend upon a willingness to adapt to the situation and recognize the ongoing and partial character of all attempts to manage or to solve.

Causes of Poor Problem Solving

Look around the world, keep asking 'Why?' and 'Why not?', and you will soon see new opportunities.

Centre for Good Governance (2017) explained in the Hand Book of Problem Solving skills the following causes for poor problem solving-

Ineffective or poor problem-solving can be the result of any of the following factors. These factors act like blinkers, constricting the perspective of person in the process of problem-solving.

1. Bounded Rationality: Propounded by Simon (1972), the concept of bounded rationality assumes that individuals make decisions by constructing simplified models that extract the essential features from problems without capturing all their complexity. Simon remarks that majorities of the people is only partly rational, and are in fact emotional/ irrational in the remaining part of their actions. He indicates two major causes of bounded rationality:

a. Limitations of the human mind

b. The structure within which the mind operates

He states that boundedly rational people experience limits in formulating and solving problems. As a result, when calculating expected utility, people do not make the best choices. For example, a person may choose to buy a particular brand of new cell-phone, based on the information he gathered from advertisements and friends. Constrained by bounded rationality, he will turn down even if he is offered a better bargain. Often, bounded rationality could also be caused by "inverted intelligence" - clever people who can easily argue that the information must be wrong.

2. Satisfying: Satisfying implies identifying and implementing a solution that is "good enough." According to Herb Simon, who coined the term, the tendency to 'satisfied' results in solving problems which do not lead to optimal solutions. Most often, people look for solutions that had worked for them before. There may be better ways to reach the outcome, but they simply ignore them. Searching for alternative and superior solutions might entail an extra cost. The alternative solution might not prove worthy enough, if the extra costs are not justified. On the other hand, the implicit costs of ignoring the alternative solution can be relatively greater if the chosen solution, based on prior experience, fails to deliver the expected outcome.

Slote (1983) gives the following examples of satisfying. One involves a fairy-tale hero who, when rewarded by the gods with whatever he asks for, just asks for himself and his family to be comfortably well-off. Another involves a motel owner who gives some stranded motorists the first available room rather than the best available room.

3. Group Think: 'Groupthink' is a term coined by psychologist Janis (1982). According to him, 'Group think' is a phenomenon in which the norm for consensus overrides the realistic appraisal of alternative courses of action. It describes situations in which group pressures for conformity discourage the group from critically appraising unusual, minority, or unpopular views. 'Groupthink' is a bug that strikes groups and can dramatically hinder their performance.

Some of the symptoms of 'Groupthink' as observed by Janis(1982) are

- Illusion of Invulnerability: Members ignore obvious danger, take extreme risk and are overly optimistic.
- Collective Rationalization: Members discredit and explain away warning contrary to group thinking.
- Illusion of Morality: Members believe their decisions are morally correct, ignoring the ethical consequences of their decisions.
- Excessive Stereotyping: The group constructs negative stereotypes of rivals outside the group.
- Pressure for Conformity: Members pressure any in the group who express arguments against the group's stereotypes, illusions, or commitments, viewing such opposition as disloyalty.
- Self-Censorship: Members withhold their dissenting views and counter arguments.
- Illusion of Unanimity: Members perceive falsely that everyone agrees with the group's decision; silence is seen as consent.
- Mind guards: Some members appoint themselves to the role of protecting the group from adverse information that might threaten group complacency.

4. Group shift: 'Group shift' is a phenomenon in which the initial positions of individual members of a group are exaggerated toward a more extreme position. More often, however, the shift is toward greater risk. What happens in groups is that the discussion leads to a significant shift in the positions of members toward a more extreme position in the direction in which they were already leaning before the discussion. Conservatives become more cautious, and the more aggressive take on more risk. The 'Group shift' can be viewed as actually a special case of 'groupthink'. The decision of the group reflects the dominant decision-making norm that develops during the group's discussion. The greater occurrence of the shift toward risk can be due to any of the following reasons:

- Discussion creates familiarization among the members. As they become more comfortable with each other, they also become more bold and daring.
- People admire individuals who are willing to take risks. Group discussion motivates members to show that they are at least as willing as their peers in terms of taking risks.
- The most plausible explanation of the shift toward risk, however, seems to be that the group diffuses responsibility.
- Group decisions free any single member from accountability for the group's final choice.

5. Conformation Bias: Conformation bias is the tendency on the part of the people to search for only for that information that supports their perceived notions. Initial perceptions and ideas of people about a problem often shape the search process for information. It is important to maintain objectivity in evaluating ideas so that they are not biased toward their initial perceptions. The possible solutions include:

- Considering alternative hypotheses - view the problem from different perspectives.
- Looking for evidence to disprove their ideas - showing that a particular idea is incorrect is as important as showing an idea is correct.
- Maintain objectivity while evaluating ideas to minimize personal bias.
- Drawing conclusions based upon the evidence, not upon their personal beliefs.

6. Insufficiency of Hypotheses: Often, while solving problems, a solver seizes upon the first explanation that comes to mind and stops thinking about the problem. This difficulty is related to confirmation bias, but reflects insufficient thought applied to a problem. Many times, the immediate answer is sufficient. Other times, however, only a careful analysis of a situation beyond the immediate response is necessary to ensure a correct solution. To avoid poor problem-solving resulting from insufficiency of hypothesis, people should develop alternative ideas, rather than seizing upon the first idea as the solution. They should spend time thinking about the issues - allow time for reflection and avoid framing the problem so that only one idea emerges.

7. Fixation: Fixation is the inability to see a problem from a fresh perspective. Again, initial perceptions and structuring of a problem often determine the approaches people use to solve that problem. Structuring a problem incorrectly is a prime contributor to the inability to solve a problem correctly. To overcome fixation, people should see the problem with "fresh eyes" - allow time for reflection and incubation. They should focus on other issues, and then return to the original problem. Time away from a problem allows one to forget incorrect solutions and focus on developing new ideas.

8. Other Obstacles: Problem-solving can be impaired by biases of personal beliefs, a misunderstanding of information relevant to solving problems, and over confidence. The solution is to study a problem objectively with all available accurate information and use objective reasoning to achieve a reasonable, sound decision. People should be sure that they understand the problem and find what constitutes a solution. They should obtain as much accurate and comprehensive information from unbiased sources possible and maintain objectivity in evaluating ideas to minimize personal bias. They should assess their decisions critically and be able to defend their ideas.

Problem solving steps

There is a variety of problem-solving processes. But each process consists of a series of steps - identifying the problem, searching for possible solutions, selecting the most optimal solution and implementing a possible solution. It is useful to view problem solving as a cycle because, sometimes, a problem needs several attempts to solve it or the problem changes. The diagram below shows a seven-step problem solving process as given by Centre for Good governance (2017).

1. Identifying the Problem: The first step in the problem solving process is sizing up the situation to identify the problem. That sounds simple enough, but sometimes managers might be uncertain about what the problem is; they might just feel general anxiety or be confused about what is getting in the way of their objectives. If that is the case, they can ask themselves or their friends or a professional expert. Other useful techniques for identifying the problem include-

- Comparison with others
- Monitor for weak signals
- Comparison of current performance with objectives or past performance
- Checklists
- Brainstorming
- Listing complaints
- Role playing

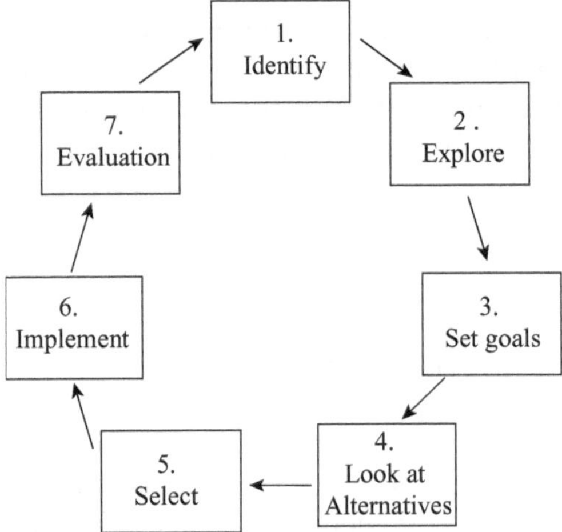

Figure 1: Problem solving steps

2. Exploring the Problem: Having identified the problem, managers should analyze it to see what the root cause is. Often people get caught up in symptoms or effects of a problem or issue and never get down to the real cause. They get mad at someone's attitude, anger, or actions, which are not the cause of the problem. The key here is to focus on analyzing the problem for the real cause without being affected by emotional issues. Seeing answers for questions such as the following will help explore the problem:

Identify the Problem – Ask Who?

- Who says that this is a problem?
- Who caused or is causing the problem?
- Whom does it or will it affect?
- Who has done something about the problem?

Identify the Problem – Ask What?

- What happened or will happen?
- What are the symptoms?
- What are the consequences for others?
- What circumstances surround the occurrence of the problem?
- What is not functioning as desired?

Identify the Problem – Ask When?

- Did it or will it happen?
- Why did it happen?
- When did it first occur?

Identify the Problem – Ask Where?

- Where is the problem occurring?
- Did it or will it have an impact?
- Where did it have an impact?

Identify the Problem – Ask Why?

- Why is this, a problem?
- Did it or will it occur?
- Why did it occur?
- Why was nothing done to prevent the problem from occurring?
- Why did no one recognize and do something about the problem at the earliest?
- Why is a response needed now?

Identify the Problem – Ask How?

- How should the process be working?
- How are others dealing with this or similar problems?
- How do you know this is a problem; what supporting information do you have?

Once the cause is found, plans can be made to fix it. Analyzing implies gathering information. If there is not enough information, they should figure out how to research and collect it

3. Set Goals: Having explored and analyzed the problem, managers should be able to write a goal statement that focuses on what is the successful end of the process.

Making and writing down a goal statement:

- helps them to clarify the direction to take in solving the problem; and
- gives them something definite to focus on

That is, what will occur as a result of the solution? This whole process is about closing or fixing the gap between the problem and the goal. Writing down the problem ensures that they are not side-tracking from, but addressing the problem.

4. Look at alternatives: Now that the problem has been analyzed, the managers can begin to develop possible solutions. This is a creative as well as practical step where every possible solution is identified. *They should identify the various alternative solutions available to them through such techniques as –*

- Analysis of past solutions
- Reading
- Researching
- Thinking
- Asking Questions
- Discussing
- Viewing the problem with fresh eyes
- Brainstorming
- Sleeping on it

The idea is to collect as many alternative solutions as possible.

Mind mapping is another technique that can be used for identifying alternative solutions. Developed by Tony Buzan in the 1970's, mind mapping uses pictures and/or word phrases to organize and develop thoughts in a non-linear fashion. It helps people "see" a problem and its solution. Here's how to do mind mapping (Buzan, 1993):

- Take a sheet of plain paper and turn it sideways (if using flipchart paper you don't need to turn it sideways - it is large enough); Using colored felt pens, draw a small picture (or write a phrase) in the centre of the paper representing the issue you want to solve; Draw lines out from the main problem (it helps to use different colors for each line).
- Each line should represent a different aspect of your problem or issue;
- Write down what each line represents either on top of or on the line;
- Add other lines flowing off these main lines;
- Write a word or short phrase on the smaller lines indicating what each new line represents (you may find that mind mapping works best for you if you write down the phrases or draw the images first and then connect them with the lines); and
- If you want, add images next to your main line that illustrate what each line means to you (some people think better with pictures, others with words).

5. Select the best solution: Now that there are a wide variety of possible solutions, it is time to select the best solution to fix the problem, given the circumstances, resources and other considerations. Here the managers are trying to figure out exactly what would work best given the nature of the problem. There are always a number of things that can affect a solution, for instance, money, time, people, procedures, policies, rules, and so on. All of these factors must be thought about. Managers should prioritize the solutions by their effectiveness. This is a slow process of elimination. There may be some possible suggestions that are immediately eliminated. Eventually, managers should narrow down the choices to one best possible solution which will promise the best or optimal outcomes.

6. Implementation: Implementation is a crucial part of problem-solving process. In order to implement the solution chosen, managers must have an action plan and communicate it to those directly and indirectly affected. Gemmy Allen ("Problem-Solving& Decision-Making") says that communication is most effective when it precedes action and events. In this way, events conform to plans and events happen when, and in the way, they should happen. Managers should answer the vital questions before they are asked, like –

- What should be communicated?
- What is the reason for the decision?
- Whom will it affect and how?

- What are the benefits expected for the individual, the department, and the organization?
- What adjustments will be required in terms of how work will be done?
- What, specifically, is each individual's role in implementing the decision?
- What results are expected from each individual?
- When does the action called for by the decision go into effect?

Communicating answers to these questions can overcome any resistance that otherwise might be encountered.

7. Evaluation: This is the final step in the problem-solving process. Managers should review the effectiveness of the solution against desired outcomes. Did the solution work? If not, why not? What went right, and what went wrong? What adjustments do they have to make to ensure that the solution works better? This stage requires careful analysis that improves upon the best solution. The review of your progress can help a manager identify any problem. Steps may need to be revised or new steps added. One may need to consider a different solution, if the current one, he/she has been working with, is not helping.

Essentials of Effective Problem Solving

- A clear description of the problem
- A description of the limiting (or negative) factors involved in the problem
- A description of the constructive (or positive) factors involved in the problem
- **A clear delineation of the "ownership" of the problem** - Whose problem is it: mine, yours, the other guy's, my boss', my spouse's, my child's, my parents', my teacher's?
- **A clear description of the scope of the problem: How extensive a problem is it?** How long has this problem existed? How many people are affected? What else is affected by this problem?
- **A clear description of the consequences if the problem were not solved** - What is the possible impact on my family, job, life in this community, etc., if this problem isn't solved? What is the worst possible thing that could happen if this problem isn't solved?

Personality Types and Problem solving Techniques

William G. Huitt(2005) lists out the following sixteen problem-solving techniques, which focus more on logic and critical thinking, especially within the context of applying the scientific approach:

(a) Means-End Analysis: In means-ends analysis, the problem solver compares the present situation with the goal, detects a difference between them, and then searches memory for actions that are likely to reduce the difference.

- **A list of brainstormed solutions to the problem**, with each alternative analyzed as to its reality, its benefits, and the consequences for following each one.
- **A system of ranking each solution to finalize the decision-making process** - A rating system for analyzing each solution is developed, e.g., 100% chance of success, 75% chance of success, 50% chance of success.
- **A clear description of myself as a problem-solver** - When it comes to this problem, am I procrastinating? Am I avoiding the problem? Am I denying the problem? Am I shutting down or blocking my creativity on this problem? Am I ignoring it, hoping it will go away? Am I using magical and/or fantasy thinking in addressing the problem?
- **Determination to follow through on the solution decided upon jointly**. This involves full motivation to "take the risk" and pursue the solution to its fullest likely to reduce the difference.

(b) Backwards Planning: The strategy of working backwards entails starting with the end results and reversing the steps you need to get those results, in order to figure out the answer to the problem.

(c) Categorizing/Classifying: It is the process of grouping objects or events together on the basis of a logical rationale. There are two kinds of categorizing, grouping and classifying. Grouping is putting together objects on the basis of a single property. Files might be grouped on the basis of "urgent" and "not-urgent". Grouping is useful in revealing similarities and differences that otherwise might go unnoticed. Classifying involves putting items together on the basis of more than a single property at a time.

(d) Challenging Assumptions: It involves the direct confrontation of ideas, opinions, or attitudes that have previously been taken for granted. The purpose is to identify the fallacies, consistencies and inconsistencies in the problem-solving process.

(e) Evaluating/Judging: It involves the comparison with a standard and making a qualitative or quantitative judgment of value or worth. Good evaluations of problem solving are generally based on multiple sources of assessment information.

(f) Inductive/Deductive Reasoning: Reasoning is the systematic and logical development of rules or concepts from specific instances or the identification of cases based on a general principle or proposition using generalization and inference.

(g) Thinking Aloud: It is the process of verbalizing about a problem and its solution while a partner listens in detail for errors in thinking or understanding.

(h) Network Analysis: It is a systems approach to project planning and management where relationships among activities, events, resources, and timelines are developed and charted. Specific examples include Program Evaluation and Review Technique and Critical Path Method.

(i) Plus-Minus-Interesting (PMI): It involves considering the positive, negative, and interesting or thought-provoking aspects of an idea or alternative using a balance sheet grid where plus and minus refer to criteria identified in the second step of the problem solving process.

(j) Task analysis: It is the consideration of skills and knowledge required to learn or perform a specific task.

Now let us take a look at Huitt's list of problem-solving techniques that conform to creative, lateral, or divergent thinking. Following is the list of problem-solving techniques;

(a) **Brainstorming:** It is attempting to spontaneously generate as many ideas on a subject as possible; ideas are not critiqued during the brainstorming process; participants are encouraged to form new ideas from ideas already stated.

(b) **Imaging/Visualization:** It is producing mental pictures of the total problem or specific parts of the problem.

(c) **Incubation:** It is putting aside the problem and doing something else to allow the mind to unconsciously consider the problem

(d) **Outcome Psychodrama:** It is enacting a scenario of alternatives or solutions through role playing.

(e) **Outrageous Provocation:** It is making a statement that is known to be incorrect (e.g., the brain is made of charcoal) and then considering it; used as a bridge to a new idea.

(f) **Overload:** It is considering a large number of facts and details until the logic part of the brain becomes overwhelmed and begins looking for patterns. It can also be generated by immersion in aesthetic experiences, sensitivity training or similar experiences.

(g) **Random Word Technique:** It is selecting a word randomly from the dictionary and juxtaposing it with problem statement, then brainstorming about possible relationships.

(h) **Relaxation:** It is systematically relaxing all muscles while repeating a personally meaningful focus word or phrase.

(i) **Synthesizing:** It is combining parts or elements into a new and original pattern.

(j) **Taking Another's Perspective:** It is deliberately taking another person's point of view.

(k) **Value Clarification:** It is using techniques such as role playing, simulations, self-analysis exercises, and structured controversy to gain a greater understanding of attitudes and beliefs that individuals hold important. The value clarification can provide a greater goal clarity and motivation and increase an internal locus of control for managers.

Problem Solving Tools

The following are some of the principal tools that enable managers to analyze and prioritize the root causes of identified problems and to assist in problem-solving activities. The tools outlined can also assist in identifying opportunities for improvement.

The toolkit includes:

- Cause-and-effect diagram
- Pareto chart
- Flow Charts
- Histogram
- Check Sheet
- Scatter diagram
- Brain Storming

12

Team Building and Performance Skills for Better Management in Extension

Kaushik Pradhan

Department of Agricultural Extension
Uttar Banga Krishi Viswavidyalaya, Pundibari, Coochbehar, 736165
West Bengal

In the present scenario, team formation is the key enabler for getting all sorts of benefit in organizational perspective as well as benefit sharing perspective. So, in any organizational atmosphere team plays a pivotal role in performance of human resources in organization through contributing to the organizational goal. Successful organizations today know that teams make a big difference in achieving strategic goals. Teams that are strong, flexible, and productive can be the competitive edge needed to produce better results, achieve higher quality, lower costs for the organization and the customer. With active involvement, high-performing teams can help promote employees bottom line results, as well as their adaptability, quality, service, and safety. To achieve these objectives, teams have to start doing things differently. Team members and leaders need to communicate more effectively with each other, encourage more involvement, tap into one another's creativity, overcome the group's resistance to change, and renew team spirit. But this change can also create difficulty for some who may lack the knowledge, understanding, or a mindset that is conducive to teamwork. Team Building for high performance teams is designed to provide skills and promote high levels of team performance and team member satisfaction. Consequently, team building is required for knowing each other within the organizational team, boosting morale, improving communication and relationships, making the workplace more enjoyable, motivating a team, getting everyone "onto the same page" including goal setting, teaching the team self-regulation strategies, helping participants to learn more about themselves (strengths and weaknesses), identifying and utilizing the strengths of team members, improving team productivity, identifying and developing leadership skills and practicing effective collaboration with team members. Group is a collection of two or more interacting individuals with a stable pattern of relationships among them, who share common goals and who perceive themselves as being a group. Group essentially consists of social interaction, stable structure, common interests, perceive themselves as part of group. A team is a small number of people with complementary skills who are committed to a common purpose, performance goals, and approach for which they hold themselves mutually accountable. This definition highlights the essentials of a team or in other words the team basics. Here the focus or emphasis is on three characteristics–small number, complementary skills and commitment. These are what basically differentiates a team from a group and makes a team something much more productive and result oriented than a group. Team Building is the process of enabling that group of people to reach their goal.Team building is the use of different types of team interventions that are aimed at enhancing social relations and clarifying team members' roles, as well as solving task and interpersonal problems that affect team functioning (Salas *et al*, 2009). It refers to the activities in which teams can engage to change its context, composition or team competencies to improve performance. It is distinct from team training, which is also a team-development intervention that is designed to improve team functioning and effectiveness. Team building differs from team training in a number of ways. Team building is not necessarily formal or systematic in nature, does not target skill-based competencies, and is typically done in settings that are not in the actual environment where the team works on the task. Team building generally sits within the theory and practice of organizational development, but can also be applied to sports teams, school groups, armies, flight crews and other contexts. There have been many issues in past literature about the conceptual definition of team building. However, now there is consensus and conceptual clarity about what team building constitutes exactly.

Its four components are:

- **Goal Setting:** This intervention emphasizes setting objectives and developing individual and team goals. Team members become involved in action planning to identify ways to achieve goals. It is designed to strengthen team member motivation to achieve team goals and objectives. By identifying specific outcome levels, teams can determine what future resources are needed. Individual characteristics (e.g. team member motivation) can also be altered by use of this intervention. Many organizations insist on teams negotiating a team charter between the team and responsible mangers (and union leaders) to empower the team to accomplish things on behalf of the organization. Successful goal settings help the teams to work towards the same outcomes and make them more task and action oriented.

- **Interpersonal-relationship management:** This intervention emphasizes increasing teamwork skills (i.e. mutual supportiveness, communication, and sharing of feelings). Team members develop trust in one another and confidence in the team. This is based on the assumption that teams with fewer interpersonal conflicts function more effectively than teams with greater numbers of interpersonal conflicts. It requires the use of a facilitator to develop mutual trust and open communication between team members. As team members achieve higher levels of trust, cooperation and team characteristics can be changes as well.
- **Role clarification:** This intervention emphasizes increasing communication among team members regarding their respective roles within the team. Team members improve their understanding of their own and others' respective roles and duties within the team. This intervention defines the team as comprising a set of overlapping roles. These overlapping roles are characterized as the behaviors that are expected of each individual team member. It can be used to improve team and individual characteristics (i.e. by reducing role ambiguity) and work structure by negotiating, defining, and adjusting team member roles. It includes an understanding of the talent that exists on the team, and how best to use it, allows members to understand why clear roles are important. The members should also realize that they are interdependent and the failure of one team member leads to the failure of the entire team.
- **Problem solving:** This intervention emphasizes identifying major task-related problems within the team. Team members become involved in action planning, implementing solutions to identify problems and to evaluate those solutions. They practice setting goals, developing interpersonal relations, clarifying team roles, and working to improve organizational characteristics through problem-solving tasks. This can have the added benefit of enhancing critical-thinking skills. If teams are good in problem-solving skills, they are less likely to need external interventions to solve their problems.
- **Environment:** Teams are not closed systems. It is critical that they interact effectively with their external environments. Teams need good diplomatic relationships with key managers, union officials, other teams, and the functions that affect their performance. Team members must feel free to disagree with each other during team meetings but should present a united, positive front to the rest of the organization. A productive team environment contains an atmosphere of trust and its members are completely accountable for the group's bottom line results. Its individual team members invest in the team through their actions and attitudes. They are respectful, caring, and cooperative. These high functioning teams are the mechanism by which organizations can unlock world-class results.

These team-development interventions have proven to have positive effects on cognitive, affective, process, and performance team outcomes. Team building has seen the strongest effect on affective and process outcomes. Team building is one of the most widely used group development interventions in organizations today. Of all organizational interventions, team-development interventions were found to have the largest effects on financial measures of organizational performance (Macy and Izumi, 1993).

Effective team building

According to Sanborn and Haszczo (2007), the effectiveness of team building differs substantially from one organization to another. The most effective team building efforts occur when members of the team are highly interdependent in performing the task, highly knowledgeable and experienced in the task to be accomplished, and when organizational leadership actively establishes and supports the team. Effective team building must also incorporate an awareness of the ultimate objective of the task. They must work to develop goals, roles and procedures to achieve it successfully. In addition to task-orientated team building efforts, team-building efforts must also be relationship oriented. To ensure effectiveness, team building should work towards the establishment of policies and procedures and working with the environment, including support systems. Caveats to team building effectiveness is that team building as an intervention is designed to work when the members of the team are actually involved in solving the problem and when they are already intact as a team (i.e. they worked with each other before) to be able to problem solve. The members of the team must have the willingness and ability to speak up about their needs.

Effects on performance

Team building is a specific team development intervention that has been scientifically proven to positively affect team effectiveness, when exerted with its intended purpose. Team building is aimed at specific needs, and thus has been proven to have specific outcomes on teams. Goal setting and role clarification were shown to have strongest impact on cognitive, affective, process and performance outcomes. However, they had the most powerful impact on affective and process outcomes. This implies that team building can help benefit teams experiencing issues with negative effect, such as lack of cohesion or trust. It could also improve teams suffering from process issues, such as lack of clarification in roles. Although the four approaches were useful in enhancing team functioning, goal setting and role clarification have proven to be the most impactful. This is because, drawing upon theory, providing teams with clearly set and challenging goals enhances motivation to work harder to be more effective and reduces conflict. Role clarification helps to set individual purposes, goals and motivation. Finally, larger team sizes (those with 10 or more members) appeared to benefit the most from team building interventions. That is because larger teams generally have a greater reservoir of cognitive resources and capabilities than smaller teams.

Challenges to team building

- The lack of teamwork skills in tomorrow's workforce: One of the challenges facing leaders of organizations is to find employees who have the ability to work effectively in a team environment. Most of the organizations rely on educational institutions to train their students with the skills. The students are rather encouraged to work individually for a higher grade and succeed without having to collaborate with one another. This creates an emphasis in self-interest- rather than an orientation to collaborate with others - than can work against the kinds of behavior needed for successful teamwork.
- The increasing need for teams to work together in virtual workplaces and across organizational boundaries: Organizations will find it increasingly important for individuals to work together who are not in the same physical space. Such teams will prove to be a challenge as they are unable to build concrete relationships within the team members. Face-to-face contact was a key to developing trust and this was initiated by a formal team building sessions with a facilitator to "agree to the relationship" and define the rules as to how the teams are going to work. Informal contact was also mentioned, e.g. sitting down over lunch to break barriers. Team building training will need to be suited according to virtual teams who are working in geographically distant places.
- Globalization and teamwork: the globalization of industry also will make team more challenging in the future. Teams of the future will be compared more and more of team members who have dissimilar languages, cultures, values and approaches to solving the problems. This challenge will need to be addressed by arranging more one on one meeting that have proven to be successful in some organizations. This challenge will be enhanced when combined in virtual workplaces when teams do not have the opportunity to have face to face communications. Training of understanding and communication across team members can address this issue.

Building of highly effective teams

Too often, teams are formed merely by gathering some people together and then hoping that those people somehow find a way to work together. Teams are most effective when carefully designed. To design, develop and support a highly effective team, use the following guidelines:

Step-1: Set clear goals for the results to be produced by the team

The goals should be designed to be "SMART." This is an acronym for:

- Specific
- Measurable
- Achievable
- Relevant and
- Time-bound.

As much as possible, include input from other members of the organization when designing and wording these goals. Goals might be, for example, "to produce a project report that includes a project plan, schedule and budget to develop and test a complete employee performance management system within the next year." Write these goals down for eventual communication to and discussion with all team members.

Step-2: Set clear objectives for measuring the ongoing effectiveness of the team

The objectives, that together achieve the overall goals, should also be designed to be "SMART." Objectives might be, for example, to a) to produce a draft of a project report during the first four weeks of team activities, and b) achieve Board-approval of the proposed performance management system during the next four weeks. Also, write these objectives down for eventual communication to and discussion with all team members.

Step-3: Define a mechanism for clear and consistent communications among team members

New leaders often assume that all group members know what the leaders know. Consistent communication is the most important trait of a successful group. Without communication, none of the other traits can occur. Successful groups even over-communicate, such that:

- All members regularly receive and understand similar information about the group, for example, about the group's purpose, membership, status and accomplishments.
- These communications might be delivered through regular newsletters, status reports, meetings, emails and collaboration tools.

Step-4: Define a procedure for members to make decisions and solve problems

Successful groups regularly encounter situations where they must make decisions and solve problems in a highly effective manner. Too often, the group resorts to extended discussion until members become tired and frustrated and eventually just opt for any action at all, or they count on the same person who seems to voice the strongest opinions. Instead, successful groups:

- Document a procedure whereby the group can make decisions and ensure that all members are aware of the procedure.
- The procedure might specify that decisions are made, first by aiming for consensus within a certain time frame and if consensus is not achieved, then the group resorts to a majority vote.

Step-5: Develop staffing procedures (recruiting, training, organizing, replacing)

Too often, group members are asked to join the group and somehow to "chip in." Unfortunately, that approach creates "chips," rather than valuable group members. Instead, if group members go through a somewhat organized, systematic process, then new members often believe that the group is well organized and that their role is very valuable in the group. Successful groups:

- Identify what roles and expertise are needed on the group in order to achieve the group's purpose and plans – they staff according to plans, not personalities.
- New group members go through a systematic process to join the group – they understand the group's purpose, their role, their next steps and where to get help.

Step-6: Determine the membership of the group

Consider the extent of expertise needed to achieve the goals, including areas of knowledge and skills. Include at least one person who has skills in facilitation and meeting management. Attempt to include sufficient diversity of values and perspectives to ensure robust ideas and discussion. A critical consideration is availability – members should have the time to attend every meeting and perform required tasks between meetings.

Step-7: Determine time frames for starting and terminating the team, if applicable

Now consider the expertise needed to achieve the goals of the team, and how long it might take to recruit and organize those resources. Write these times down for eventual communication to and discussion with all team members.

Step-8: Determine the membership of the team

What expertise might the team need to achieve the goals of the group? For example, an official authority to gather and allocate resources, or an expert in a certain technology. Always consider if the members will have the time and energy to actively participate in the team.

Step-9: Assign the role of leader – to ensure systems and practices are followed

The leader focuses on the systems and practices in the team, not on personalities of its members. For example, the leader makes sure that all team members: a) are successfully staffed, b) understand the purpose of the group and their role in it, c) are active toward meeting that purpose and role, and d) utilize procedures for making decisions and solving problems. (Note that the leader does not always have to be a strong, charismatic personality – while that type of personality can often be very successful at developing teams, it often can create passivity or frustration in other members over time, thereby crippling the group.)

Step-10: Assign role of communicator – communication is the life's blood of teams

Communication is the most important trait of a successful team. It cannot be left to chance. Someone should be designated to ensure that all members receive regular communications about purpose, membership, roles and status. Communications should also be with people outside the team, especially those who make decisions or determine if the team is successful or not.

Step-11: Identify needs for resources (training, materials, supplies, etc.)

Start from analysis of the purpose and goals. What is needed to achieve them? For example, members might benefit from a training that provides a brief overview of the typical stages of team development and includes packets of materials about the team's goals, structure and process to make decisions. Consider costs, such as trainers, consultants, room rental and office supplies. How will those funds be obtained and maintained?

Step-12: Identify the costs to provide necessary resources for the team

Consider costs, such as paying employees to attend the meeting, trainers, consultants, room rental and office supplies. Develop a budget that itemizes the costs associated with obtaining and supporting each of the resources. Get management approval of the budget.

Step-13: Contact each team member

Before the first meeting, invite each potential team member to be a part of the team. First, send him/her a memo, and then meet with each person individually. Communicate the goals of the project, why the person was selected, the benefit of the goals to the organization, the time frame for the team effort, and who will lead the team (at least initially). Invite the team member to the first meeting.

Step-14: Early on, plan team building activities to support trust and working relationship

Team building activities can include, for example, a retreat in which members introduce themselves, exercises in which members help each other solve a short problem or meet a specific and achievable goal, or an extended period in which members can voice their concerns and frustrations about their team assignments.

Step-15: Carefully plan the first team meeting

In the first meeting, review the goals of the team, why each member was selected, the benefit of the goals to the organization, the time frame for the team effort, who will lead the team (at least, initially), when the team might meet and where, and any changes that have occurred since the individual meetings. Have this information written down to hand out to each member. At the end of the meeting, ask each person to make a public commitment to the team effort.

Step-16: Regularly monitor and report on status of team members toward achieving the goal

It is amazing how often a team starts out with a carefully designed plan, but then abandons the plan once the initial implementation of the plan is underway. Sometimes if the plan is behind schedule, team members conclude that the project is not successful. Plans can change – just change them systematically with new dates and approval of the changes.

Step-17: Support team meetings and the members' processes in the team

At this point, it is critical that supervisors of team members remain available to provide support and resources as needed. The supervisor should regularly monitor team members' progress on achieving their goals. Provide ongoing encouragement and visibility to members. One of the most important forms of support a supervisor can provide is coordination with other supervisors to ensure that team members are freed up enough to attend meetings.

Step-18: Regularly celebrate team members' accomplishments

One of the best ways to avoid burnout is to regularly celebrate accomplishments. Otherwise, members can feel as if they are on treadmill that has no end. Keep your eye on small and recurring successes, not just the gold at the end of the rainbow.

Team leadership

A lack of leadership is often seen as a roadblock to a team's performance. Rather than focusing on ineffective teams, Larson and LaFasto (1989) looked in the opposite direction by interviewing excellent teams to gain insights as to what enables them to function to a high degree. They came away with the following conclusions:

- A clear elevating goal — they have a vision
- Results driven structure — visions have a business goal
- Competent team members with right number and mix
- Unified commitment — they are a team, not a group
- A collaborative climate — aligned towards a common purpose
- High standards of excellence — they have group norms
- Principled leadership — the central driver of excellence
- External support — they have adequate resources

Team leadership model

While there are several Team Leadership models, Hill's Team model is perhaps one of the better known ones as it provides the leader or a designated team member with a mental road map to help diagnose team problems, and then take appropriate action to correct team problems (Northouse, 2007). This Team Leadership model is built on a number of research projects. The four layers of team leadership model are:

1. *Top layer:* Effective team performance begins with leader's mental model of the situation and then determining if the situation requires **Action** or just **Monitoring?**
2. *Second Layer:* Is it at an **Internal** or **External** leadership level?
3. *Third layer:* Is it **Task, Relational**, or an **Environmental** intervention? Select a function depending on the type of intervention. See the next section for explanation of Function Interventions.
4. *Bottom layer:* Correctly performing the above three steps create high **Performance** through **Development** and **Maintenance** functions.

Conflict management

Conflict management is the practice of being able to identify and handle conflicts sensibly, fairly, and efficiently. Since conflicts in a business are a natural part of the workplace, it is important that there are people who understand conflicts and know how to resolve them. This is important in today's market more than ever. Everyone is striving to show how valuable they are to the company they work for and, at times, this can lead to disputes with other members of the team.

Conflict Management Styles

- Conflict happens and how an employee responds and resolves conflict will limit or enable that employee's success. Here are five conflict styles that a manager will follow according to Kenneth W. Thomas and Ralph H. Kilmann:

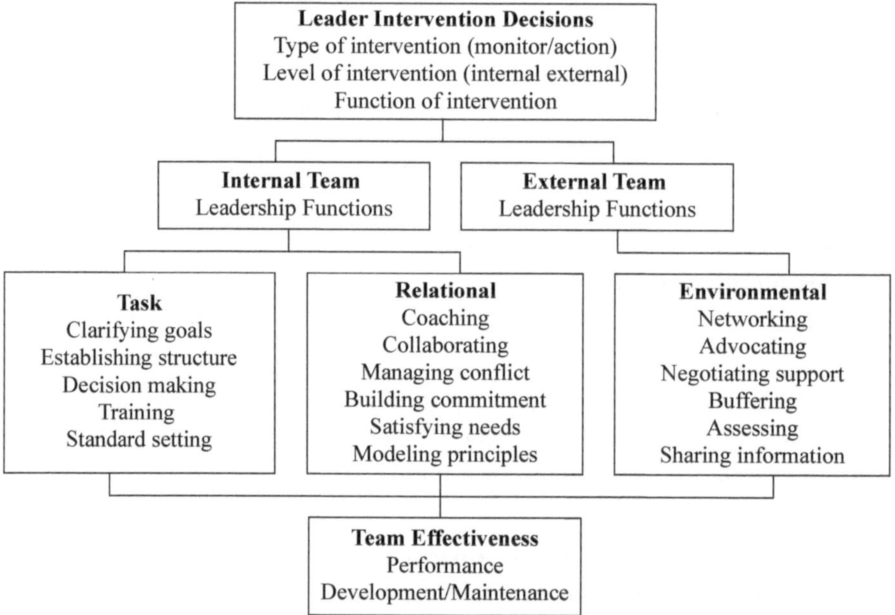

- **Accommodating:** An accommodating manager is one who cooperates to a high degree. This may be at the manager's own expense and actually work against that manager's own goals, objectives, and desired outcomes. This approach is effective when the other person is the expert or has a better solution.
- **Avoiding:** Avoiding an issue is one way a manager might attempt to resolve conflict. This type of conflict style does not help the other staff members reach their goals, and does not help the manager who is avoiding the issue assertively pursue his or her own goals. However, this works well when the issue is trivial or when the manager has no chance of winning.
- **Collaborating:** Managers become partners or pair up with the each other to achieve both of their goals in this style. This is how managers break free of

the 'win-lose' paradigm and seek the 'win-win.' This can be effective for complex scenarios where managers need to find a novel solution.

- **Competing:** This is the 'win-lose' approach. A manager is acting in a very assertive way to achieve his or her goals, without seeking to cooperate with other employees, and it may be at the expense of those other employees. This approach may be appropriate for emergencies when time is of the essence.
- **Compromising:** This is the 'lose-lose' scenario where neither person nor manager really achieves what they want. This requires a moderate level of assertiveness and cooperation. It may be appropriate for scenarios where you need a temporary solution, or where both sides have equally important goals.

13

Personal and Organizational Effectiveness by Management Tools

Sukanta Biswas and Subhransu Mohan Nanda

Department of Veterinary & Animal Husbandry Extension Education
University of Animal & Fishery Science, Kolkata-700037, West Bengal, India

The Management tools are very useful to achieve the objectives of any extension organization. There are number of management tools, which extensively used for better personal and organizational effectiveness, such as follows: Johari window, SWOT analysis, Agro-Ecosystem analysis, PRA, Transaction Analysis, etc.

- **Personal Effectiveness-Johari Window:**

The personal effectiveness is very useful for success of management in any extension organization. In Extension organization, the manager or leader has to deal with human beings to obtain the objectives' of the organization through better personal effectiveness. The basic precondition for personal effectiveness is better self-awareness but understanding one does not alone make a person effective.

The Johari Window: The simple and widely used model of self-awareness is the Johari window, developed by Joseph Luft& Harry Ingham in 1973. In this model, there are two main dimensions for understanding the self: Those aspects of a person's behavior and style that known to him(Self) and those aspects of his behavior known to those with whom he interacts(Others). A combination of these two dimensions reveals fur areas of knowledge about the self.

	Know to self	Not Known to self
Known to others	**ARENA**	**BLIND**
Not known to others	**CLOSED**	**DARK**

Johari Window

(a) ARENA: The upper left hand square is the arena of the public self that part of an individual's behavior known both to the person and to others with whom he interacts. The arena includes information such as- name, age, physical appearance and familial or organization affiliation.

(b) Blind Area: This area contains those aspects of the person's behavior and style that others know but that the person himself does not know. A person may have mannerism of which he is not aware that are perceived by others as funny, annoying or pleasing. Ex- An individual might be surprised to hear that his methods of asking questions annoys others because it is interpreted as cross examination rather than curiosity or a request for information.

(c) Closed Area: This area involves that which is known to the person but not revealed to others. Things in this area are secret. Ex- A subordinate may be, if his supervisor does not ask him to sit down during a meeting, but he will remain standing without letting the supervisors know that he is annoyed. The supervisor may think that the subordinate does not mind standing and accept his behavior as a part of their hierarchical relationship. Most of the people have many such feelings in their closed areas that they are unwilling to reveal to the persons concerned.

(d) Dark Area: This area is inaccessible both to the person and others. Some psychologist believe that, this is a very large area indeed and those certain circumstances (Ex- An accident, particular life stage or special techniques such as- psychoanalysis or psychodynamics may suddenly make a person realize some hidden aspects of himself. Because the dark area cannot be consciously controlled or changed and therefore cannot be considered in a discussion of personal effectiveness, this discussion will be limited to the arena, blind & closed areas of a personality.

Personal Effectiveness: It may be assumed that, a large arena and small blind and closed areas would be desirable and would contribute to the personal effectiveness.

This is not necessarily so, a person with a large arena may still be ineffective because a large arena is not the only factor in personal effectiveness.

Personal Effectiveness Combination

By combining high or low effectiveness with large or small area in the arena and the blind and closed areas gives 12 possible personality combinations as depicted below:

Arena	Blind Area	Closed Area	Effectiveness	Type of Person
	Large		High	Self-confident
	Large		Low	Unperceptive
	Small		High	Perceptive
	small		Low	Overly Cautious
		Large	High	Good Listener
		Large	Low	Secretive
		Small	High	Frank
		Small	Low	Ego-centric
Small			High	Task Oriented
Small			Low	Closed
Large			High	Superficial
Large			Low	Open

Self-Confident: A person with large blind area and high effectiveness is likely to be self-confident. He may not be aware of his limitations, but he may also not be aware of some of his strengths. However, he is likely to rely on his strengths and be blind to his weakness. Although his effectiveness may see him through situations, it will certainly be limited because of his lack of awareness of some of his limitations and strengths.

Unperceptive: A person with a large blind area and low effectiveness is unperceptive to the non-verbal cues that people may send about his behavior. Example- A professor who cannot see that the whole class is drowsy from a dull lecture may continue to bore the class. Unperceptive people find it difficult to realize subtle sarcasm, subdued communication of resentment and negative feelings and body language.

Perceptive: A person with a small blind area and high effectiveness is quite perceptive of verbal and non-verbal ques. This perceptiveness help him to pick up such cues quickly and use them to change his strategy of interaction and hence his effectiveness. A perceptive supervisor who sees that a subordinate about what is bothering him before pursuing task related topics. This is likely to help the subordinates become more open and relate to the supervisor more effectively.

Overly Cautious: A person with a smaller blind area knows more about his strengths and limitations. However, if such a person has low effectiveness he is more likely to be overly concerned with his weakness than he is to concentrate on his strengths. An over cautious persons finds it difficult to take the initiatives and to risk because his limitations loom large to him and may immobilize him. Just having a smaller blind area does not necessarily make a person effective.

Good Listener: A person with a large closed area and with high effectiveness is likely to be good listener. Instead of giving his own opinions, he listened to the opinions of others and makes decisions based on his own judgments. He may not share his own points of view, even if his views are not close to the views of others.

Secretive: A person with a large closed area and with low effectiveness is likely to be secretive. Other people may wonder what criteria he uses to judge them or what he expects from them. They are also not likely to know how he feels, as he will not share his feelings with others.

Frank: A person with a small closed area and with high effectiveness is likely to be quite outspoken and frank. He gives feedback and expresses his opinions and points of views without any inhibition. He shares his personal feelings, experiences, joys and sorrows as well.

Ego-centric: A person with a small closed area but with low effectiveness may tend to talk excessively about himself, his achievements, his talents, his experiences and even his personal life. He is so ego-centric that he is not likely to pay attention to others and their needs.

Task Oriented: A person with a small arena can be quite effective in a limited way. One model for a effective administrator is a person with a small arena and a high task orientation. Such a person does not relate t others o a personal or social level. He is mainly concerned with task performances and may restrict his communication and interaction with others only to the tasks involved.

Closed: A person with a small arena and low effectiveness is usually closed, neither sharing his impression nor listening to other & using feedback has he received. Such a person will be quite effective.

Superficial: A person with a large arena but with low effectiveness does not use his openness to good effect with others. He may interact with others, offer his opinions and listen to others, but these acts are usually of a superficial nature. He does not exercise has judgment about when to open and what to look for in the feedback he receives from others.

Open: A person with a large arena (the open self) and high effectiveness is open. His opinions are given freely and are well understood, he feels free to communicate his impressions and he gives feedback to others with sensitivity that they appreciate. Similarly, he is eager to receive feedback from others: he solicits it and then critically examines and uses it to good effect.

Developing Personal Effectiveness

Personal effectiveness must be viewed across 03 dimensions, such as- Openness, Perceptiveness and communication, al significant dimensions in inter personal relationship. By becoming more open, a person reduces his closed area, the blind area is reduced by increasing perceptiveness and communication can be improved in various ways. These three dimensions, however, do not function in isolation: each interacts with the others. In order to increase effectiveness, it is necessary to work on a combination of all three dimensions.

Openness: It is the extent to which one share ideas, feelings, experiences, impressions, perceptions and various other personal data with others. It is an important quality and contributes a great deal to a person's effectiveness.

Perceptiveness: The ability to pick up verbal and non-verbal cues from others indicates perceptiveness. This should be combined with other two dimensions. It can be increased by checking with others about their reactions to what has been said. If a person does not do so this he may become overly concerned about the cues receives.

Communications: It is an important decision to increase the personal effectiveness and it should be combined with others two for higher effectiveness in personality & persons.

SWOT Analysis: SWOT analysis is an extremely useful tool for understanding and decision making for all sorts of situation in business and farm organization.

SWOT is an acronym for Strength, Weakness, Opportunities and Threats and these 04 attributes are also called SWOT parameters.

Strengths: It is the basic asset of the organization that would provide competitive advantage for its growth and development, eg. Patents, strong brand names, god reputation among customers, cost advantages from proprietary know-how, exclusive accesses to high natural resources, favorable access to distribution networks.

What advantages do you have? What do you do well? What relevant resources do you have access to? What do other people see as your strengths?

Consider this from your own point of view and from the point of view of the people you deal with. Don't be modest, be realistic. If you are having any difficulty with this, try writing down a list of your characteristics. Some of these will hopefully be strengths.

In looking at our strength, think about them in relation to our competitors- For

Example, if all our competitors provide high quality products, the high quality production process is not strength in the market, it is a necessity.

Weakness: Absence of certain strength may be viewed as a weakness. It is the inability of an organization that can create a state of time and situation, specific advantage for its growth and development, eg. Lack of patent protection, a weak brand name, poor reputation among customers, high cost structure, lack of access to the best natural resources, lack of access to key distribution channels. What could we improve? What do we do badly? What should we avoid?

Again consider this from an internal and external basis: Do other people seem to perceive weakness that we do not see? Are our competitors doing any better than me? It is best to be realistic now, and face any unpleasant truths as soon as possible.

Opportunities: It is the ability f an organization to grow and achieve its specific objectives in a given situation, eg. An unfulfilled customer needs arrival of new technologies, loosening of regulations and removal of international trade barriers.

Where are the good opportunities facing you? What are the interesting trends you are aware of?

Useful opportunities can come from such things as:

Changes in technologies and markets on both, abroad and a narrow scale.

Changes in Govt. policies related to you filed.

Changes in social patterns, population profiles, life style changes etc.

A useful application to looking to opportunities is to look at your strength and ask yourself whether these open up any opportunities. Alternatively, look at your weakness and ask yourself whether you could open up opportunities by eliminating them.

Threats: It is a situation that blocks the abilities of the extension organization to grow and develop for meeting its ultimate goals, Eg-shift in consumer tastes away from the firm's products, emergence of substitute products, new regulations, increased trade barriers. What obstacles do you face? What are your competitors doing? Are the required specifications from your job products or services changing? Is changing technology threatening your position? Do you have bad debt or cash flow problems?

Could any of your weakness seriously threaten your business?

Carrying out this analysis will often be illumination-both in terms of pointing out what needs to be done and in putting problems into perspectives.

Strength and weakness are the corporate, organizational characteristics in nature which are internal. Opportunity and threat are external in nature.

Internal	**External**
Share holders	Government
Employees	Customers
Product qualities	Economic/Political situation
Price of the products	Price policy of the Govt.

Examples of SWOT

A Start up small consultancy business might carry out following SWOT Analysis:

Strengths

We are above to responds very quickly as we have no red tape. No need for higher mgmt. approval etc.

We are able to give really good customer care, as the current small amount of work means we have plenty of time to devote to customers.

Ur lead consultants has strong reputation within the market

We can change direction quickly if we find that our marketing is not working.

We have little overhead charges so we can offer good value to customers.

Weakness

Our farm has to market prestige or reputation

We have a small staff with shallow skills base in many years

We are vulnerable to vital staff being sick, leaving etc.

Our cash flow will be unreliable in the early stages.

Opportunities

Our business sectors are expanding with many futures opportunities for success.

Our local council wants to encourage local businesses with work where possible.

Our competitors may be slow to adopt new technologies.

Threats

Will developments in technology change this market beyond our ability to adapt?

A small change in focus of a large competitor might wipe out any market position we achieve.

The consultancy might therefore decide to specialize in rapid response, good value services to local business. Marketing would be in selected local publications, to get the greatest possible market presence for a set advertising budget. The consultancy should keep up t date with changes in technology where possible.

Uses of SWOT Analysis

(a) It plays an important role in understanding the management problems at all stages irrespective of the type of organization.

(b) It helps in taking appropriate decisions for development of an organization in a particular operational environment.

(c) It is useful for increasing competitive abilities of scientist and organizations.

(d) It helps to bring out the relevant changes in projects and organizations.

(e) It gives the scope for safety and security t every organization without facing hurdles in running the organization profitably.

(f) SWOT analysis is a frame work for analyzing our strength and weakness and opportunities and threats we face.

(g) It helps to focus our strength. Minimize weakness and take the greatest possible advantage of opportunities available.

Application Of SWOT: *Examples of what a SWOT analysis can be used to assess, as follows:*

(i) Industry: Many industrial scientist, managers and technical personnel applied the SWOT analysis frequently on systems and organizations for taking appropriate decisions for their smooth running. SWOT application was first used in 1910 in European and other developed countries.

(ii) Strategic Management & Planning: It is a continuous process of effectively relating the organizations objectives and resources to the opportunities in the environment. SWOT analysis helps policy makers and managers in shaping the strategic directions of a specific agency operating within a given situations or context.

(Besides industry, the SWOT analysis in general is applicable in many walks of life as follows:

Individual/Household or families/ Private or Govt. organizations/Politics/

A Company/ A methods of sales distribution/ a product or bran/ a business idea/

A strategic options/ an opportunity to make an acquisition/A potential partnership

A Changing a supplier/ Outsourcing a service, activity or resources/ An investment opportunity etc.

14

Conflicts and Stress Management for Optimum Efficiency in Organization

Rakesh Roy

Malda Krishi Vigyan Kendra
Uttar Banga Krishi Vishwavidyalaya, Pundibari, West Bengal 736165

A conflict is a fight or a clash of interest, opinion, or even principles. Conflict can never be eliminated from the society; as there are different reasons of conflict. It may vary from personal, racial, class, caste, political, international and many more.

Conflict in a group often follows a specific course. Routine group interaction is first disrupted by an initial conflict within the group. It is often caused by internal differences of opinion, disagreements between its members, or scarcity of resources available to the group. Some of the common sorts of conflicts are:

- *Inter-group conflict* is conflict between two or more groups.
- *Organization conflict* is discord caused by opposition of needs, values, and interests between people working together.
- *Role conflict* involves incompatible demands placed upon a person in a manner that makes accomplishing both troublesome.
- *Social conflict* is the struggle for supremacy or autonomy between social classes.
- *Conflict of interest* is involvement in multiple interests which could possibly corrupt the motivation or decision-making.
- *Cultural conflict* is a type of conflict that occurs due to the difference in cultural values and beliefs.
- *Ethic conflict* is conflict between two or more contending ethnic groups.
- *Work-family conflict* involves incompatible demands between the work and family roles of an individual.

Conflicts may be both constructive and destructive but conflict is rarely seen as constructive. However in certain contexts, moderate levels of conflict can be seen as being mutually beneficial, facilitating understanding, tolerance, learning, and effectiveness. In a team setting, the group can learn to overcome intra-group conflict which would conclude to minimizing negative outcomes.

With minimizing negative outcomes, positive outcomes will grow with increase of teamwork, working as a group, and an increase of understanding and cooperation with teammates which eventually leads to the control on intra-group conflict.

From the various conflict and conflict management theories, the process of conflict management can be understood in a new conceptual model, the Construction Conflict Management Model (CCM Model) shown in Fig. 1. It shows that it would link the pre-conflict/causal factors through to its comprehensive management within the environment of construction firms.

This is intended to explore the causal factors taking into consideration the internal and external factors and level and type of these factors, the conflict process and the outcomes with a view to effectively identify and manage conflicts in construction firms.

This integrative model looks at the causal factors (pre-conflict) underlying conflict situations, taking into consideration the Push and Pull factors which causes it to come into being, how the conflict situation changes with time and the mechanisms for the multi –level management of conflict.

Conflict Management

Conflict management is the practice of being able to recognize and handle conflicts sensibly, fairly, and efficiently. Since conflicts in organization are very natural in workplace, it is essential to have managers who realize conflicts and know how to resolve them. There are different types of conflicts and its management styles and techniques depend both on the style of managers and the types of conflicts.

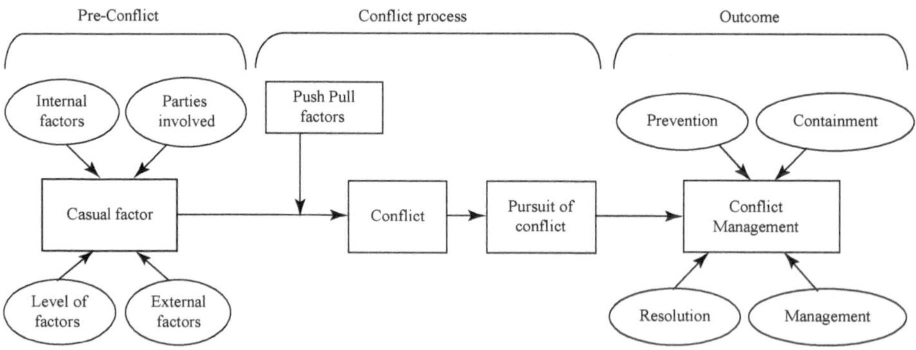

Fig 1. The "CCM" Model (Adapted from Kelly and Nicholson (1980) and Lynch (2001)).

Organizational conflicts

In this chapter, we will mainly focus on organizational conflicts and its managements.

Intrapersonal conflict

The name simply gives the idea that a conflict which occurs within a person, often involves some form of goal conflict or cognitive conflict. Goal conflict exists for individuals when their behavior will result in outcomes that are mutually exclusive or have compatible elements (both positive and negative outcomes).

- **Approach-approach conflict** is a circumstance where a person has an option between two or more alternatives with positive outcomes, e.g., a person can choose between two equally attractive jobs.
- **Avoidance - avoidance conflict** is a situation in which a person must choose between two or more alternatives, and they all have negative outcome, e.g., employees may be threatened with punishment in the form of demotion unless they do something they dislike spend much time travelling on their job.
- **Approach-avoidance conflict** is a situation in which a person must choose whether to do something that had both positive and negative outcomes, e.g., being offered a good job in a bad location.

Interpersonal Conflict

Interpersonal conflict refers to any types of conflict involving two or more people. Mild or severe interpersonal conflict is a natural outcome of human interaction. When you work or interact with someone who doesn't share opinions or goals, conflict can arise. The types of interpersonal conflicts may be classified as follows.

- ***Pseudo conflict***: A pseudo conflict usually happens due of the following circumstances:
- People involved in the conflict believe that they have different goals whereas in reality, they have similar goals.
- When one person involved in the conflict mocks or taunts the others and therefore conflict arises.
- A simple misunderstanding leads to a difference of opinion and therefore a conflict arises.

These types of pseudo conflicts can be resolved without too much difficulty. It just takes a bit of clarification about what you actually meant or some further exploration of how your goals actually do align.

- ***Fact conflict*:** Fact conflict happens when two or more people disagree over information or the truth of something. As this kind of conflict involves facts, it can be resolved easily. All that is to be done is to check a credible source for the truth.
- ***Value conflict*:** This kind of conflict comes up when different personal values lead to disagreement and hence conflict arises. Value conflict doesn't always have a comprehensible path to resolution. People can have such widely varying personal values and beliefs, so we may find it helpful to just acknowledge our opposing viewpoints respectfully and accept that we likely won't change each other's minds.
- ***Policy conflict*:** This conflict happens when people can't agree on a problem-solving strategy or action plan in a given situation. Personality, upbringing, education, and any number of other factors might have an impact on someone's approach to policy, or problem-solving, so this kind of conflict isn't unusual. As for instance, it might happen when parents disagree on the most effective way to discipline a child.
- ***Ego conflict*:** In an argument where neither you nor the other person involved could back down or accept a loss. Ego conflict often develops alongside other types of conflict, and it can make any disagreement trickier to navigate. It commonly happens when conflict gets personal.

***Meta conflict*:** Meta conflict happens when you have conflict about your conflicts. Some of the common examples of Meta conflict are:

- That's so unfair. That's not what we're talking about at all.
- You always nod along, but you never actually hear what I'm saying!
- You're too worked up. I can't deal with you when you're like this.
- We need to communicate clearly to resolve this conflict. Meta conflict might bring up issues with communication; it often does so in unhelpful ways.

Intra-Organizational Conflict

There are mainly four types of intra-organizational conflict in an organization. Although these types of conflict can overlie, especially with role conflict, each has distinctive characteristics.

(i) **Vertical conflict:** Vertical conflict refers to any conflict between levels in an organization, e.g., superior-subordinate conflict. This conflict generally arises during the situation when the superiors who want to control their subordinates and subordinates don't want to be under their command.

(ii) **Horizontal conflict:** Horizontal Conflict refers to conflict between employees or departments as the same hierarchical level in an organization.

(iii) **Line-staff conflict:** Most organizations have staff departments to assist the line departments. The line-staff relationship frequently involves conflict. Staff managers and line managers typically have different personal characteristics. Staff employees tend to have a higher level of education, come from different backgrounds, and are younger than line employees. These different personal characteristics are frequently associated with different values and beliefs, and the surfacing of these different values tends to create conflict.

(iv) **Role conflict:** A role is the cluster of activities that others expect individuals to perform in their position. A role frequently involves conflict.

Constructive and Destructive Conflicts

Except in very few situations where the conflict is constructive that can lead to competition and creativity so that in such situations the conflict can be encouraged, in all other cases where conflict is destructive in nature, it should be resolved as soon after it has developed as possible, but all efforts should be made to prevent it from developing.

Strategies to encourage constructive conflict

There could not be a fixed strategy for all organization. The strategies to encourage constructive conflict in an organization may be as follows.

- **Goal structure:** Goals should be clearly defined and the role and contribution of each unit towards the organizational goal must be clearly identified. Each unit and the individuals in these units must be aware of the importance of their role and such importance must be fully recognized.
- **Co-ordination:** Properly coordinated activities reduce conflict. Wherever there are problems in co-ordination, a special liaison office should be established to assist such co-ordination for better communication.
- **Trust and communication:** Greater trust among the members of unit, lead to more honest and open the communication among them. Individuals and units should be encouraged to communicate openly with each other so that they can all understand each other, understand each other's problems and help each other when necessary.
- **Reward System:** The compensation system should be such that it does not create individual competition or conflict within the unit. It should be appropriate and proportionate to the group effort and reflect the degree of interdependence among units where necessary.

Strategies to resolve destructive conflict

Conflicts usually happen, but the approach an employee takes and further responds and resolves these conflicts will limit or enable that employee's success. Here are five conflict styles that a manager will follow according to Kenneth W. Thomas and Ralph H. Kilmann (Fig 2.).

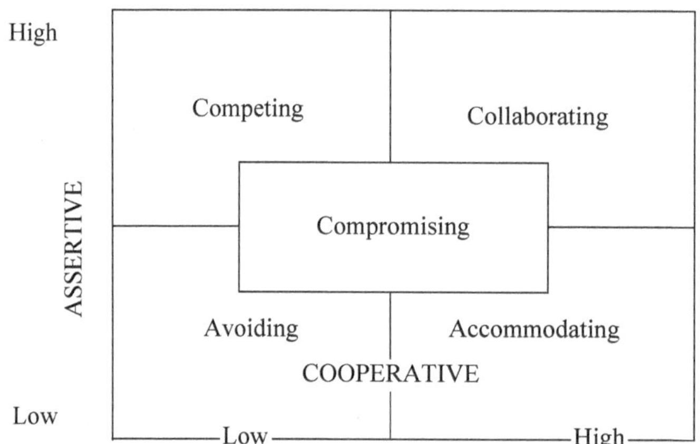

Fig. 2. Strategies to resolve destructive conflicts

- **Avoiding**. In certain circumstances, it may perhaps be sensible to take a passive role and avoid it all together. In some situations getting involved by a manager would provoke further controversy or in some cases conflict is so trivial in nature that it would not be worth to get involved and try to solve it. It could also be that the conflict is so fundamental to the position of the parties involved that it may be best either to leave it to them to solve it or to let events take their own course.
- **Accommodating:** It simply means covering up the conflict by appealing for the need for unity rather than addressing the issue of conflict itself. If two parties have a conflict within the organization, the supervisor may try to calm things down by being understanding and supportive to both parties and appealing them for co-operation. The supervisor does not ignore or withdraw from the conflict nor does he try to address and resolve the conflict but expresses hope that everything will work out for the best of all. Thus, accommodating provides only a temporary solution and conflict may resurface again in the course of time. Smoothing is more sensitive approach than avoiding in that as long as the parties agree that not showing conflict has more benefits than showing conflicts, the conflict can be avoided.
- **Compromising**: A compromise in the conflict is reached by balancing the demands of the conflicting parties and bargaining to reach a solution. Each

party gives up something and also gains something. The technique of conflict resolution is very common in negotiations between the labour unions and management. Through the process of negotiating and bargaining, mostly in the presence of arbitrators, they reach a solution by compromising. This type of compromise is known as integrative bargaining in which both sides win in a way.

- **Competing**: The simplest feasible resolution is the elimination of the other party – to force opponent to flee and give up the fight – or abolish them. This is technique of domination where the dominator has the power and authority to enforce his own views over the opposing conflicting party. This technique is potentially effective in situations such as a president of a company firing a manager because he is considered as a trouble-maker and conflict creator. This technique always ends up in one party being a loser and the other party being a clear winner.
- **Collaborating**: This method involves confronting the conflict in order to seek the best solution to the problem. This approach objectively assumes that in all organizations even though it is well managed, there will be differences of opinions which must be resolved through discussions and respect for differing viewpoints. In general, this technique is very useful in resolving conflicts arising out of semantic misunderstandings.

Stress

In an organizational perspective, stress may be defined as the reactions of individuals to new or threatening factors in their work environments.

Types of stress

Stress can be either positive or negative. Some new work situations can bring us positive challenges and excitement, while others are very threatening and anxiety-arousing. As for example, the depression in the economy can create negative stress for sales personnel, as they will be much more anxious about making sales quotas and its commissions. On the other hand, promotions to new jobs present employees with positive stress. While employees may feel anxious about their new work assignments, they also anticipate them eagerly and look forward to the additional challenges, rewards, and excitement. In these cases, the new and uncertain job situations create positive stress (also called eustress).

There is an optimum level of stress for every individual under which he or she will perform to full capacity. If the stress experienced is below this optimum level, then the individual gets bored, the motivational level to work reaches a low point, and apathy sets in. If one operates in a very low stress environment and constantly experiences boredom, the person is likely to psychologically or physically withdraw from work. Psychological withdrawal will result in careless mistakes being frequently made, forgetting to do things, and thinking of things other than work during work hours. Physical withdrawal will manifest itself in increased rates of tardiness and absenteeism which may ultimately lead to turnover. Though the optimum stress level is different for different individuals, each individual can sense and determine how much stress is functional for him or her to operate in a productive manner. The relationship between stress and performance is explained (Fig 3.).

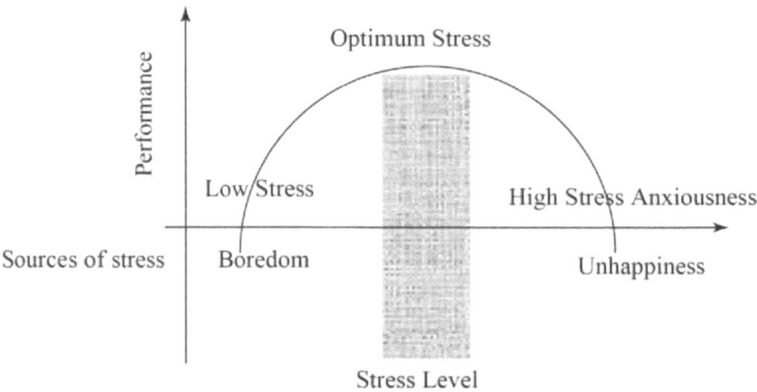

Fig 3. Relationship between Stress and Performance

Sources of Stress

Stress is a must in our daily life. Both stresses and strains come from our work and non-work lives which we experienced in one domain are carried over to the other. Thus, it can be seen very often that due to distress at work, that stress will be carried over to the home, which will intensify the sense of awareness of even small distresses experienced in the family sphere.

One major source of job stress is the job itself. The way the job is designed, the amount of time pressure an individual faces, and the number of expectations others have of a person at work can all lead to job stress. Interpersonal relationships are a second source of job stress. How much contact an individual has with coworkers and bosses, how much time he or she deals with clients or consumers, and how pleasant those interactions are all influence how much stress an individual experiences at work. Third, problems in personal lives can spill over into the work environment, adding further tension to an already stressful work situation.

Sources of Job Stress

Job Characteristics

- Role ambiguity

- Role conflict
- Role overload or under load
- Ethical dilemmas

Interpersonal Relationships

- Organizational climate
- Amount of contact with others
- Dealing with people in other departments

Organizational Factors

- Personal Factors
- Career concerns
- Rate of life change
- Geographical mobility

Consequences of job stress for an individual

The impact of distress on individuals has subjective, cognitive, physiological, behavioral and health facets to it.

- The *subjective or intrapersonal effects* of stress are feelings of anxiety, boredom, apathy, nervousness, depression, fatigue, anger, irritability and sometimes aggressive behaviors on the part of the individual experiencing the stress.
- The *cognitive* effects include poor concentration, short attention span, mental blocks and inability to make decisions.
- The *physiological* effects can be seen in increased heart and pulse rate, high blood pressure, dryness of throat, and excessive sweating.
- The *behavioral* consequences are manifest in such things as accident proneness, drinking; excessive eating, smoking, impulsive behaviors, depression, and withdrawal behaviors.
- The manifest *health* effects could be stomach disorders, asthma, eczema, and other psychosomatic disorders. In addition, the mental health, i.e. the ability to function effectively in one's daily life, will also decline as excessive stress is experienced.

Consequences for the family

Distress which is handled by individuals in dysfunctional ways, such as reasoning to drinking or withdrawal behaviors, will have an adverse effect on their home life. Spouse abuse, child abuse, alienation from family members, and even divorce could result from dysfunctional coping mechanisms.

Consequences to organizations

The organizational effects of employee stress are many. The adverse consequences include low performance and productivity, high rates of absenteeism and turnover, poor decision-making, lost customers because of poor worker attitudes, increased alienation of the worker from the job, and even destructive and aggressive behaviors resulting in strikes and sabotage. The stresses experienced by employees who take on critical roles and are responsible for safety can sometimes be detrimental to the public.

Management of Stress

Stress is a factor that everybody has to contend with on a daily basis both in the work and non-work spheres of life. Since the body has only a limited capacity to respond to stress, it is important for individuals to optimally manage their stress to operate as fully functioning human beings. There are several ways in which stress can be handled so that the dysfunctional consequences of stress are dissipated. Some of them are:

- **Role analysis technique:** The role analysis technique as it is referred to help both the manager and the employee to analyze what the job entails and what the expectations are. Breaking down the job to its various components clarifies the role of the job incumbent for the entire system. This helps to eliminate imposing overload can thus be considerably reduced through this technique and stress levels lowered for the individual.
- **Job relocation:** Job relocation assistance is offered to employees who are transferred, by finding alternative employment for the spouses of the transferred employees and getting admissions in schools for their children in the new place. These arrangements help to reduce the anxiety and stress for the moving family.
- **Recreational programme:** Providing recreational facilities, arranging group meditation programmes, help to reduce the stress levels of the employees.
- **Employee assistance programme:** Another widely used strategy is the employee assistance programmes which offer a variety of assistance to employees.
- **Career counseling:** Career Counseling helps the employee to obtain professional advice regarding career paths that would help the individual to achieve personal goals. It also makes the employees aware of what additional educational qualifications or specialized technical training, if any, that they should acquire.

- **Time management:** Time management is an effective way to manage with stress. People should learn to get better organized so that they can do their work more competently and fritter away less time needlessly.
- **Delegation:** Delegation some responsibilities to others can directly decrease work demands put upon the manager and helps to reduce the stress.
- **Supervisor training:** Supervisor training is a type of stress management programme that are being conducted by the organizations so that the supervisors can prevent job stress. Managers are trained to give better performance appraisals, to listen to employees' problems more effectively, and to communicate job assignments and instructions more clearly.
- **Individual stress reduction workshops:** Some organizations have also sponsored individual stress reduction workshops for their employees. These programs have run the gamut from bio-feedback, sensitivity groups and transcendental meditation to career counseling, time management and interpersonal skills workshops.

15

Negotiation Skill and Decision Support Systems in Extension Communication

Partha Pratim Pal
ICAR-ATARI, Kolkata, India

Madhumita Jena
Kalahandi KVK, OUAT, Odisha, India

Swayambhu Ghosh
ICAR-ATARI, Kolkata
ICAR-Agricultural Technology Application & Research Institute, Kolkata, India

Negotiation is a communication and problem-solving process built on a broad foundation of skills and knowledge. It is also one of the most popular and effective means of resolving conflicts and misunderstandings. Negotiation is back and forth communication designed to reach agreement while leaving the other side intact and positive.

Basic principle, without which negotiation is impossible

Successful negotiation requires compromise from both sides. Both parties must gain something, and both parties must lose something. You must be prepared to give something up to which you believe you are entitled. You cannot expect to defeat your opponent or "win" a negotiation by either the power of your negotiating skills or the compelling force of your logic. This is not to say that good negotiating ability is irrelevant. In most cases, a range of possible outcomes exists. A skilled negotiator often can achieve a settlement near the top of the range.

Benefits of negotiation skills

Negotiation is a coveted leadership skill which helps businesses reach their business objective. Here are a few reasons negotiation skills are essential in the workplace

- **Builds a relationship:** Despite the difference in opinion, negotiation skills help strike a solution and focus more on creating goodwill and value. This builds a long-term relationship.

- **Delivers excellent solutions:** Good negotiation skills ensure that solutions to the conflicts are not short-term. It focuses on creating long-lasting solutions because both parties make a concession only when the solution is satisfactory.
- **Avoids future conflicts:** As both parties agree to a common solution, the chances of future conflicts reduce to a great extent.
- **Create an environment of business success:** Good negotiation skills ensure the accomplishment of business goals, which creates an environment of business success. This also increases the chances of future business transaction.

Qualities that a negotiator must have

1. Create a friendly atmosphere
2. Build up good rapport with the individual / party that they are negotiating with
3. Are firm about their stand
4. Keep the interest of both sides in mind
5. Look for immediate gains
6. Are willing to make concessions
7. Are persuasive
8. Are articulate
9. Are good listeners
10. Frequently check to confirm that everything has been correctly understood by both parties

Phases in a negotiation

1. **The preparation phase:** this is where you identify your purpose and set your priorities. You must also decide in advance what the lowest deal is or offer that you will be willing to accept. Have all information that you are likely to need available with you.
2. **The debating phase:** negotiation is a process of give and take where you give a little and get a little at the same time. Here you try to find out what the person or party you are negotiating with wants. During this phase you must state what you want but do not spell out all the conditions yet. Use open questions and be willing to listen to the other person too. Try to find out how much the other person is willing to move from his/her stand.

3. **The proposal stage:** This is where you suggest the concessions you are willing to make. Formulate your proposals with if……, then………. Listen to the other side's proposals too. Build on common ground.
4. **The bargaining phase:** This is the part where you spell out what it is that you will actually trade. Accept and confirm details agreed upon by repeating them. Summarize the proposal in a few words. End positively by looking ahead

Elements of Negotiation

Negotiation

↓

Process + Behaviour + Substance (Agenda)

Process: The way individuals negotiate with each other is called the process of negotiation. The process includes the various techniques and strategies employed to negotiate and reach to a solution.

Behaviour: How two parties behave with each other during the process of negotiation is referred to as behavior. The way they interact with each other, the way they communicate with each other to make their points clear all come under behaviour.

Substance: There has to be an agenda on which individuals negotiate. A topic is important for negotiation. In the first situation, going for the late night movie was the agenda on which you wanted to negotiate with your parents as well as your friends.

Negotiation is simply a technique, a discussion among individuals to reach to a mutual agreement where everyone gains something or the other and conflicts are avoided.

Negotiation, however, may not be the only way to achieve your aim. People negotiate only when they believe they will fare worse if they adopt other approaches. In spite of this, they may choose not to negotiate, and instead choose other approaches. Such an alternative course of action is referred to as an ATNA (Alternative to a Negotiated Agreement).

A BATNA (Best Alternative to a Negotiated Agreement) is another choice or substitute action that may produce an outcome superior to any outcome we might gain from a negotiation process.

A WATNA (Worst Alternative to a Negotiated Agreement) is another choice or substitute action that may produce an outcome inferior to any outcome we might gain from a negotiation process.

We win with BATNAs and lose with WATNAs. BATNAs are a source of power, while WATNAs are a source of weakness. The more likely that a side's WATNA will happen, the *more* likely it is that that side will negotiate. The more likely that a side's BATNA will happen, the *less* likely it is that that side will negotiate.

In other words: *if BATNAs are likely, don't negotiate; if WATNAs are likely, negotiate*.

Situation	Watna	Batna
A person is thinking of buying a used car from a car yard.	Keep driving current faulty vehicle until it breaks down	Buy direct from other owners who advertise their vehicles in newspapers or online, cutting out the cost of the middleman
Country A receives military threats from country B.	Country A is invaded and occupied permanently by country B.	Country B depends on oil revenues to wage war. The price of oil declines dramatically, as country A's intelligence predicted. Country B stops making threats.
Union wants a 30 per cent wage increase.	Union goes on strike, even though strike fund has been Embezzled by corrupt official.	Market value of company stock suddenly rises. All employees have stock, so become wealthier as a result. Union representatives decide to defer claims until better organized and resourced.
Two lovers cannot agree over who is to pay a restaurant bill.	No-one pays and the restaurant owner calls the police.	The restaurant owner, a romantic at heart, tells them the food is on the house

Negotiation Approaches

1. Distributive negotiation

Distributive negotiation, sometimes called zero-sum negotiation or win-lose negotiation, is a bargaining approach in which one person succeeds only if another person loses. A distributive negotiation usually involves discussion of a single issue.

Tips for success in a distributive negotiation:

Be persistent. When you're taking a distributive approach to a negotiation, persistence and polite assertiveness can help you fulfill your interests.

Make the first offer. In a distributive negotiation, you can make the first offer to begin the bargaining in your favour.

Don't communicate your minimum favorable outcome. It's important to aim high in distributive negotiations to ensure successful bargaining. You can withhold any information on the minimum you're willing to accept from bargaining for the best results.

2. Integrative negotiation

Integrative negotiation, sometimes called win-win negotiation or collaborative negotiation, is a bargaining approaches where negotiating parties' attempts to reach a mutually beneficial solution. Unlike distributive negotiations, integrative negotiations can involve multiple issues.

Tips you can use in an integrative negotiation:

Take a principled approach. You can discuss your principles during an integrative negotiation to build trust with the other party.

Discuss your needs and interests openly. Communicating about your goals in an integrative negotiation can promote transparency and enable a positive relationship.

Use bargaining to solve problems. In an integrative negotiation, both parties can use negotiations as an opportunity for collaborative problem-solving

Different ways to negotiate

"In a world deluged by irrelevant information, clarity is power." Negotiation is a method that transforms your demand in a sharp and crisp way to other party. In this age of information and overuse of gadgets, any party has much lesser time for focusing on what other party is demanding. The humankind has been gradually engrossed in the social media and it's glittering content. As a result, a negotiable party like a job-hiring manager can afford only 6 seconds to go through a resume, leading to much lesser scope for an applicant to negotiate. That has forced the people to invent several techniques of negotiation so that under any constrain the negotiation can happen. We will come to that later. But now it is needed to elaborate the types of negotiation that occurs in society.

a. Distributive negotiation: When a party thinks his/her loss will necessarily benefit other party such type of negotiation takes place. Only a single conflict can be the interest of communication. For an example, when a mushroom producer approaches the customer, he or she feels lowering the price may cause benefit to customer, whereas the other party thinks the mushroom growers is simply overcharging for its products.

b. **Integrative negotiation:** Such type of negotiation can occur when both parties realizes the possibility of a win-win situation. In this interest-based bargaining, it asserts that both parties can gain something and create value by offering trade-offs. For an example, the mushroom grower can lower the price slightly and convinced the customer to pay slightly higher than their proposed price and that leads to a successful trade with mutual benefit.

c. Inter-class negotiation: The class in our society exists from very beginning of the civilization. The class occurs when a disparity in power, position or possession comes into picture; however, the class also forces one party to get deprived and broadening the disparity. Such examples may be noted as, sharecropper and established farmer or an employee and management. Often, people has to negotiate with such senior-level people for their job duties and salary benefits or gross margins. This is a crucial workplace negotiation because their job satisfaction depends on it. Therefore, when negotiating about their salary or wages and other perks, clear as well as polite communication is **needed.**

d. Intra-class negotiation: Your job may require working closely with different departments and without strong negotiation skills, it might be difficult for you to reach your goals. For example, two croppers having adjacent land may be cultivating different crops. If one tea grower sprays pesticide on its plants, that sprayed poison may cause harm to the silkworms of a person practicing sericulture in a nearby field. In those cases, a degree of negotiation can save the second farmer. That may be done through dialog, or legal action.

Stages of the Negotiation Process

While there are many approaches to negotiation tactics, there are five common steps that most effective negotiations follow to achieve a successful outcome:

1. **Prepare:** Negotiation preparation is easy to ignore, but it's a vital first stage of the negotiating process. To prepare, research both sides of the discussion, identify any possible trade-offs, determine your most-desired and least-desired possible outcomes. Then, make a list of what concessions you're willing to put on the bargaining table, understand who in your organization has the decision-making power, know the relationship that you want to build or maintain with the other party, and prepare your BATNA ("best alternative to a negotiated agreement"). Preparation can also include the definition of the ground rules: determining where, when, with whom, and under what time constraints the negotiations will take place.

   The first thing that a person must focus on is a strategy before starting negotiation. There may be instances where the other party may disagree with the solution one provides. Good negotiators often come with one or more backup plans. For example, if a farmer is planning to sell his products in local market he should be prepared with a backup plan of selling at other districts or at any other market.

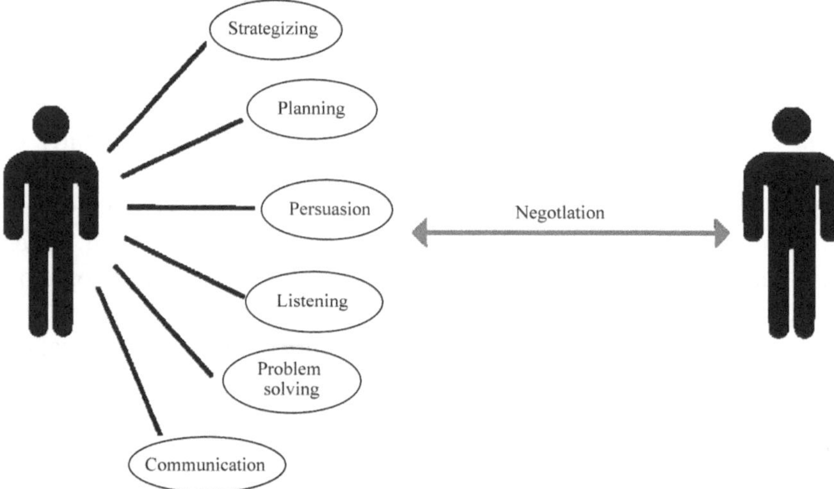

2. **Exchange information:** This is the part of the negotiation when both parties exchange their initial positions. Each side should be allowed to share their underlying interests and concerns uninterrupted, including what they aim to receive at the end of the negotiation and why they feel the way they do.

3. **Clarify:** During the clarification step, both sides continue the discussion that they began when exchanging information by justifying and bolstering their claims. If one side disagrees with something the other side is saying, they should discuss that disagreement in calm terms to reach a point of understanding.

4. **Bargain and problem-solve:** This step is the meat of the process of negotiation, during which both sides begin give-and-take. After the initial first offer, each negotiating party should propose different counter-offers for the problem, all the while making and managing their concessions. During the bargaining process, keep your emotions in check; the best negotiators use strong verbal communication skills (active listening and calm feedback; in face-to-face negotiation, this also includes body language). The goal of this step is to emerge with a win-win outcome—a positive course of action.

5. **Conclude and implement:** Once an acceptable solution has been agreed upon, both sides should thank each other for the discussion, no matter the outcome of the negotiation; successful negotiations are all about creating and maintaining good long-term relationships. Then they should outline the expectations of each party and ensure that the compromise will be implemented effectively. This step often includes a written contract and a follow-up to confirm the implementation is going smoothly.

Once someone has chalked out the backup plan or a strategy, he/she can prepare a plan. The planning helps them to be prepared for the challenges. Also, on the contrary to that, it must be mentioned that, sticking to a plan strictly may have an adverse effect in communication. After this stage the verbal or non-verbal communication starts.

Aristotle's Theory of Persuading People

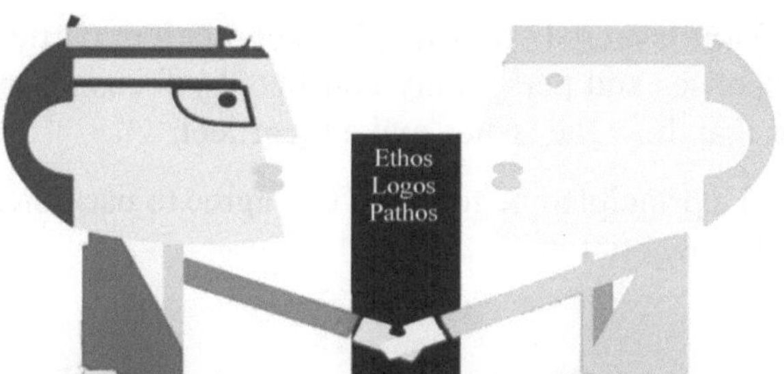

But, the objective of this communication has to be persuading the other party for agreeing to the given terms. The persuading is a well discussed skill in several professions. The public speakers, cold readers depend on persuasion more than any other skills. Mastering the persuasion helps a person bring out a positive reply easily from other party. In this limited space the art of persuasion may not be discussed, however, three parts of persuasion by Aristotle may give a brief idea to adopt the skill. According to Aristotle, ethos, logos and pathos are the pillar of persuading people. Ethos refers to ethics, when a farmer comes with product that has clarity and quality his chances of persuading his audience. Logos refers to logic and reason, the ability to explain the product, the added values and benefits helps the audience to overlook the gross margin and focus on the product only. Pathos refers to emotions and feelings. The product boosted with emotion helps the buyer get persuaded easily. All of these parts combine and make a better persuasion.

Types of Negotiation

1. **Principled negotiation**

   Principled negotiation is a type of bargaining that uses parties' principles and interests to reach an agreement. This type of negotiation often focuses on conflict resolution. This type of bargaining uses an integrative negotiation approach to serve the interests of both parties. There are four elements to a principled negotiation:

   Mutual gain: The integrative approach to a principled negotiation invites parties to focus on finding mutually beneficial outcomes through bargaining.

   Focus on interests: Negotiators can identify and communicate their motivations, interests and needs in a principled negotiation.

   Separate emotions from issues: In a principled negotiation, parties can reduce emotional responses and personality conflicts by focusing on the issues at hand, rather than how the issues make them feel.

   Objectivity: Parties in a principled negotiation can agree to use objective criteria as a baseline for negotiations

2. **Team negotiation**

   In a team negotiation, multiple people bargain toward an agreement on each side of the negotiation. Team negotiations are common with large business deals. There are several personality roles on a negotiation team. In some cases, one person may perform more than one role. Here are some common roles on negotiation teams:

   Leader: Members of each team in a negotiation usually appoint a leader to make the final decisions during negotiations.

   Observer: The observer pays attention to the other party's team during a negotiation, discussing their observations with the leader.

   Relater: A relater on a negotiation team works on building relationships with members of the other team during bargaining.

   Recorder: A recorder on a negotiating team can take notes on the discussions of a negotiation meeting.

   Critic: While this may sound like a negative role, having a critic on the team during negotiations can help you ensure you understand the concessions and other negative results of an agreement.

Builder: A builder on a negotiation team creates the deal or package for a bargaining team. They can perform financial functions during negotiations, calculating the cost of an agreement.

3. **Multiparty negotiation**

A multiparty negotiation is a type of bargaining where more than two parties negotiate toward an agreement. An example of a multiparty negotiation is bargaining between multiple department leaders in a large company. Here are a few of the challenges of multiparty negotiations:

Fluctuating BATNAs: BATNA stands for best alternative to a negotiated agreement. With multiple parties in a negotiation, each party's BATNA is more likely to change, which can make it harder for parties to agree. Each party can evaluate their BATNA at each stage in negotiations to understand the results of a proposed agreement.

Coalition formation: Another challenge of multiparty negotiations is the possibility for different parties to form coalitions, or alliances. These alliances can add to the complexity of bargaining. Coalitions can agree to a specific set of terms to help all parties reach an agreement.

Process-management issues: Managing the negotiation process between multiple parties can lead to a lack of governance and miscommunications. People in multiparty negotiations can avoid these issues by choosing a leader who's willing to collaborate with others toward an agreement.

4. **Adversarial Negotiation**

An adversarial negotiation is a distributive approach in which the most aggressive party in a negotiation achieves an agreement that serves their interests. Here are a few examples of adversarial negotiation tactics:

Hard bargaining: Hard bargaining is a strategy in which one party refuses to compromise in an agreement.

Future promise: A person using this tactic can promise the other party a future benefit in exchange for current concessions. You can counteract this tactic by asking for the future promise in writing.

Loss of interest: Another adversarial negotiation tactic is loss of interest, in which one party pretends they've lost their interest in pursuing an agreement.

Models of Negotiation

Negotiation is defined as a discussion among individuals to reach to a conclusion acceptable to one and all. It is a process where people rather than fighting among themselves sit together, evaluate the pros and cons and then come out with an alternative which would be a win win situation for all.

1. **Win-Win Model:** In this model, each and every individual involved in negotiation wins. Nobody is at loss in this model and everyone is benefited out of the negotiation. This is the most accepted model of negotiation. Let us understand it with the help of an example: Daniel wanted to buy a laptop but it was an expensive model. He went to the outlet and negotiated with the shopkeeper to lower the price. Initially the shopkeeper was reluctant but after several rounds of discussions and persuasion, he quoted a price best suited to him as well as Daniel. Daniel was extremely satisfied as he could now purchase the laptop without burning a hole in his pocket. The negotiation also benefited the store owner as he could earn his profits and also gained a loyal customer who would come again in future

2. **Win-Lose Model:** In this model one party wins and the other party loses. In such a model, after several rounds of discussions and negotiations, one party benefits while the party remains dissatisfied. Please refer to the above example once again where Daniel wanted to buy a laptop. In this example, both Daniel and the store owner were benefited out of the deal. Let us suppose Daniel could not even afford the price quoted by the storeowner and requests him to further lower the price. If the store owner further lowers the price, he would not be able to earn his profits but Daniel would be very happy. Thus, after the negotiation, Daniel would be satisfied but the shopkeeper wouldn't. In a win lose model, both the two parties are not satisfied, only one of the two walks away with the benefit.

3. **Lose-Lose Model:** As the name suggests, in this model, the outcome of negotiation is zero. No party is benefited out of this model. Had Daniel not purchased the laptop after several rounds of negotiation, neither he nor the store owner would have got anything out of the deal. Daniel would return empty handed and the store owner would obviously not earn anything. In this model, generally the two parties are not willing to accept each other's views and are reluctant to compromise. No discussions help.

4. **RADPAC Model of Negotiation:** RADPAC Model of Negotiation is a widely used model of negotiation incorporates. Every alphabet in this model signifies something

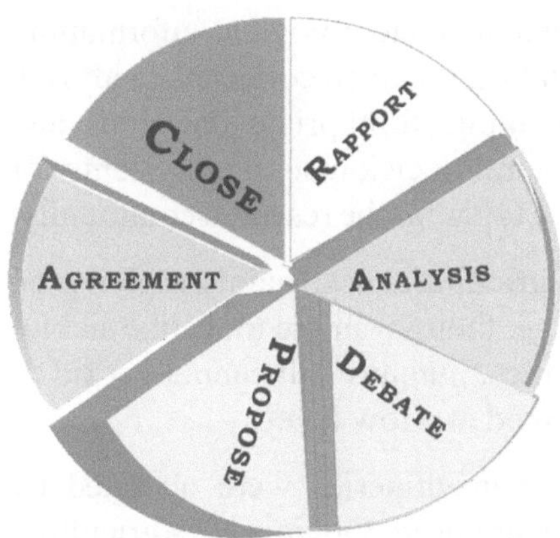

R - Rapport: As the name suggests, it signifies the relation between parties involved in negotiation. The parties involved in negotiation ideally should be comfortable with each other and share a good rapport with each other

A - Analysis: One party must understand the second party well. It is important that the individual understand each other's needs and interest. The shopkeeper must understand the customer's needs and pocket, in the same way the customer mustn't ignore the shopkeeper's profits as well. People must listen to each other attentively

D-Debate: Nothing can be achieved without discussions. This round includes discussing issues among the parties involved in negotiation. The pros and cons of an idea are evaluated in this round. People debate with each other and each one tries to convince the other. One must not lose his temper in this round but remain calm and composed.

P-Propose: Each individual proposes his best idea in this round. Each one tries his level best to come up with the best possible idea and reach to a conclusion acceptable by all.

A -Agreement: Individuals conclude at this stage and agree to the best possible alternative.

C -Close: The negotiation is complete and individuals return back satisfied.

Decision Support Systems in extension communication

Undoubtedly, high demands for food from the world-wide growing population are impacting the environment and putting many pressures on agricultural productivity. Agriculture 4.0, as the fourth evolution in the farming technology, puts forward four essential requirements: increasing productivity, allocating resources reasonably, adapting to climate change, and avoiding food waste. As advanced information systems and Internet technologies are adopted in

Agriculture 4.0, enormous farming data, such as meteorological information, soil conditions, marketing demands, and land uses, can be collected, analyzed, and processed for assisting farmers in making appropriate decisions and obtaining higher profits. Therefore, agricultural decision support systems for Agriculture 4.0 have become a very attractive topic for the research community.

Agriculture 1.0 refers to the traditional agricultural era, mainly replying on the manpower and animal forces. In this stage, though simple tools like sickles and shovels were used in agricultural activities, humans still cannot get rid of heavy manual labour, so productivity remained at a low level.

Agriculture2.0 when various agricultural machineries were operated by farmers manually and plenty of chemicals were used. Obviously, Agriculture 2.0 significantly increased the efficiency and productivity of farm works.

Agriculture 3.0 emerged from the rapid development of computing and electronics. Computer programs and robotic techniques allowed agricultural machineries to perform operations efficiently and intelligently

Nowadays, the evolution of agriculture steps into Agriculture 4.0, thanks to the employment of current technologies like Internet of Things, Big Data, Artificial Intelligence, Cloud Computing, Remote Sensing, etc. The applications of these technologies can improve the efficiency of agricultural activities significantly. it is worth mentioning that data from all fields are gathered and processed, providing a clear view for farmers. Stakeholders and farmers may encounter difficulties in making proper decisions about agricultural management with the explosive amount of information because it is much challenging to transfer these data into practical knowledge/utility.

Thus, platforms like decision support systems (DSSs) are needed in order to assist them in making evidence-based and precise decisions. Decision Support System (DSS) offers a framework within which complex systems can be represented in a structured way, allowing them to be more easily understood and helping to draw out additional information and new insights. It is an interactive computer based expert system that helps decision makers to utilize data and models to solve unstructured problems. The applicable use of successful decision support can assist in the sustainability of agricultural resources. Based on the important parameters in agriculture such as type of soil, seed, irrigation, fertilizers, and climatic data the activities in agriculture management can be classified into different categories. For effective and sustainable agriculture management decision support system at each of these activities is very much essential.

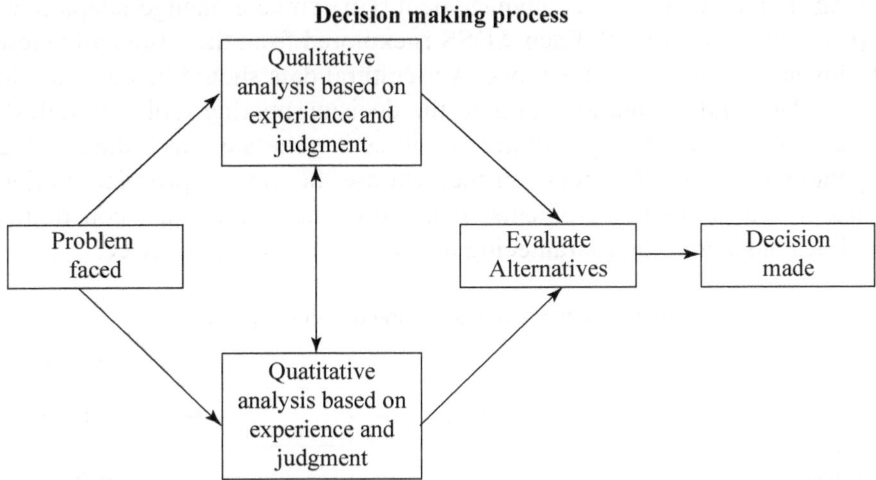

We are faced with decision making every day. From something as simple as deciding what to wear in the morning, to something as complex as deciding what career to follow, decision making invokes certain similar cognitive processes. Decision making is based on a combination of experience, empirical data, and analysis of the situation at hand. We make decisions based on a qualitative approach, a quantitative approach, or some combination of the two. A simple task may require only past experience and a bit of knowledge of the current situation to make a final decision. A decision support system (DSS) is a computer-based program that assists with the decision making process. The program can be quantitative, qualitative, or a combination of both. These programs are important because agricultural production and processing systems are complex due to the many biological, chemical, and physical processes involved, and require a great deal of information to be processed for proper management.

Structure of a Decision Support System

When a decision-maker is faced with a problem that cannot be easily solved based on experience and judgment alone, the DSS is utilized. The DSS will ask questions that help determine the nature of the problem and the resources that need to be used. These resources may include quantitative modules (simulation, optimization), or rule bases (heuristics).Decision support systems (DSSs) are used in agriculture to collect and analyze data from a variety of sources with the ultimate goal of providing end users with insight into their critical decision-making process. In particular, in the agriculture domain, these systems help farmers to solve complex issues related to crop production. The selected ADSSs have covered the agricultural applications in: (i) mission planning; (ii) water resources management; (iii) climate change adaptation; and (iv) food waste control. Each ADSS is explored from the systematic view by following the general framework. Agricultural data should be collected in the first place and treated as inputs to the decision-making tools (modules). Advice about managing agricultural activities is generated according to the computational results. Farmers can then choose the most appropriate option and adopt it to solve the problems. It is worth mentioning that constraints should be considered for guaranteeing the quality of provided advice.

A general framework of agricultural decision support

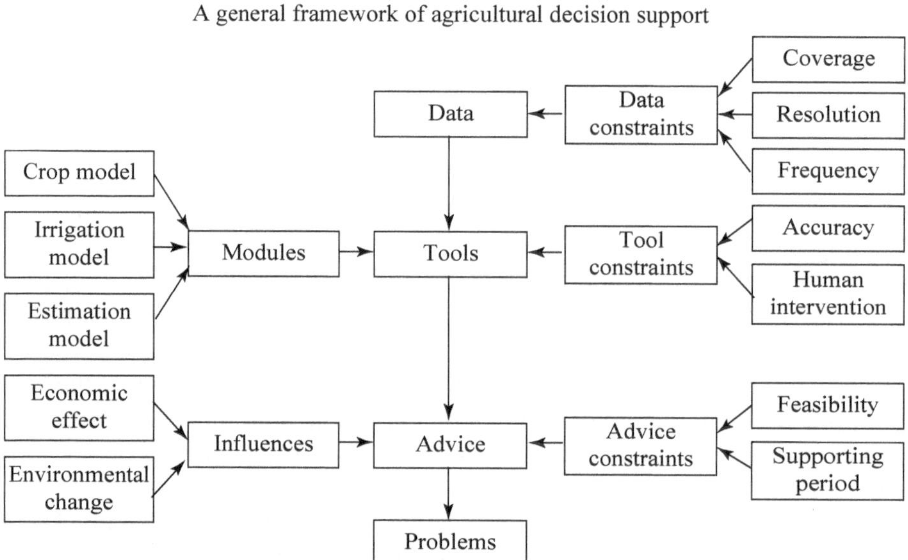

The methodological elements **Decision Support System** (DSS)

- **User communication channel**: The communication channel through which the user inputs the required data about the field of interest and the constraints about the available soil management measures. This information channel provides also the outputs from the DSS to the end-users. The textual and graphical form of the input and output information are provided in a user-friendly form.
- **Steering information channel**: The information entered by the end-user through the interface are sent to the decision support models, where the modelling constraints and operations are set, and the data required for the performance of the demanding modelling tasks are selected.
- **Data flow**: Flow of data that are transformed according to the requirements of the individual decision models.

- **Raw data flow:** Information for the required data are sent to the data and knowledge bases and available data are sent back to the data transformation part for their further formatting in order to be used in the decision support models.
- **Flow of modelling results:** Outputs from the individual decision support models are sent for further meta-analysis and translation into a set of applicable measures.
- **Output information flow:** Information about the proposed management measures are sent back to the user interface and are communicated to the end-users

Overview of Decision Support Systems

- The first DSS for agriculture cited in the literature is Televise, which was developed by Norway in 1957 for plant protection. Another such system named as Guntz Divoux was developed by France in 1963. Use of computerized quantitative models to assist in decision-making and planning was started systematically during this period.
- First computer-aided DSS for production scheduling was investigated, which was running on IBM 7049. Development of the IBM system 360 and other more powerful mainframe systems made it practical and cost-effective to develop Management Information System (MIS) for large companies. These early MIS focused on providing managers with structured periodic reports primarily for accounting and transaction processing.
- Decision Support System was first used by Gory and Scott Morton in their review in "Sloan Management" wherein they argued that MIS primarily focused on structured decisions and suggested that information systems supporting semi-structural and unstructured decisions should be termed as "Decision Support System "DSS gained high reputation during 1980s when Ralph Sprague and Eric Carlson's book "Building Effective Decision Support System" further explained the framework of database, model base, dialog generation and software management. It provides a practical and understandable overview of how organization could or should build DSS.
- In 2000, Application Service Providers (ASPs) began hosting the application software and technical infrastructure for decision support capabilities. Emergence of enterprise knowledge portals, knowledge management, business intelligence and communication lead DSS to an integrated environment.

Difference between Decision Support System and Expert system

Decision Support System is a computer-based system that aids the process of decision making. It is an interactive, flexible and adaptable computer system.

It is especially developed for supporting the solution of a non-structured management problem for improved decision making

Expert system is a computer program that is designed to mimic the decision-making ability of a decision-maker. It organizes a set of knowledge about a particular subject. It contains facts and judgmental knowledge which gives it the ability to guess like a human. There are set of rules on which it makes decisions using if-else structure. The inference engine does reason by manipulating the knowledge base. The user interface represents questions and information to the operator and also receives answers from the operator.

Difference Between DSS and Expert System

Decision Support System	Expert system
It facilitates decision-making.	It automates decision-making.
The decision environment is unstructured.	The decision environment has structure.
It extracts or gains knowledge from a computer system.	Inject expert knowledge in to a computer system.
Characteristics of the problem domain are complex and broad.	In this, it is limited and specialised.
Type of data manipulation is numeric.	Type of data manipulation is symbolic.
It has limited capacity.	It has a full capacity.
It uses goals and system data to establish alternatives and outcomes, so a good decision can be made.	The expert system can eventually replace the human decision maker.

DSS in agriculture in an Indian context

Application of DSS in the area of agriculture takes the form of integrated crop management decision support and encompasses fertilizer management, weed management, water management, plant protection, soil erosion, land use planning, drought management, pollution control, etc. These systems are addressing problems related to conservation and improving soil fertility, local water balance, efficient agronomical practices, canopy management, pest and insect management, reducing pre- and post-harvest losses, conservation of forests and global environment change etc. Thus, the quality of decision-making can play an important role in complex and uncertain situations. Empirical evidence reveals that human judgment and decision-making can be far from optimal and could even deteriorate further with added complexity and stress. Therefore, aiding the deficiencies of human judgment and quality decision making has been a major focus of research throughout the history particularly with the advancement in electronic processing of data and design of Decision Support System (DSS). DSS can help to reduce uncertainty and improve the decision making process by providing access to data through procedures and analytical reasoning. Computerized decision support for sustainable agriculture is not new. These systems have been designed to address complex tasks involving agronomic, economic, regulatory, climate change and pollution control, enabling us to match the biological requirements of crop to the physical characteristics of land so that the objective specified by the user is obtained. Most agricultural DSSs aim to help stakeholders realize their strategic aim of securing a competitive advantage through timely decision-making. DSSs are widely used and known with agriculture and they have proved to be important tools in the decision-making process from farm to fork.

DSS in crop productivity improvement

DSS is widely applied in various parts of India for different agricultural management activities. Crop productivity being one such activity, it has given considerably good results with the use of DSS. The DSS named as "Crop Environment Resource Synthesis (CERES) -Wheat", is a part of DSSAT which was successfully applied to simulate the crop growth and development of wheat under variable climatic, water and nitrogen levels in semi-arid and subtropical regions of Punjab for five cropping seasons from 2000-2001 to 2004-2005. The model results concluded that grain yield and water productivity are affected by water holding capacity of the soils. This model was then extended with Cropping System Model (CSM) named as "DSSAT-CSM-CERES-Wheat 4.0". It was calibrated and validated on 13 different datasets of different farms of Ludhiana and Phillaur, Punjab collected between 2002-2006 to predict and increase crop yield and for irrigation scheduling. The model helped for estimating crop yield, evapotranspiration, crop water productivity (CWP) and Irrigation Water Productivity (IWP)

Cropping System Simulation Model (Crop Syst) is another simulation based DSS model linked with Geographical Information System (GIS). It uses the identical approach to simulate the growth and development of all herbaceous crops using periodic biomass and Leaf Area Index (LAI). It helped to decide water saving and water productivity policy for rice crop in Punjab by integrating crop management practices such as transplanting date, type of seed and irrigation. Indian Agriculture Research Institute (IARI) then evaluated Crop Syst and CERES models, and results of evaluation demonstrated that these models can be effectively applied for on farm management activities such as irrigation and soil nitrogen management. The CROPGRO - Soybean model is a part of DSSAT, which was used to successfully simulate climatic change, growth and yield of soybean for four major states as Madhya Pradesh,

Maharashtra, Rajasthan and Karnataka which together contribute 98% of soybean area in India. It was also used to estimate the potential yields in water limiting and water non-limiting areas and also to estimate yield gaps for major soybean regions of India

DSS in crop water requirements management

DSS is also applied to careful management of water resources, crop water requirements. Crop water requirements depend on the factors such as evaporation, evapo-transpiration, meteorological factors such as solar radiation, air temperature, humidity, wind speed etc. CROPWAT DSS helped to decide irrigation scheduling for different crop patterns and to calculate crop water requirements in eastern Godavari Delta, Andhra Pradesh. Along with climatic data it helped in assessment of reference evapo-transpiration under temperature conditions of Kashmir Valley. It also gave good results when applied to simulate different crop water requirements as per the need of crop under different planting dates and probable canal water supplies for No-par distributaries' of Western Yamuna Canal system. Along with the GIS mapping model it was used to spatially analyze and study crop water requirements of rice in the eastern part of India. It also helped to study the spatial variation of climatic water balance, probabilistic monthly monsoon rainfall and mapping of cold periods in the region.

DSS in irrigation scheduling

Irrigation scheduling is one of the important activities in agriculture. A DSS tool for Simulation of Water and SALT (SWASALT) was calibrated and validated for irrigated areas in the semi - arid region of Haryana. It helped to prevent on farm water logging and soil salinization because of canal irrigation. This model was also used to calculate Water Management Response Indicators (WMRI) which helped to optimize the on-farm irrigation schedule by minimizing the percolation losses to ground water for different soil types. GIS based integrated model of rainfall, soil, water use, canal flow model, soil water balance model and groundwater flow model is used as an effective DSS tool. It helped to increase crop production for different cropping pattern as per the groundwater availability for Godavari Delta Central Canal Irrigation Project in Andhra Pradesh.

DSS based on climatic data

Climatic parameters such as temperature, rainfall, sunshine hours play a very important role in crop production. DSSAT-Cropping System Model (DSSAT-CSM) was also applied to study impact of climatic parameters in rice-wheat system productivity over the Indo-Gangetic plains of India. The comparison of observed and simulated rice and wheat yield showed that, along with climatic parameters crop productivity can be improved by integrating biotechnological advancements and precision farming. A simulation based multi-year, multi-crop and daily time step cropping based model called as "Crop Production and Management (CROPMAN)" model was used in Punjab to study the effects of different dates of transplanting and weather parameters on yield, evapo-transpiration and water productivity. It was also simulated to study grain yield of chickpea crop for semi-texture soil of Punjab for rice-cheek pea cropping pattern. It was observed that grain yield is increased with rice-chickpea cropping pattern than rice-wheat pattern. It also successfully concluded that irrigation water requirement is more in the environments of low rainfall and coarse-textured soils compared to medium-textured soil and high rainfall areas. The DSS is helpful as a research and teaching tool and intermediate parameter estimation and for missing data estimation

DSS based on Nutrient Management

Application of fertilizers is increasing day by day to get higher-yield and good-quality crops. To maximize profits and avoid waste, farmers need to plan their use of nutrients for each field crop in each year. Nutrient management can play an important role in farm related management, and can protect, restore and enhance the status and diversity of all surface water ecosystems and ensure the progressive reduction of groundwater pollution. For Nutrient management, different DSSs have been designed to recommend site-specific and need-based parameters that result in an optimized fertilizer management strategy. DSS for Planning Land Applications of Nutrients for Efficiency and the Environment (PLANET) provides best management practice tool for farmers and their advisors to adopt in the use of organic manure and fertilizers. Fertilizer recommendations for field are calculated based on the precious cropping fertilizer and organic manure application. To encourage maximum uptake of DSS by the farming community, the logic to generate fertilizer recommendations based on input data was developed and made available to commercial agriculture software developers for integration within their systems, which are being widely used by farmers.

DSS in advisory system

Advisory DSS is playing extremely important role in Indian agriculture. e-Sagu, farm specific DSS developed by IIT, Hyderabad, and Media Lab Asia under the aegis of Media Lab Asia which helped to improve farm productivity by delivering high-quality farm specific agro-expert decisions in a timely manner to each farm at the farmer's doorsteps. The advice was provided at all stages of cultivation of crops from sowing to harvesting, which reduces the cost of cultivation and increases farm productivity as well as quality of Agricultural commodities. "m-KRISHITM" DSS tool developed by Tata Consultancy Services and was deployed in Borgaon village, Maharashtra, for proper nutrient and pest management advice for grape farms through mobile phones. Integrated Pest Management is an important parameter in agriculture. An Integrated Pest Management (IPM) DSS called as "Cell Phone" was developed for sustainable plant protection of south 24 paraganas, West Bengal. The DSS helped for sustainable IPM by creating continuous awareness among farmers and in turn to improve crop productivity.

Comparison of Results of different DSS in Indian Context

S. No	Name of DSS	Parameters Considered	Region in India	Scenario before implementation of DSS	Results after implementation
1.	DSSAT –CERES (Wheat)	Climate, Water and Different Nitrogen Levels	Semiarid and Sub Tropical region of Punjab	Crop productivity was affected due to increase in depth of quality ground water.	Improved water productivity under dry land and limited water environments
2.	Crop Syst	Deep alluvial loamy sand typic Ustripsamment soils under hyperthermic regime	Ludhiana Punjab	Earlier the transplanting dates of crops were in May which required frequent irrigation, to meet the crop requirement.	Calibrated the model for shifting of transplanting dates of rice from May to June, which helped to increase the effective water utilization and in turn improved grain yield.
3.	CROPGRO-Soybean Model	Climatic Data	Madhya Pradesh, Maharashtra, Rajasthan and Karnataka	Soybean grain yield was affected by temporal variations of rainfall.	Calibrated model helped to increase soybean yield in water limiting environment based on climatic data

(Contd.)

S. No	Name of DSS	Parameters Considered	Region in India	Scenario before implementation of DSS	Results after implementation
4.	CROPWAT	Climatic and crop data	Andra Pradesh, Kashmir, West Bengal	Conventional irrigation scheduling was affecting crop water requirements and thus crop yield.	Helped to estimate crop water requirements to improve irrigation scheduling and in turn to increase a crop yield.
5.	SWASALT	Soil and irrigation data	Haryana	Canal irrigation increased the percolation losses which resulted water logging and soil salinization.	Prevented Water logging and soil salinization which helped for effective utilization of water resources.
6.	DSSAT-CSM	Climatic Data	Punjab	Only climatic parameters were considered for crop productivity improvement.	Model results indicated that there is a need integrate biotechnological techniques and precision farming.
7.	CROPMAN	Site Specific Climatic Data	Punjab	Crop productivity was affected by incorrect transplanting dates which increased soil evapo-transpiration and reduced water produced.	A yield can be increased by shifting of transplanting from mid May to lower June onward

S. No	Name of DSS	Parameters Considered	Region in India	Scenario before implementation of DSS	Results after implementation
8.	e-Sagu	Climatic Data, Farm specific crop details	Tamilnadu	There was a need to provide the farm specific pest management and other advice.	Helped farmers for farm specific agro-expert decisions to the farmers to increase the crop yield
9.	m KRISHITM	Climatic Data, Farm specific crop details	Maharashtra	There was a need to bridge the gap between farmers and agriculture expert for proper nutrient and pest management.	Helped farmers for nutrient and pest management for Grape farms.
10.	IPM	Climatic Data, Farm specific crop details	West Bengal	No support for effective Pest Management for crops.	Assisted farmers increase awareness about pest management.

Though ADSSs are quite helpful in farm management, the unwelcome fact is that the use of ADSSs has been limited due to some critical issues

- Farmers seldom have experiences or knowledge of using ADSSs. The typical graphical interface of ADSSs is sometimes not user-friendly and it may be confusing for farmers to perform desired operations.

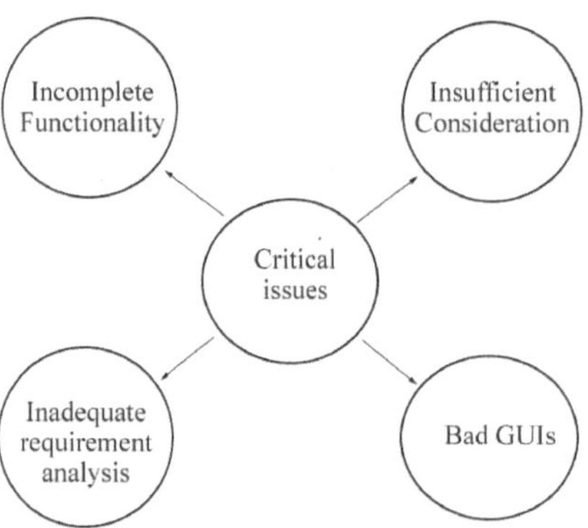

- ADSS developers may ignore the requirement analyses from the end users, leading to the fact that inputs and outputs of ADSSs may not fit farmers' needs and decision-making styles.
- The functionalities of current ADSSs are limited and task-specific. An ADSS may only focus on a single perspective. As a consequence, farmers have to use several ADSSs to manage agricultural activities.
- When generating the advice, current ADSSs may miss some fundamental factors, such as climate change, soil spatial variability, crop disease, etc. The lack of these considerations may result in imprecise outputs from ADSSs.

Conclusion

It is observed that in India, simulation-based techniques are widely applied in different areas of agriculture such as to increase crop yield, crop water requirements, on farm irrigation scheduling, and to study the impact of climatic parameters. Information Communication Technology based advisory systems are also playing an important role in Indian scenario. In India majority of the rural population lives in rain-fed regions, therefore challenge before Indian agriculture is to transform rain-fed farming into more sustainable and productive systems to better support the population dependent on it. Unfortunately, ease of use, low adoption, failure to show cost benefits, complexity and user inputs, distrust for the output, lack of field testing, lack of integration among heterogeneous components, success measurements, non-involvement of end-user before and after development stages and under-definition of beneficiaries are some issues that need to be addressed. But keeping the amount of input data required as small as possible; keeping the system itself as flexible as possible; providing users with default values; ensured involvement of users from basic development stage; greater user involvement through participatory learning approaches; interactive prototyping as well as keeping DSS development manageable and small in scope can provide avenues for improvement in DSS research and development. The effectiveness of decision making in agriculture domain can surely be improved by advanced information technology techniques in recent years. It is promising to see that future ADSSs can better serve Agriculture 4.0 by overcoming these challenges.

16

Market Led Extension: Role in Empowerment of Livestock & Allied Farm Stakeholders

Sangeeta Bhattacharyya

(Agricultural Extension) & VO, Mobile Veterinary Clinic Department of ARD, GOWB, India

Bikash Santra

ICAR-Central Citrus Research Institute, Nagpur-440033 Maharashtra, India

Introduction

As India was struggling to feed her population through "ship-to-mouth" strategy, the agricultural scientists focused on the enhancing the food grain production of India so that the country became self-sufficient. Through tireless efforts our country ushered into Green Revolution which marked the beginning of the era of self-sufficiency for India. The efforts of researchers were seamlessly taken to fields and communicated to masses by the efficient extension professionals of our country. The focus of extension was "Production Led". But as time passed, India became self-sufficient in major food crops, the farmers started facing problems of marketing their surplus produce. Market gluts, non-remunerative prices, distress sales and emergence of exploitative middle men made farmers all the more helpless. It was at this time when the concept of "Production Led Extension" was thought of being reformed to "Market Led Extension" (MLE). As of today, MLE has helped many farmers market their produce easily and fetch remunerative prices of the produce. Agricultural, livestock, fisheries and all allied sectors have received benefit from this approach of extension.

Definition of Market–led Extension

If we break the word market led extension, we get 2 words: market and extension. By market we mean a congregation of prospective buyers & sellers with a common motive of trading a particular commodity. By extension we mean reaching out to the mass. Hence market led extension can be explained as agriculture & economics coupled with extension and it is the perfect blend for reaching at the door steps of common man with the help of technology. In other words market led extension is the market ward orientation of agriculture through extension.

Challenges in Agricultural Marketing System

There existed and even till date exists, various challenges in agricultural marketing system of India. The numerous challenges triggered the emergence of the concept of MLE. Some of these challenges have been enlisted below.

- Market size is large and continuously expanding, but marketing system did not keep pace
- Private trade is 80% marketed surplus
- Direct marketing "farmer – consumer" is negligible
- 85% of the 27,294 rural periodic market, facilities for efficient trade is still almost absent
- 7161 market yards/sub yards is inadequate, ill equipped and mismanaged
- Due to lack of proper handling at farm gate lead to 30 % F&V, 7% grains, 10% spices loss before reaching market
- Rs 50,000 crores /year lost due to poor marketing chain
- Low risk bearing capabilities
- Lack of storage of farm produce
- Poor grading and standardization
- Lack of processing facilities
- Quality differences in agricultural products
- Sporadic success stories of using information technology by farmers are publicized
- Market intelligence: As far as is possible marketing decisions should be based on sound information. The process of collecting, interpreting, and disseminating information relevant to marketing decisions is known as market intelligence.
- Financing
- Facilitating Functions: It includes product standardization, financing, risk bearing and market intelligence. Facilitating functions are those activities which enable the exchange process to take place.

- Overburdened extension system

Enhanced Roles of Agricultural Extension Personnel in Light of Market Led Extension

With the focus now shifting towards MLE, extension professionals have a big role to play. The enhanced roles of extension professionals will be:

- SWOT analysis of the market: Strengths (demand, high marketability, good price etc.), Weaknesses (the reverse of the above), Opportunities (export to other places, appropriate time of selling etc.) and Threats (imports and perishability of the products etc.) need to be analyzed about the markets. Accordingly, the farmers need to be made aware of this analysis for planning production and marketing.
- Organization of Farmers' Interest Groups (FIGs) on commodity basis and building their capabilities with regard to management of their farm enterprise.
- Supporting and enhancing the capacities of locally established groups under various schemes / programmers like watershed committees, users groups, SHGs, water users' associations, thrift and credit groups. These groups need to be educated on the importance, utility and benefit of self-help action.
- Enhancing the interactive and communication skills of the farmers to exchange their views with customers and other market forces (middlemen) for getting feedback and gain the bargaining during direct marketing ex. Rythu Bazars, Agri-mandi and Uzavar Santhaigal etc.
- Establishing marketing and agro-processing linkages between farmers' groups, markets and private processors
- Advice on product planning: selection of crops to be grown and varieties suiting the land holding and marketability of produce will be the starting point of Agri-enterprise. Extension system plays an important role in providing information in this
- Educating the farming community: to treat agriculture as an entrepreneurial activity and accordingly plan various phases of crop production and marketing
- Direct marketing: farmers need to be informed about the benefits of direct marketing. In some of the states, Rytu Bazars in AP, Apni Mandis in Punjab and Haryan and Uzavar Santhaigal in Tamilnadu have shown success
- Capacity building of FIGs in terms of improved production, post-harvest operations, storage and transport and marketing
- Acquiring complete market intelligence regularly on various aspects of markets
- Regular usage of internet facility through computers to get updated on market

intelligence

- Publication of agricultural market information in news papers, radio and Television besides internet
- Organization of study tours of FIGS: to the successful farmers/ FIGs for various operations with similar socio-economic and farming systems as the farmers learn more from each other
- Production of video films of success stories of commodity specific farmers
- Creation of websites of successful FIGs in the field of agribusiness management with all the information to help other FIGs achieve success

Required information to extension system and farmers

Farmers now require a different set of information in the era of MLE and the increasing relevance of marketing rather than production. This information set includes inputs on:

- Present agricultural scenario and land use pattern
- Suitability of land holding to various crops/enterprises
- Crops in demand in near future
- Market prices of crops
- Availability of inputs
- Usage of inputs
- Credit facilities
- Desired qualities of the products by consumers
- Market network of the local area and the price differences in various markets
- Network of storage and warehouse facilities available
- Transport facilities
- Regular updating of market intelligence
- Production technologies like improved varieties, organic farming, usage of bio-fertilizers and bio-pesticides, IPM, INM, and right methods of harvesting etc.
- Post-harvest management like processing, grading, standardization of produce, value addition, packaging, storage, certification, etc. with reference to food grains, fruits and vegetables, eggs, poultry, fish, etc.
- Contract farming
- Private modern terminal markets
- Food retail chains
- Food safety and quality standard

- Certification
- WTO regulations

Paradigm Shift from Production-led Extension to Market Led Extension

A paradigm shift has occurred from PLE to MLE and the major changes have been highlighted below in Table 1.

Table 1: Paradigm Shift from Production-led Extension to Market Led Extension

Aspects	Production-led extension	Market-led extension
Purpose/objective	Transfer of technologies	Optimum returns
Expected end results	Adoption of package of practices	High returns
Farmers seen as	Progressive farmers	Entrepreneur: "Agri-preneur"
Focus	"Seed to seed"	"Rupee to Rupee"
Technology	Fixed package for an agro-climatic zone	Baskets of package of practices to different farming systems
Extensionists' interactions	Training\Motivation	Joint analysis of the problems
Linkages/liaison	Research-Extension- Farmer	Research-Extension-Market-Farmer
Extensionists' role	Delivery mode and feedback to research system	Establishment of marketing and agro-processing linkages
Maintenance of Records	Not much important	Very important to understand the CB ratio
IT support	Emphasis on production technologies	MI – price trends, demand position, current prices, market practices

Market Research

The terminologies often used in market research are as follows. The differences between market data, market information, and intelligence can be subtle, but very real.

- **Market Data:** Unconnected pieces of information (Prices for our products have dropped by 5 percent).
- **Market Information:** Increased knowledge derived by understanding the relationships of data (New offshore facilities have lower labour costs).
- **Market Intelligence:** Organizing the information to fully appreciate the implications and impact on the organization (Our key competitor is about to acquire a facility in India that will)

Sources of Market Data

Technology plays an essential role in market research and MLE. Several platforms have been created for bringing market data to doorsteps of producers.

Some of these are:

- NETVET- for Veterinary assistance
- For agriculture data:
  - Agrisurf
  - Agriwatch
  - Commodity India
  - Agfind
  - Agmarknet
  - Agricoop
- Global ones: www.fao.org
- National ones: eNAM, mKisan
- Organizations: NHB, APEDA, NAFED, NMCE, Trade NIC Online
- Institutional ones: NIAM, MANAGE etc..

ICT initiatives of Govt.: A step towards MLE

Government has also created several ICT platforms for not only helping farmers access their desired information online but also facilitating market research. Some of these are:

AGRISNET: An infrastructure network up to block level agricultural offices facilitating agricultural extension services and agribusiness activities to usher in rural prosperity

AGMARKNET: With a road map to network 7000 agricultural produce wholesale markets and 32000 rural markets

ARISNET: Agricultural Research Information System Network

Seed NET: Seed Informatics Network

Coop Net: To network 93000 Agricultural Primary Credit Societies (PACS) and Agricultural Cooperative Marketing Societies to usher in ICT enabled services and rural transformation

HORTNET: Horticultural Informatics Network

FERTNET: Fertilizers (Chemical, Bio and Organic Manure) Informatics Network facilitating "Integrating Nutrient Management" at farm level

VISTARNET: Agricultural Extension Information System Network

PPIN: Plant Protection Informatics Network

APHNET: Animal production and Health Informatics Network networking about 42000 Animal Primary Health Centers

FISHNET: Fisheries Informatics Network

LISNET: Land Information System network linking all institutions involved in land and water management for agricultural productivity and production systems, which has now evolved as "Agricultural Resources Information System" project during the Tenth Plan is being implemented through NIC.

AFPINET: Agricultural and Food Processing Industries Informatics Network

ARINET: Agricultural and Rural Industries Information System Network to strengthen Small and Micro Enterprises (SMEs)

NDMNET: Natural Disaster Management Knowledge Network

Weather NET: Weather Resource System of India

Potential of Market Led Extension in Dairy Sector

India's marketing year (MY) 2022 (January-December) fluid milk production is forecast higher at 203.5 million metric tons (MMT) based on a relatively normal June-September monsoon season. Today India is not only the global leading milk producer, but it has also become the largest consumer of milk. FAS New Delhi forecasts India's fluid milk consumption in 2022 at 85 MMT, up by 2.5 percent from the USDA official 2021 figure of 83 MMT. Approximately, 46 percent of the milk produced is consumed either at the producer level or sold to non-producers in rural areas. Fifty-four percent of milk production is marketed through milk cooperatives and/or unorganized players such as milkmen and contractors.

A key Indian demand driver for fluid milk consumption is India's demographics. About a third of the national population is under 14 years-of-age, a cohort inclined to consume higher quantities of milk. Dual income households, rapid digitization of commerce (e-platforms), increasing disposable incomes, growing urbanization, changing consumer lifestyles, and other demographic shifts are helping to pump up demand for processed, value-added dairy products. India's growing organized retail sector is driving value added dairy product sales with 15-20 percent annual growth.

Strategies for MLE in Dairy Sector

There are a number of technologies, which can be conveniently applied by the rural mass to increase farm income.

For instance, SHGs may be formed to start preparation of paneer from cow milk or goat milk. Around this core activity, several supporting activities may be initiated by the enterprising rural youths. They may find opportunities ranging from supply of basic inputs to services, information, market integration, and marketing, *etc.*

Traditional dairy products like sweets, dahi, lassi, etc. are other products, which can be undertaken as small viable businesses and produced hygienically by customized small-scale machines and technologies.

Enterprises producing khoa, paneer, whey based RTS beverages, fermented milk products, kulfi etc can develop as lucrative options for rural youth.

MLE in Fisheries Sector

The inland aquatic resources in India comprise of 2.433 million hectares (m ha) of ponds and tanks, 2.906 m ha of reservoirs, 0.798 m ha of floodplain lakes and derelict water, 0.195 million km of river and canals.

Fisheries sector together with subsidiary industries also provides employment to a large section of the economically backward population of the country apart from providing the cheap and nutritious protein source for the people.

Freshwater pond fish culture, Resource utilization from open water bodies, Coastal and marine aquaculture, Processing and value addition, Value added sea food products and Value added fish based products can be possible strategies for streamlining MLE in fisheries sector.

Agri-entrepreneurship: a MLE strategy

This refers to an individual's characteristic by virtue of which he has an intense desire and will power to achieve the goal of earning most benefit by undertaking innovative activities of agriculture and allied enterprises including the work of agri-value addition in order to improve one's livelihood/ lifestyle by dint of actively engaging oneself in profitable and innovative agricultural enterprises warranting consistent hard work and adequate risk bearing ability.

For bringing about agri-entrepreneurship, farmers must adopt strategies such as (1) changing the method (do how) of agriculture by the sustainable adoption of technology, (2) changing the dimension of agriculture through the strategy of market led crop diversification or farm diversification or occupational/role diversification or a feasible and convenient combination of all the three strategies, and (3) changing their mindset/attitude (self-reform).

Options: ARYA, DAESI, VATICA, BPD units of ICAR

Integrated Farming System Model: a step towards MLE

A success story of IFS is from Sri Lalisahni, a farmer of Chakramdas village in Vaishali district who is practicing family farming in his half acre of land with a family size of seven members. Based on data collected from farmers' field and cost-benefit analysis, showed seven to eight-fold increase in income **(Rs. 55,578/- annum)** from the same land.

Other MLE Strategies

Public Private Partnerships: The Canadian Council for Public Private Partnerships defines Public Private Partnerships as a cooperative venture between the public and private sectors, built on the expertise of each partner that best meets clearly defined public needs through the appropriate allocation of resources, risks and rewards.

Contract farming: Gurdev Singh (2005) provides a universal definition of contract farming. "Contract farming is a form of vertical coordination between the producers (farmers) and the contractor (processor or marketing firm or a third party such as input manufacturer or service provider) where the latter directly influences the production decisions and exercises some control at the production point under the obligation of purchasing certain quantity of produce at specific price from the producer. The quantity and price relate to delivery of specific quality produce at designated location and for a period of time."

Cooperative Marketing: by forming farmers' cooperatives- AMUL Model, Sundarini Naturals

Impacts of PPP in Agri Marketing

Knowledge management: Farmers obtained an average net income of ` 22 000/ ha by diversifying from groundnut and paddy to maize in Chittoor district of Andhra Pradesh and also expanded maize area from 60 ha to 1150 ha (Srinath and Ponnusamy 2011).

Development of high end technologies: Commercialization of Bt maize varieties based on partnership between Agricultural Genetic Engineering Institute (AGERI) of Egypt and Pioneer Hi-Bred Company (Khush 2005).

Reduction of risks and uncertainties: John Deere, a leading farm implements manufacturing company has helped to promote mechanized farming in tribal region of Gujarat by establishing 8 Agricultural Implements Resource Centers each covering 600 acres of cultivated land through PPP (Reddy and Rao, 2011).

Productivity enhancement: MAHYCO going into partnership with Monsanto, which finally resulted in the introduction of Bt cotton in India (APCoAB 2007). The country experienced an unprecedented increase in Bt cotton acreage, productivity and reduction in real cost of production bringing in more equality in farm-income distribution (Morse et al. 2007).

Economic empowerment of farm women: The PPP between Cadbury India, Kerala Agricultural University and DBT during past 23 years trained 250 women and established 28 cocoa chocolate units in different parts of Kerala. *PPP in vegetable marketing in* Coimbatore district of Tamil Nadu, enhanced the income level of farmwomen by 20 per cent (Thangamani *et al 2012).*

Gender mainstreaming in agriculture: Better market linkage of women vegetable growers with Annapoorna hotel in Coimbatore district of Tamil Nadu resulted in higher income (Thangamani et.al. 2012).

Success Stories of Contract Farming

In 1970s, WIMCO, a Swedish multinational company involved in mechanized match manufacturing, initiated contract farming for Poplar, an exotic plant variety in Punjab, Haryana and Uttar Pradesh. It received good farmer response.

In 1990s, Pepsico set up a tomato processing plant as joint venture with Haryana Agro Industries Corporation. It needed about 40,000 MT of tomato per season. It introduced tomato on a large scale in a non-traditional area, Punjab and Haryana with purchase contracts backed by research and extension support. The scheme met with enthusiastic farmer response and Punjab is now a major tomato growing area.

Some other success stories are: Seed multiplication in Marathawada and Andhra Pradesh, Tea and coffee in Karnataka, Kerala and Tamil Nadu, Rubber and Pepper in Kerala, Poplars in Uttar Pradesh, Haryana and Punjab, Medicinal plants in Uttar Pradesh, Castor, Isabgol, cumin and aniseed in North Gujarat, Jute in West Bengal, Tomato and chilies in Punjab, Andhra Pradesh and Karnataka, Mangoes in Andhra Pradesh, Tamil Nadu and Maharashtra.

AMUL Model: the success story of MLE in Dairy Sector

The AMUL Model famous worldwide for its cooperative structure operates in 3 stages as follows:

1. Formation of Primary milk-producers cooperatives (PMPC) at village level. Milk collection centre at village level is operated by paid PMPC secretary. Collection of milk is done twice daily. Farmers bring milk at the collection centre, where after weighing and quality check entries are made in the farmers' books as well as in record register of the centre.

Quality check includes separation of cows and buffalo's milk and fat content (on the basis of which payment is made at predetermined price). Payments are made to the farmers regularly.

2. Union of PMPS at district level procures raw milk from member societies; manages milk and milk product processing plants, cattle feed plant; marketing of milk and milk products; extension services related to animal husbandry and fodder crops; cattle and human insurance. It also provides family welfare, health and hygiene related services at village level through such schemes as pipe water scheme and bio-gas plants.
3. For procurement of milk from nearly 800 villages twice daily, the Union has milk tankers which collect milk twice a day from PMPS and depending on the distance of the PMPS, delivery it to chilling plants at intermediary level or directly to Union milk processing plant. The logistics is worked out to minimize cost as well as time since milk is a perishable commodity.

Sundarini Naturals: Milestone Achievement in MLE

Sundarban Cooperative Milk and Livestock Producers' Union Ltd. is a producer cooperative affiliated to West Bengal Cooperative Milk Producers' Federation Ltd. The operational area of the Cooperative is South 24 Parganas district of West Bengal. Brand name is Sundarini. It is run by 5000 women of Sundarban. It was registered in 1997 and brand launched in 2015.

Objective of the cooperative is to empower marginalized women farmers of Sundarban Islands for better life and livelihood, provide certified & tested chemical-free food for farmers and consumers with utmost transparency.

USP of Sundarini are: 100% automation and instant testing facilities at village level Dairy Cooperative Societies, 100% farmers' database in Central Server System, 100% Cashless Payment through individual bank account of farmers, participation in social activities like Mangrove Plantation, Cleanliness Drive, Awareness Programmes etc. Representatives from Management Committee (MCM) of various village-level Women Dairy Cooperative Societies take part in decision making at district level along with professionals, technical experts of the organization and district administration.

It received organic certification on Wild Sundarban Honey, Cow Milk & Milk Products and Agricultural Produce (in Conversion) as per guidelines of National Programme for Organic Production (NPOP), APEDA, Ministry of Commerce & Industries, Government of India from Rajasthan State Organic Certification Agency, Government of Rajasthan, Jaipur. It received several awards and recognitions

Sundarini is engaged in several profit making ventures such as: Certified Organic Cow Milk Production, Milk Processing for Bilona Cultured Cow Ghee, Certified Organic Cow Ghee, Certified Organic Malai Paneer & Delicious, Healthy, Chemical-free, Traditional Bengali Sweets, Organic Agriculture & Biodynamic Farming: Farmers have been meticulously trained on Biodynamic Farming at Bhaikaka Krishi Kendra, Anand, Gujarat under complete guidance and support from National Dairy Development Board (NDDB), Processing for Unpolished, Organically Grown, Chemical-free, Pesticide-free Dudheswar Rice, Aromatic Gobindobhog Rice, Aromatic Radhatilak Rice, Kalabhat (Black Rice), Laal Dudheswar (Red Rice) & Sona Moong Dal, Certified Organic Wild Sundarban Honey Collection.

Challenges in MLE

The notable challenges surrounding MLE are:

1. Rapid changes in the information tech and need for collection of relevant information
2. Generation of data on Market intelligence – interlinking of marketing and Agricultural line departments
3. Reorganization of extension system
4. Strong communication skills with credibility

Conclusion

Amidst challenges and constraints, the Indian extension system is always striving towards excellence in same vigor as pre Green Revolution to this post-Green Revolution Era. But the focus of the extension functionaries needs to be extended beyond production. Farmers' sensitization on various aspects on quality, consumer's preference, market intelligence, processing and value addition and other marketing information are now the need of the hour. And necessary capacity building of extension functionaries needs to be done for this purpose.

17

Managerial Skill and Performance Appraisal for Better Extension Organization

Malay Kumar Mandal

Department of Dairy Business Management
F/O- Dairy Technology, WBUAFS, Mohanpur, Nadia, West Bengal

Managerial skills and performance appraisal system is the right instrument that plays a vital role directly or indirectly in achieving the goals of an organization. It improves the interpersonal relationship among the employees and employers in the organization. It reflects an evaluative judgment of the traits, characteristics and the work performance of the employees on jobs. Management skills are also known as leadership skills and involve planning, decision making, delegation, time management and time management to ensure optimum organization in focus and the technical of how and why of accomplishing tasks. Managers who are expected to carry out performance appraisal should have some appropriate training. This should include the reasons the organization carries out appraisals, and the skills of performance appraisal. Managers need to appreciate how the process fits into the wider strategic process of performance management, and how the data collected contributes to an analysis of the organization's human resources, and its capability to contribute to business strategy and value.

What are Management Skills?

Management skills can be defined as certain attributes or abilities that an executive should possess in order to fulfill specific tasks in an organization. They include the capacity to perform executive duties in an organization while avoiding crisis situations and promptly solving problems when they occur. Management skills can be developed through learning and practical experience as a manager. The skills help the manager to relate with their fellow co-workers and know how to deal well with their subordinates, which allows for the easy flow of activities in the organization.

Good management skills are vital for any organization to succeed and achieve its goals and objectives. A manager who fosters good management skills is able to the achieve the goals forward with fewer hurdles and objections from internal and external sources.

Types of Management Skills

According to Robert Katz, the three basic types of management skills include:

1. **Technical Skills**

   Technical skills involve skills that give the managers the ability and the knowledge to use a variety of techniques to achieve their objectives.

2. **Conceptual Skills**

   These involve the skills managers present in terms of the knowledge and ability for abstract thinking and formulating ideas. The manager is able to see an entire concept, analyze and diagnose a problem, and find creative solutions. This helps the manager to effectively predict hurdles their department or the business as a whole may face.

3. **Human or Interpersonal Skills**

   The human or the interpersonal skills are the skills that present the managers' ability to interact, work or relate effectively with people. These skills enable the managers to make use of human potential in the company and motivate the employees for better results.

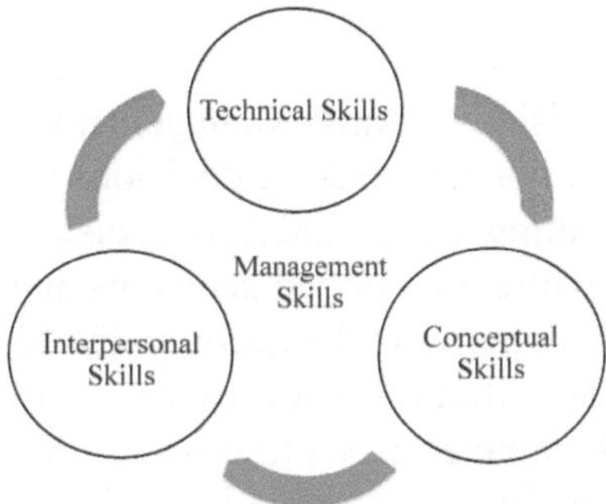

There is a wide range of other skills that management should possess to run an organization effectively and efficiently. A good manager has all the skills and can implement those skills for running the organization properly. The following are six essential management skills that any manager ought to possess for them to perform their duties:

1. **Planning**

   Planning is the first element/function in management which sets the model point in management. It is a vital aspect within an organization. It refers to one's ability to organize activities in line with set guidelines while still remaining within the limits of the available resources such as time, money, and labor. It is also the process of formulating a set of actions or one or more strategies to pursue and achieve certain goals or objectives with the available resources. The planning process includes identifying and setting achievable goals, collection and synthesis of information, developing necessary strategies, and selecting optimum course of action and schedules on how to achieve the set goals.

2. **Communication**

   Possessing great communication skills is crucial for a manager. It can determine how well information is shared throughout a team, ensuring that the group acts as a unified workforce. How well a manager communicates with the rest of his/her team also determines how well outlined procedures can be followed, how well the tasks and activities can be completed, and thus, how successful an organization will be.

   Communication involves the flow of information within the organization, whether formal or informal, verbal or written, vertical or horizontal, and it facilitates smooth functioning of the organization. Clearly established communication channels in an organization allow the manager to collaborate with the team, prevent conflicts, and resolve issues as they arise.

3. **Decision-making**

   Another important management skill is decision-making. Managers make numerous decisions, whether knowingly or not, and making decisions is a key component in a manager's success. Making proper and right decisions results in the success of the organization, while poor or bad decisions may lead to failure or poor performance. A manager must be accountable for every decision that they make and also be willing to take responsibility for the results of their decisions. A good manager needs to possess great decision-making skills, as it often dictates his/her success in achieving organizational objectives.

4. **Delegation**

   Delegation is another key management skill. Delegation is the act of passing on work-related tasks and/or authorities to other employees or subordinates. It involves the process of allowing your tasks or those of your employees to be reassigned or reallocated to other employees depending on current workloads. A manager with good delegation skills is able to effectively and efficiently reassign tasks and give authority to the right employees. When delegation is carried out effectively, it helps facilitate efficient task completion. Delegation helps the manager to avoid wastage of time, optimizes productivity, and ensures responsibility and accountability on the part of employees. Every manager must have good delegation abilities to achieve optimal results and accomplish the required productivity results.

5. **Problem-solving**

   Problem-solving is another essential skill. A good manager must have the ability to tackle and solve the frequent problems that can arise in a typical workday. Problem-solving in management involves identifying a certain problem or situation and then finding the best way to handle the problem and get the best solution. It is the ability to sort things out even when the prevailing conditions are not right. When it is clear that a manager has great problem-solving skills, it differentiates him/her from the rest of the team and gives subordinates confidence in his/her managerial skills.

6. **Motivating**

   The ability to motivate is another important skill in an organization. Motivation helps bring forth a desired behavior or response from the employees or certain stakeholders. There are numerous motivation tactics that managers can use, and choosing the right ones can depend on characteristics such as company and team culture, team personalities, and more. There are two primary types of motivation that a manager can use. These are intrinsic and extrinsic motivation.

What is a Performance Appraisal?

A performance appraisal system plays a significant role in the development of an organization together with the employee's growth. The appraisal of the employee must be used as a means to achieve organizational development. The performance appraisal system must be conceived as a means to develop and implement strategies that will enable the employee to acquire higher competencies, develop a creative attitude and achieve growth by contributing to the organizational growth.

Performance appraisal is the periodic assessment of an employee's job performance as measured by the competency expectations set out by the organization. The performance assessment often includes both the core competencies required by the organization and also the competencies specific to the employee's job. The appraiser, often a supervisor or manager, will provide the employee with constructive, actionable feedback based on the assessment. This in turn provides the employee with the direction needed to improve and develop in their job.

Based on the type of feedback, a performance appraisal is also an opportunity for the organization to recognize employee achievements and future potential.

Purpose of performance appraisal

The purpose of performance appraisal is two-fold.

1. It helps the organization to determine the value and productivity that employees contribute.
2. It also helps employees to develop in their own roles.

Benefit for organization

Performance appraisal of Employee can make a difference in the performance of an organization. They provide insight into how employees are contributing and enable organizations to:

- Identify where management can improve working conditions in order to increase productivity and work quality.
- Encourage employees to contribute more by recognizing their talents and skills
- Support employees in skill and career development
- Improve strategic decision-making in situations that require layoffs, succession planning, or filling open roles internally

Benefit for employee

Performance appraisals are meant to provide a positive outcome for employees. The insights gained from assessing and discussing an employee's performance can help:

- Recognize and acknowledge the achievements and contributions made by an employee.
- Recognize the opportunity for promotion or bonus.
- Identify and support the need for additional training or education to continue career development.
- Determine the specific areas where skills can be improved.
- Motivate an employee and help them feel involved and invested in their career development.

Performance Appraisal Methods

There are various methods that are used by managers and employers to evaluate the performance of the employees, but they can be put into two categories:

1. **Traditional Methods**

   (a).Ranking method

   (b). Paired comparison

   (c). Grading methods

   (d). Forced distribution method

   (e). Forced choice method

   (f). Check-list method

   (g). Critical incidents methods

   (h). Graphic rating scale method

   (i). Essay method

   (j). Field review method

   (k). Confidential report method

2. **Modern Methods**

   (a).Management by objectives (MBO)

   (b). Behaviorally Anchored rating scales (BARS)

   (c). Assessment centre

   (d). 360- Degree appraisal

   (e). Human resource accounting

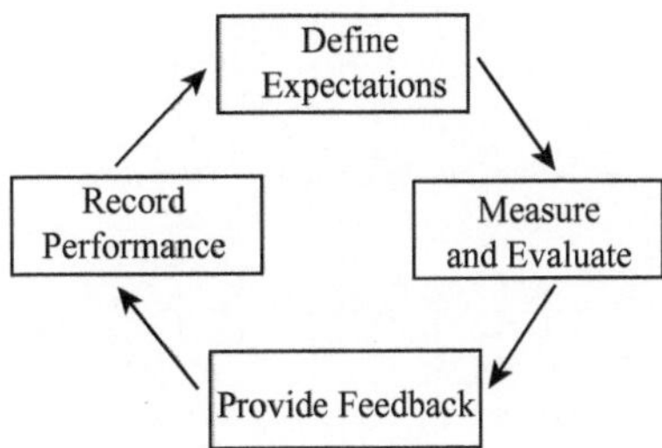

Conclusion

Management is universal in the modern World. Every organization whether formal or informal is required to make decisions, co-ordinate its activities, handle people, evaluate performance and direct the people towards goal or group objectives. Management in extension is more important as extension is becoming more and more specialized and the scale of operation is ever increasing. It is a continuous process to reach the desirous goal of not only the organization but also the employees.

18

Capacity Building Concept, Design and Model for Extension Personnel

Debasish Saha

Department of Veterinary and Animal Husbandry Extension Education
F/O: Veterinary and Animal Sciences, WBUAFS, Kolkata- 700037
West Bengal

Capacity Building is the improvement in an individual or organization's facility or capability to produce and perform. Since the year 1950s, international organizations, governments, non-governmental organizations and communities use the concept of capacity building as part of *"social and economic development* " in states and national plans. The Agriculture Sector in India occupies the centre stage to promote inclusive growth, enhance rural income and sustain food and nutritional security. To spur growth in this sector Government of India intends to follow massive Agricultural Production, reduction in wastage of produce, credit support to farmers and a thrust to the food processing sector. Indeed, Agriculture continues to be a way of life in our Country, it provides employment to around 60% of the work force and contributes almost 18% to our Gross Domestic Products (GDP). With more than 6 lakh villages, home to millions of farmers and farm workers, it is very difficult to visualize a prosperous India without Agriculture and Rural Development.

Empowerment of our farmers is important for our progress. In this context, we need to look at Agricultural Strategies that maximize productivity and generate income and employment for the rural population. This task can be accomplished by strengthening the capacity building of Agricultural Extension Personnel through allocation of funds to this sector. This initiative will be an integral part of the flagship Programme. The all out development in agriculture sector belongs to the farmers, the Agriculturist, the entrepreneur and the investor.

The major function of extension is accomplished through dissemination of farm information, training of farmers and extension functionaries, educating the farmers through field activities such as demonstration, field visit, field days, farm advisory service, exposure visit and capacity building of extension personnel etc. The farming community can avail the services of the extension machinery to get the solutions to their farming problems and to increase their economic status. As a component of capacity building, training & exposure visits have been assumed greater significance in recent times. Training of agricultural extension professionals has emerged as an important intervention to improve their competencies, capacity building and increase in productivity with a purpose to accelerate the rate of agricultural development.

Definitions of Capacity Building

Capacity Building can be defined as "activities which strengthen the knowledge, abilities, skills and behavior of individuals and improve institutional structures and processes such that the organization can efficiently meet its mission and goals in a sustainable way. Training is one of the essential components of capacity building.

Capacity is the mean or the ability, to fulfill a task or meet an objective effectively. It refers to the skills of staff and strength of specific organizations; thus, training of staff and creating or strengthening single organizations is equal with capacity building.

Capacity building means a new build-up of capabilities. Capacity building also increases the abilities and resources of persons, communities and organizations to manage change. Capacity building refers to activities that improve an organization's ability to achieve its mission or a person's ability to define and realize his/her goals or to do his/her job more effectively. Capacity building is as important as capital investment and infrastructure.

According to UNESCO (2006), capacity building focuses on increasing an individual and organization's abilities to perform core functions, solve problems, and objectively deal with developmental needs.

Capacity building is improving or upgrading the ability of the person, team and institutions to implement their functions and achieve goals over time. Capacity building is important for all levels, from individuals to national organizations. Capacity building also suggests to building the organizational capacities of communities and supports the formation of non-profit organizations.

Functions of Capacity Building: *Capacity building helps as follows -*

- To enhance the performance level of various factors involved in Extension setup for better management of Agricultural Technology System.
- To adopt new technologies for increasing production and productivity.

- To share their experience with other farmers regarding technology adoption.
- To improve the techno- managerial skills of the extension professionals.
- To improve knowledge, attitude and practice of extension professionals on the management skills like planning, communication, motivation, leadership, time management etc.
- To enable the extension functionaries for effective and efficient dissemination of technology to the farming community.
- To redefine the role and responsibilities of the Agriculture Extension Machinery by suitably up-scaling the up-to-date technical knowhow of the field extension set up
- To enhance the sustainable net income of the farmer by taking all the enterprises on the farm into consideration, integrating them and treating the whole farm as one unit.

Capacity building methods used for staff involved in Rural Development and Extension:

Capacity building methods may include conferences, workshops, consultations, study tours, participatory research and extension, on-the job training, demonstration plots, coaching and mentoring. Providing formal and non-formal training, meeting, seminars, cross visits etc, are the main methods to build the capacity of extension staff to guarantee a good mix of theory and practice.

There are three main tools for the development of capacities: information dissemination through training, facilitation and mentoring, networking and feedback to promote learning from experience. Each has advantages and disadvantages.

Training is often used as the main capacity building method in developing countries or any regions. Training, on-the-job training and workshops are important activities of capacity building in the field of agricultural research, extension and development.

Training has become an inseparable part of HRD. It has become one of the components, which enables any institution to churn out its employees as the most productive and most suitable ones.

Training – Definitions

1. Training is the art of increasing the knowledge and skill of an employee for doing a particular job.
2. Training is a learning process, which seeks a relatively permanent change in behavior that occurs as a result of experience.

3. Training is the process of aiding employees to gain effectiveness in their present or future work through the development of appropriate habits of thought, action, skills, knowledge and attitude (Milton Mall, 1980).
4. Training is the process of changing employee behavior, attitudes, or opinion through some type of guided experience (Krietner, 1989).
5. Training is a systematic process of changing the behavior, knowledge and or motivation of present employees to improve the match between employee characteristic and employment requirement (Milkovich and Boudreau, 1997)

Need for training

The process of training has caught up mainly in industries. This can be attributed to the sudden and competitive change that is occurring in the world. However, the needs for training can be fixed down to the following:

1. Rapid changes in technologies and jobs people do.
2. Immediate and long term skill shortage.
3. Changes in the expectation and composition of work force.
4. Competition and market pressure for improvement in quality of products and services.

Types of training given to extension personnel – This is of broadly two types

1. Pre-service Training

It is a process through which the individuals are made ready to enter a certain kind professional job, as in agriculture, medicine or engineering. It is a professional training prior to any appointment, oriented to make an individual prepared to enter into a new profession. **Swanson (1984)** defines it as a programme of training activities that prepares an individual for a career in extension, and usually leads to some type of diploma, certificate, degree, or other qualification in one or more of the following agriculture, fisheries, forestry, animal and/ or veterinary science or home science. The state departments of Agriculture now prefer University graduates for entry into their extension services and similarly the Veterinary department prefers to take only Veterinary graduates released from the Universities.

2. In-Service Training

It is meant for in service candidates who are on the job. In-service training is a process of staff development for the purpose of improving the performance of an incumbent holding a position with assigned job responsibilities. It promotes the professional growth of individuals. In-service training is a problem centered, learner oriented and time-bound series of activities, which provide the opportunity to develop a sense of purpose. Broaden perception of the participants and increase their capacity to gain knowledge and mastery of techniques. According to Arnon (1987), even for the University graduate, learning cannot cease on completion of formal studies. He said that the in-service training is given with the following objectives

1. To keep up with research by regular meetings between researchers and extension workers, joint colloquia etc.
2. To impart basic knowledge not only in the fields directly related to agriculture, but also in sociology, economics, psychology etc.
3. To improve extension methods, by constant evaluation of methods, the joint study of research findings and extension methods, exchange of experiences.

In-Service training is of different types, some of them are as follows:

i. Orientation Training

This training is given usually to newly appointed extension personnel. It provides an introduction to public employment and provides answers to questions which a newly recruited person is likely to ask. This term is also used for training in-service extension personnel in a new responsibility like a new operational programme so that personnel are appropriately oriented towards meeting the requirements of new situation.

ii. Induction / portal / vestibule Training

Induction training is given to new extension personnel immediately after they have been employed and before they are assigned to work in particular area usually as an Assistant Agriculture Officer or Agriculture Officer, or Extension Officer.

iii. Maintenance or refresher training

This training is originally started for trainers of the training institutes and Universities for refreshing their knowledge and skills for imparting them to trainees. The term indicates any new training for updating professional competence of extension personnel notably in the subject matter area of specialization. This training is usually imparted in the later career of extension personnel. This training is having considerable importance to extension personnel as it relates to updating to technical knowledge and competence of extension personnel. This deals with new information and new methods and review of older materials. This type of training is given to the employees to keep them at their peak performance level and also prevent them from getting into a rut.

iv. Retraining

It refers to the efforts designed to prepare an individual for a new assignment or a broadened aspect of the old specialty.

v. Career or development training / Training for professional qualification

This type of training is designed to upgrade the knowledge, skills and ability of employees to help them assume greater responsibility in higher positions. This training may lead to the acquisition of higher degree (undergraduate or postgraduate) or diploma by the employees, to motivate them to move up higher levels of administrative hierarchy (promotions) The Directorate of Extension is operating such a scheme on an yearly basis under which, in addition to salary and allowances which personnel get from their own employing organizations, it pays fixed monthly stipends to extension personnel to cover their cost of boarding, lodging and tuition fees. Only meritorious extension personnel and that too below the age of 45 years are eligible for such courses.

vi. Training to Farmers: There is a regular farmer training programme in all agricultural universities. There are training centers for young farmers. In some states, they also arrange short courses for the farmers. The training includes crop raising, animal feeding and management, plant protection. For such training the following points should be considered. a) Time of holding the training b) Duration of course c) Venue of course and d) Production cum demonstration camps and discussion groups of the farmers:

Training Process

In case of training, the focus will be on a person-on-the job-in the organization. Whereas in the case of training process, the focus will be both at the starting point and at the end with difference. The application of what a person has learned during training process is called the effectiveness of training.

The training process has three phases as follows:

- Pre-training
- Training
- Post-training

I. Pre-training phase

- Pre-training process starts with understanding the situation, which calls for behavior that is more effective.

- Key aspect of the process is analysis of situation and job on which improved performance is to be achieved.
- Pre-training begins with description of the job to be changed by it.
- The technical requirement of the job is not enough but also knowledge on operational description of the job is required so that the training programme can be designed to meet out those requirements.

II. Training phase

- Most of the training programmes would be for a session or an evening course or a residential program.
- In the training program, the trainee is exposed to a new subject matter, new people, new atmosphere and the participant would be at unease for a while, later when the subject which would be useful and stimulating is taught the participant would focus his attention on the subject of his interest and would be in line with other participants.
- There would be several questions in his mind, such that he is lacking, the skill required for his job or is it an opportunity given for his sincere work in the organization or is it a plan of the organization to keep him away from the organization so that it would implement the programme which he had strongly opposed.
- With all such questions in his mind, there will be no guarantee that the trainee will learn what he has chosen to learn. His mind would deviate and he would learn something of his interest from the training program provided. This error in selection would be due to the lack of necessary capabilities of the trainee or irrelevant training design and methodology followed by that training institution etc.,
- Finally after overcoming all the hurdles in the initial stage of training programme, the participant would explore in training situation what interests him the more. After exploring, if he finds it useful he tries it again and checks for its effectiveness and satisfaction. There would be several trials repeatedly.
- If he is satisfied with the results, he decides to incorporate it in his organization, but if he finds it to be not useful he discards it and tries some other variant, in some cases he may discontinue his learning.

III. Post-training phase

- Here the situation changes, the participant goes back to his work place, meets his colleagues, family members etc. He goes prepared with some anticipation; as he had been away from them for a while and also had come back learning some new ideas.

- Newly learned skills undergo modifications to fit in with the work situation. If the organization were encouraging and helping, the participant would use his training for the betterment of his organization. Some organization would offer support to the participants to have contact with the training institution even after the training program.
- On the other hand, if the organization resented his absence and if his table is loaded with work, he would feel extra burden and would work to make up for lost time. He would loose his interest to make use of his training and the contact with the training institution is also broken off.

Training Models

There are several models for training processes, of which there are three important models.

1. Simple model of training process
2. Elaborated model of training process
3. Spiral model of training process

1. **Simple Model of the Training Process:** More effective behavior of people-on-the-job-in-the-organization is the primary objective of the training process as well a whole. In the simple training process, improvement is dependent variable and participants and organizations independent variables. A model of training in its simplest form is presented in fig 1.

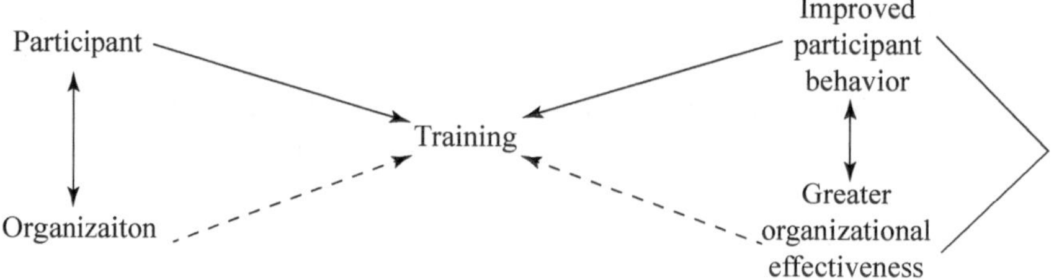

Fig.1. Simple Model of the Training Process

2. **Elaborated model of training process:** Training is actually a more complex process than figure 2 suggests. In the first place, the training system itself needs to be included. It may be temporary system, such as an occasional program, or a permanent institution, such as training department. In either case, the trainers-in-the-system also learns through the various opportunities available for checking their effectiveness, i.e. through feedback. Thus the independent and intervening variables become dependent variables. This elaboration is shown in figure

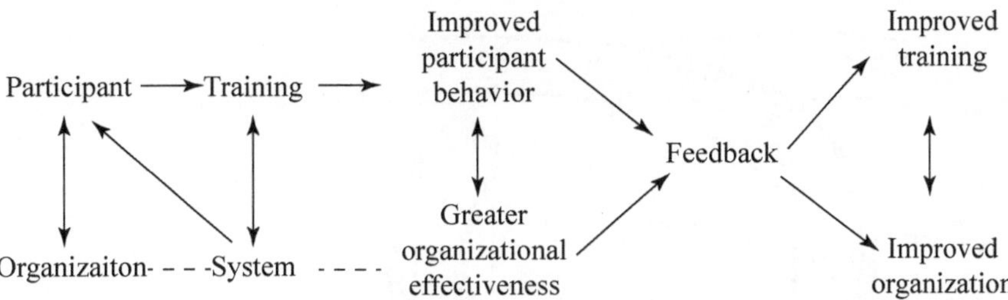

Fig. 2. Elaborated Model of the Training Process

3. **Spiral Model:** The process as a whole, with its three partners and three stages, is depicted in figure 3. It is a spiral model, overlapping the people-on-the-job-in-the-organization. This spiral model is useful in visualizing a training program as an entity, as well as each event and series of events that make up the program. For instance, the phase of actual acquisition and development of new knowledge and skills.

The spiral model in the figure 3 shows the phases through which participants pass as they learn, then return to their jobs. At various stages in the process the other two partners contribute "inputs" to assist the participants. These inputs are shown as arrows: arrows originating inside the spiral depict inputs of the work organization; arrows originating outside the spiral, inputs of the training institutions. The arrows are merely visual conveniences. The large spiral itself comprises spiral feedback system. We will use this spiral model to explicate the training process, further focusing turn on participants, work organizations.

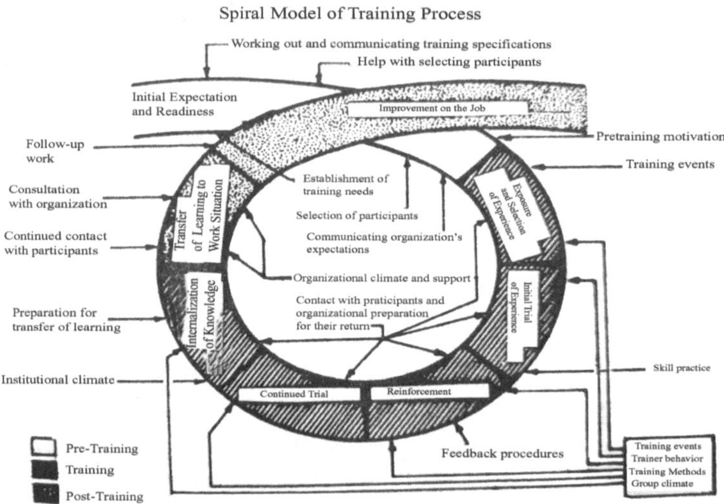

Fig. 3. Spiral Model of the Training Process

Designing Extension Training Programmes

While a training plan provides a structure for training, the design of a training programme provides its content. A training plan provides broad parameters within which training is required to take place in accordance with the assessed training needs of extension personnel within the frame work of extension training policy. The design of the training programme operationalizes the training plan and provides actual training. A well designed training programme will go a long way in ensuring success of training intervention. As a corollary, an ill-designed training programme is deemed to be a failure. The following are the steps in designing a training programme:

A. Objectives of training programmes

The first step in the design of a training programme is a clear statement of the objectives of the training programme. These objectives have to be based on the Training Needs Assessment (TNA) of extension personnel and stated, in order of priority, from general to specific objectives. These objectives have to be stated in terms of knowledge, Skills, Attitudes and Attributes, which the trainee will gain at the end of the training programme. A clear enunciation of objectives of training programme will enable the trainees to have a clear idea as to what should they expect from training.

At a simple level of treatment the objectives of a training programme fall under two categories, namely, General behavioral objectives, and Specific Behavioral objectives. Both types of objectives are required to be stated in the objectives of a training programme. At a more sophisticated level of treatment, following the Bloom's taxonomy of educational objectives, the training objectives can be classified into three classes of Cognitive Objectives, Psycho-Motor Objectives, and Affective Objectives, and their sub-classes. If the design of a training programme is conceptualized to consist of (a) objectives, (b) learning experience and (c) evaluation, then the objectives provide the base upon which subsequent edifice of learning experience and evaluation could be built and hence their importance in the design of a training programme.

B. Skill - Mix

The second step in the design of training programme is determination of appropriate skill-mix for different levels of extension personnel.

Katz postulate three types of skills for a manager, namely (i) Technical Skills, (ii) Human Skills, and (iii) Conceptual Skills as proposed by Misra (1990).

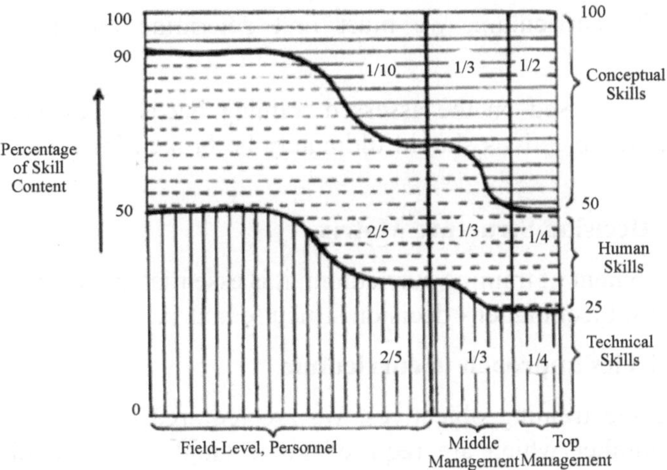

Skill Mixes for Different Level of Extension Personnel.

Fig.4. Skill mixes for the different levels of Extension Personnel

For example, field-level personnel like Village Level Extension workers and Agricultural Extension Officers require technical skills in ample measure, human skills in fairly good measure and conceptual skills in moderate measure.

C. Curriculum Development

The next step in the design of a training programme is development of appropriate training curriculum. Curriculum is required to be developed for two reasons. Specific curriculum is required to be developed for a specific training course which is organized in response to assessed training needs of extension personnel which emerges out of the changing needs of farmers.

Since no readymade curriculum exists for the purpose, specific curriculum is required to be developed for a specific training course which has a specific target group. Its challenge lies in the fact that it is interdisciplinary. Curriculum development is required to anticipate future needs.

Components of a Standard Curriculum

- Course objectives
- Achievement Targets
- Course Structure
- Assessment
- Course Contents

Developing Standard Curriculum

Objective

While developing the curriculum, we must first determine the training objectives -

General and specific based on the assessed training needs of extension personnel. The specific objectives should ultimately be broken into specific information units.

a. Subject Matter - Decision Structure Matrix

For determining the content of training curriculum, it is essential that the target group is located on a subject matter - decision structure matrix.

b. The concentric circles approach to curriculum

Thirdly, for making the training objectives, we are required to decide the subjects and their number which are required to be taught. This requires prioritization of subjects.

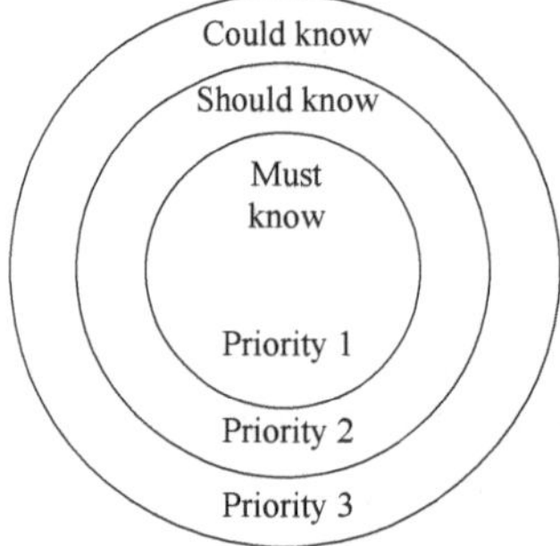

Fig. 5: The Concentric Circles Approach to Curriculum

The 'Concentric Circles Approach to Curriculum' divides the subjects into three categories of what must be known, should be known, and could be known. It is essential to concentrate the efforts on the inner circle of 'must know' not to drift to middle or outer circles at the cost of inner circle as has often been observed in practice.

c. The information unit

An information unit is a definition or a description of a single idea. Every aspect of the subject matter is expressed in terms of an identifiable technical unit which may be analyzed, improved and linked to others in logical or psychological sequence. This breaking down of all the subject matter for each activity into information units makes it easy for it to be updated and objectives combined in order to obtain new training responses.

d. Training Methodology

If curriculum is the 'heart' of a training programme, training methods could be described as the 'arteries' and 'veins' of the training system through which training messages reach the trainees and trainees and trainers receive concurrent feedback on the training programme from the trainees. The choice of appropriate training method is required to be guided by the level and background of trainees as well as by the training curriculum and the time available for training.

While the appropriate choice of the training methods will certainly enhance the effectiveness of a training programme, an inappropriate choice of training methods is equally likely to mar or reduce the effectiveness of a training programme.

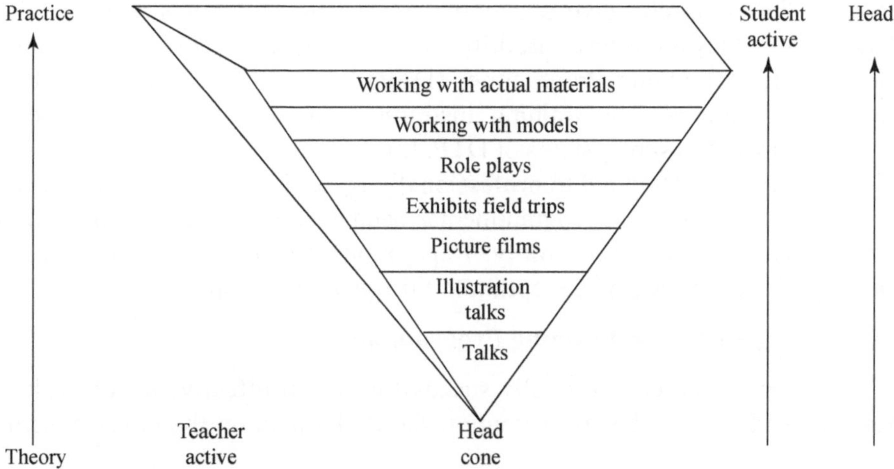

Source: Misra, D.C. 1990. New Direction in Extentension Training

Fig. 6. The Extension Training Methodology Cone

A training method should never be forgotten. It is only a means, for attainment of training objectives. It should never be treated as an end, and an end in itself. In training practice, such a tendency is often noticed and is required to be curbed as such a tendency displaces the training objectives reducing the effectiveness of a training programme. The detail of training methodology is illustrated in the Fig. 6.

e. Training media

1. Non-Projected media - Including books, hand-outs, graphics, flipcharts, photographic prints and other printed materials, real objectives, specimens, models and simulation devices, chalkboards, and magnetic and flannel boards.
2. Projected media - Including opaque projector (epidiascope), projection, slides and filmstrips, microfilm, movie films, broadcast television, closed circuit television video tape.
3. Sound media - such as broadcast radio, reel and cassette tapes, records and public address system. The choices of appropriate training media will not only depend upon the nature of audience and the training objectives but also upon the training methods. For group discussion, chalkboard and overhead projector may be adequate but may also be supported by handouts. Training media should be used only when required and not used because they are there.

f. Training manuals and handbooks

The training manuals and hand-books, in their coverage and content, lie in between the comprehensive text books and scattered leaflets and bulletins. Additionally, they focus on a carefully selected subject matter of specialization. The Design of Training Programmes (DTP) falls within the purview of the training institutions. The training institutions are required to pay special attention to various sub-systems of DTP. It is only when different sub-systems of DTP have been attended to professionally by a training institution, it could be claimed that a training programme has been designed. Training institutions have to realize this responsibility. Reputations are built the hard way and training institutions are no exception to this general precept.

Conducting an Active Training Programme

A training program can be totally successful only if effective exercises have been worked out previously. Attention should be paid on the physical setup, rapport building and content of the program. Programs that look gorgeous on paper are worthless if the trainer doesn't have delivery skills to carry out the design requirements.

Steps To Conduct an Active Training Programme

1. Preparing yourself mentally

Feeling comfort with the course content. Thorough preparation well in advance Preparation of material activities for training program Course materials, manuals, rooms, audio visual equipments etc. and get connected with the participants. If a question is asked and you do not know the answer give it as a group exercise; another way is to write them down and promise to find the answer.

Repeating a course may be a bored one to the trainer but not to a new trainee - Focus your attention on the participants and not on oneself and make opportunities to learn from their experience through discussions.

2. Arranging the physical environment

The physical set up at first the participants receive will create permanent impressions of the program. The seating arrangements should depend on many factors like number of participants, method of speech, and the like. In case the program has little of writing work, the participants can get rid of tables and they can arrange the chairs to their comfort.

In other case, if small subgroups should be formed, care should be taken to leave enough space so that one group does not disturb another group. A well-known arrangement is horseshoe type. This can be modified into a square or a circle. All these arrangements favor group discussions with face to face contact with each participant. These arrangements can be formed with the help of the participants themselves for their own comfort.

3. Greeting participants and establishing program

The best and most desired start is a good welcome address. The trainer should be able to reach the mind of each person, make each feel good in the new situation, and allow his feelings to flow without any hesitation. Hence a trainer should ensure that his program should have a good greet and hence to build rapport with the participants.

A short refreshment before the actual training enables participants to mix well among themselves. Trainer himself can build relationship by knowing their names and making them feel comfortable. During the opening session he/she should introduce the participants to each of them and he himself should be introduced with a touch of un boastful higher knowledge. There are number of wordings which can be addressed. To mention a few 'I have got something for you' this should make a feeling among the participants that they have a person with much greater knowledge and experience to his credit. "I've been through this too" This makes a 'we' feeling among the participants and the trainer. The participants feel that the trainer can understand one's problems and this workload so this helps to bring out their own experience in this field. "I admire you" This greeting puts the participants on a higher stand. This is the way one can express one's admiration over the participant's qualities and deed. It may be on very simple actions of theirs but such an admiration heartens the people to a much higher extent.

4. Getting the best from the first 30 minutes of trainers

The first 30 minutes of any classroom period is the most crucial period which a trainer should not trample upon. It is called the 'grave period' according to Napien and Gershenfeld (1983) during which any over hostility or antagonism will be submerged under a veneer of politeness, watchfulness and reserve. It is during this time that the participants perceive what role they expect to play during the training program, what they intent to accomplish during the course.

Begin the class at the time intended without creating impatience among the participants, once competence should be made known to the members. One should make himself compatible with the group and create trust. The trainee should be clear on what activities are there for the participants and how and when they can get connected to their home town.

5. Reviewing the agenda

In the beginning moments of the program, one should be made clear of what is going to be done i.e. What is expected of the programme and What is expected of the participants. The training objectives should be given in writing and these should be explained clearly. The list of what is to be accomplished should also be presented. They should be informed of how the program will be done with indications of the stay place, food arrangements, telephone messages etc. A content outline and a description of the activities designed should also be given.

6. Inviting feedback

After reviewing the agenda, one must not fail to get the feedback on the agenda. This gives the participants an opportunity to give their views or to tell what they expect more of the programs. The simplest approach is to ask directly "Does this m match what you hope to gain from this program?""Is there anything you would like to add to it?". The feedback helps the trainer to change his program if feasible to the requirements of the participants and remains compatible with them. Otherwise, the programme will be a waste with a content not interested to the participants. After all these steps, one can readily and confidently enter into the actual training programme.

B. Experiential learning is a very powerful method and appropriate for people who work with groups. It is an excellent way to develop good insights into the ways groups work [54]. Demonstration plots, cross visits, study tours and Farmer Field School are useful methods to transfer information and technology to staff and farmers, particularly in remote areas. The advantages of FFS are that both farmers and staff are able to gain knowledge, skills, good relationships, facilitator skills, communication skills and experiences.

C. Mentoring is an important method for capacity building in extension. Mentors are senior research and extension staff who are experienced persons. Mentors are people who have more experience in livestock production and extension methodology. Mentoring involves passing on skills, attitudes and knowledge from experienced staff to newer extension workers. Hopkins-Thomson asserted that "mentoring and coaching processes can serve to augment the succession planning and professional development of districts." Millar & Connell stated that building the technical and extension skills of staff using experienced people as mentors is a key element of scaling out impacts. They can provide the support trainees need in order to become responsible as they acquire new skills and adapt to change. Mentors should be highly skilled in communicating, listening, analyzing, providing feedback and negotiating with less experienced persons. Nowadays, mentoring is commonly used for academic, job and personal development.

Conclusion

The needs of farmers are constantly changing with time and farmers' socio-economic attributes. The implication of this is that extension needs to periodically upgrade in knowledge, skills and attitudes in order to keep pace with the emerging challenges and dynamics of extension work. Capacity building is essential in ensuring that the initial extension job training is provided as well as ensuring coping to the job changes and the varied needs of the clients. The overhead cost and demands of follow-up session should be embedded in the training programme such that the same training facilitators are engaged to carry out the follow-up session in order to ensure stability and continuity.

Funding of extension training programmes by the government, organizations intervention agencies and private extension organizations should be made adequate and steady. Existing training facilities across institutions and

19

Motivation for Improved Performance of Veterinarians and Livestock Farmers for Sustainable Development

N.K. Sudeep Kumar

Extension Education, Tamil Nadu Veterinary and Animal Sciences University, Chennai - 600 051, Tamil Nadu, India

Motivation of staff both in private and public organizations, leads to greater effectively leading to higher productivity and better performance. Motivation is the performance or procedure of presenting an intention that leads a person to capture some accomplishment (Quratul, 2011). Veterinary institutions like other organizations also seek to achieve better performance level. This requires providing motivation as an incentive or within the veterinarian as an individual to be self-motivated. There is a good scope for veterinarians to be more committed to work. McGregor argued that management has the responsibility to ensure that the productive elements of the enterprises are organized, such as money, materials and people with the purpose of meeting economic ends. People have an inborn dislike to work and tend to avoid it whenever an opportunity arises. It is also observed that people are born selfish; indifferent to the needs of the organization; hence people's efforts need to be directed through coercion, controlling their action and modification of their behaviors to attain organizational goals. Hence, people in the organization need to be directed to take responsibility. To achieve organizational objectives, people need to be persuaded, rewarded, coerced, controlled, directed or threatened with punishment. While another theory is opposable to it. It is believed that if vets are motivated they would reach greatest potential. As extension specialist we need to motivate our peer and farmers aiming to improve performance and increased satisfaction.

Human Development

Human development focuses on improving the lives of the people for greater wellbeing. In effect, human development means developing people's abilities for improved performance. It is about providing people with opportunities, not insisting that they make use of them. The process of human development should at least create an environment for people, individually and collectively, to develop to their full potential and to have a reasonable chance of leading productive and creative lives that they value.

Sustainable development

The concept of sustainable development was described by the Bruntland Commission Report (1987) as "development that meets the needs of the present without compromising the ability of future generations to meet their own needs." Sustainable development binds together concern for the carrying capacity of natural systems with the social, political and economic challenges faced by humanity. There are four dimensions to sustainable development – society, environment, culture and economy – which are intertwined in which environmental, societal and economic considerations are balanced in search of an improved quality of life.

Role of veterinarians and livestock farmers

Agriculture (inclusive of Livestock) contributes 15 to 16 % of GDP. Livestock sub-sector contributes 4.11% GDP and 25.6% of total Agriculture GDP. Livestock contributed 16% to the income of small farm households as against an average of 14% for all rural households. Livestock provides livelihood to two-thirds of rural community. It also provides employment to about 8.8 % of the population in India. There are 67,784 registered veterinary practitioners as on 31.03.2015, as per the entries made in the Indian Veterinary Practitioners' Register (IVPR) maintained by Veterinary Council of India. The production and health aspects of livestock species are taken care by the field veterinarians and at the same time suitable need based technologies are developed by the research scientist. Farmers and farm women are the backbone for livestock rearing involved in farming activities which are economical, environment friendly and easily marketable. A combination of dedicated veterinarians and hard working farmers can improve livestock contribution to the national economy. The veterinarians have a pivotal role in improving the livelihood of livestock farmers. In this context it is essential to keep the veterinarians motivated to support the farmers at their best for improved farm health and increased productivity of their animals and birds

Why motivation

Motivation in any organization is to improve the performance level, change attitude of employees and leads to stability of work force. For an individual, motivation will help to achieve personal goals, get job satisfaction, self-development and always gain by working with a dynamic team. Further, motivation is very important because it puts human resource into action, improves level of efficiency of employees, leads to achievement of goals, builds friendly relationship and finally leads to stability of the work force helping in achieving the vision and mission of any organization.

Significance of motivation on performance of the job

Only motivated individuals are prepared to be consistent in their performance and work hard; consequently, it increases their productivity and performance while meeting the organizational target. The employees should be motivated so that they take more interest as well as make significant efforts to carry out their duty productively. Like job security, training and salary, motivation is also a critical variable that can have a significant impact on the performance of employees and quality of service.

Motivation intends to encourage behavioural alteration. Motivation is used as an important force to empower an individual to meet specific objectives. Several research on employee motivation, states that motivation helps to enhance profitability, execution, and constancy. Comparing to highly motivated employees, less motivated employees are more inclined towards freedom and self-reliance along with more self-propelled impetus towards their job. Comparing to less motivated employees, employee responsibility towards their work also increases in case of highly motivated employees'. Based on the nature of the organization or business, motivation is the most important factor to achieve organizational goal and objectives.

What is motivation?

The word '**motivation**' has its origin in the Latin word '*movere*,' meaning "**to move**." Psychologically, it means an inner or environmental stimulus to action, forces or the factors that are responsible for initiation, sustaining (and restraining/abstaining from) behavior.

- Motivations may be diverse, multiple and dynamic.
- It is the **process of stimulating people to actions to accomplish the goals**.
- It's the crucial element in setting and attaining our objectives.
- It fuels competition and sparks social connection.
- Motivation encompasses the desire to continue striving toward meaning, purpose, and a life worth living.

In the work goal context the psychological factors stimulating the people's behaviour can be -

- desire for money

- success
- recognition
- job-satisfaction
- team work, etc.

Where does motivation come from?

Motivation can stem from a variety of sources. People may be motivated by external incentives, such as the motivation to work for compensation, or internal enjoyment, such as the motivation to create artwork in one's spare time. Other sources of motivation include curiosity, autonomy, validation of one's identity and beliefs, creating a positive self-image, and the desire to avoid potential losses.

What is intrinsic motivation?

Intrinsic motivation is a drive that comes purely from within; it's not due to any anticipated reward, deadline, or outside pressure. For example, people who are intrinsically motivated to run do so because they love the feeling of running itself, and it's an important part of their identity. Extrinsic motivation can increase motivation in the short term, but over time it can wear down or even backfire. By contrast, intrinsic motivation is powerful because it is integrated into identity and serves as a continuous source of motivation.

What is extrinsic motivation?

Extrinsic motivation is the reason someone does work other than the joy of doing the work itself. Anything promised for completing the task or received as a result of completing the task are extrinsic motivators. An extrinsic motivator needs three elements to be successful, according to research by psychologist Victor Vroom: expectancy (believing that increased effort will lead to increased performance), instrumentality (believing that a better performance will be noticed and rewarded), and valence (wanting the reward that is promised).

How can I stop procrastinating?

Procrastination is often driven by underlying feelings of distress or anxiety elicited by a given task. But there are ways to navigate the discomfort and beat procrastination. You can break the project into small, more manageable pieces; accomplishing one step will fuel your motivation for the next. You can set limits for the time spent preparing to begin, or aim to complete tasks as quickly as possible. You can also set a reward that you'll get after completing the task or a part of it.

How can companies motivate their employees?

Companies have the opportunity to motivate employees with incentives, but they also need to be mindful that incentives can backfire- as in the case of the Wells Fargo scandal. Employees are motivated by external rewards when they believe that working harder will lead to a better performance that they'll be rewarded for a better performance, and they appreciate the reward, such as a bonus or time off. It can be difficult to meet those criteria - "Will my hard work really be noticed?" "Does my contribution really matter since I'm on a large team? - So companies should tailor incentives to each unique team and role.

Tools to improve motivation

Reward

A thoughtfully created employee rewards scheme can go a long way to motivating your team and increasing productivity. While there are number of common ways companies reward employees (Staff outing, staff lunch etc.) a rewards scheme is not a one-size fits all policy. Instead, think about what works best for your team specifically, make them inclusive and appropriately sized.

Whether they are geared towards personal goals or embodying company values, chances are you'll see your team reinforcing your company values and better teamwork. Don't sleep on small rewards either; a hand-written note or a shout-out at a team meeting can ensure your team stays motivated.

Trust

Employees want to know you have their best interests at heart while employers want to know they can trust employees to do a job well. Building a culture around trust creates a positive atmosphere which motivates your staff and benefits productivity.

Recognition

It's simple but recognizing an employee's hard work can have a tremendous impact. It can also spur them on to achieve more. Recognition can take many forms from an informal "thank you" or Kudos to a glitzier employee of the month or year award.

Career advancement

One study found that the number one reason for employees leaving their jobs was career development. It makes sense - employees want to use their skills.

They also want to learn new skills. If your company doesn't offer a clear career development path, they may leave. And if they don't leave, they'll be far from productive. Combat this by talking to your employees about their career expectations and by building career development into your business.

Purpose

Increasing numbers of employees want more from their jobs than a pay cheque. Organizational is a strong motivator for many workers-especially younger employees. Engaging your staff with your business's purpose can help increase commitment to your business and improve motivation.

Office environment

The likelihood that someone is going to love their job 100% of the time is slim. There will always be the occasional down day where people simply won't feel as capable to perform in their role. It's just as important to motivate your team on a bad day as it is a good one. Thankfully, one way you can tackle this is by creating an office environment that is pleasant to be in. Studies have shown that plants are a cost-effective way to improve office life and increase positivity and motivation.

Feedback

Everyone likes to hear that they've done a good job, but unfortunately not everyone is given the opportunity. The benefits of giving feedback to your team and employees are numerous, and improved motivation is one of them.

Employees want to develop and improve and giving regular feedback enables them to see what they're doing and how well they're doing it.

The same works for the inverse too, if someone is not performing optimally in their position, feedback enables them to address their issues and perform better. It also makes them feel valued, and when employees feel valued they're more likely to take ownership and responsibility on projects.

Talk and listen

Whether it's at a performance management meeting, formalized in a company survey or in the kitchen making a drink, talking with your team is the best way to understand what motivates them. Good communication is an effective tool that can be used to boost morale and employee value.

Take the time to listen to what your team has to say and come up with ways to address their concerns. Ask what they want, but be prepared that different generations may want different things from their job and the workplace.

Theories of Motivation

1. Maslow's Hierarchy of Needs

Abraham Maslow is among the most prominent psychologists of the 20th century and the hierarchy of needs, accompanied by the pyramid representing how human needs are ranked, is an image familiar to most business students and managers. Maslow's theory is based on a simple premise: Human beings have needs that are hierarchically ranked. There are some needs that are basic to all human beings, and in their absence, nothing else matters. As we satisfy these basic needs, we start looking to satisfy higher-order needs. Once a lower-level need is satisfied, it no longer serves as a motivator.

The most basic of Maslow's needs are physiological needs. Physiological needs refer to the need for air, food, and water. Imagine being very hungry. At that point, all your behavior may be directed at finding food. Once you eat, though, the search for food ceases and the promise of food no longer serves as a motivator. Once physiological needs are satisfied, people tend to become concerned about safety. Are they safe from danger, pain, or an uncertain future? One level up, social needs refer to the need to bond with other human beings, to be loved, and to form lasting attachments. In fact, having no attachments can negatively affect health and well-being. The satisfaction of social needs makes esteem needs more salient. Esteem needs refer to the desire to be respected by one's peers, feeling important, and being appreciated. Finally, at the highest level of the hierarchy, the need for self-actualization refers to "becoming all you are capable of becoming." This need manifests itself by acquiring new skills, taking on new challenges, and behaving in a way that will lead to the satisfaction of one's life goals.

Maslow's hierarchy is a systematic way of thinking about the different needs employees may have at any given point and explains different reactions they may have to similar treatment. An employee who is trying to satisfy her esteem needs may feel gratified when her supervisor praises her. However, another employee who is trying to satisfy his social needs may resent being praised by upper management in front of peers if the praise sets him apart from the rest of the group.

Maslow's Hierarchy of Needs

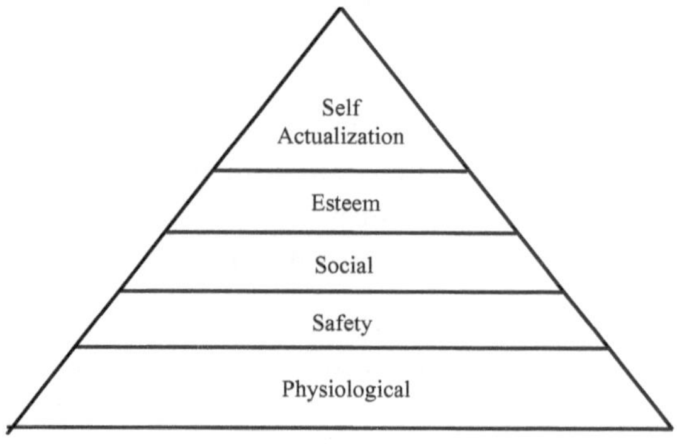

So, how can organizations satisfy their employees' various needs? By leveraging the various facets of the planning-organizing-leading-controlling (P-O-L-C) functions. In the long run, physiological needs may be satisfied by the person's pay check, but it is important to remember that pay may satisfy other needs such as safety and esteem as well. Providing generous benefits, including health insurance and company-sponsored retirement plans, as well as offering a measure of job security, will help satisfy safety needs. Social needs may be satisfied by having a friendly environment, providing a workplace conducive to collaboration and communication with others. Company picnics and other social get-togethers may also be helpful if the majority of employees are motivated primarily by social needs (but may cause resentment if they are not and if they have to sacrifice a Sunday afternoon for a company picnic). Providing promotion opportunities at work, recognizing a person's accomplishments verbally or through more formal reward systems, job titles that communicate to the employee that one has achieved high status within the organization are among the ways of satisfying esteem needs. Finally, self-actualization needs may be satisfied by providing development and growth opportunities on or off the job, as well as by assigning interesting and challenging work. By making the effort to satisfy the different needs each employee may have at a given time, organizations may ensure a more highly motivated workforce.

2. Existence, Relatedness, and Growth (ERG) Theory

ERG theory of Clayton Alderfer is a modification of Maslow's hierarchy of needs. Instead of the five needs that are hierarchically organized, Alderfer proposed that basic human needs may be grouped under three categories; namely, Existence, Relatedness, and Growth (see the following figure). Existence need corresponds to Maslow's physiological and safety needs, relatedness corresponds to social needs, and growth need refers to Maslow's esteem and self-actualization.

ERG Theory

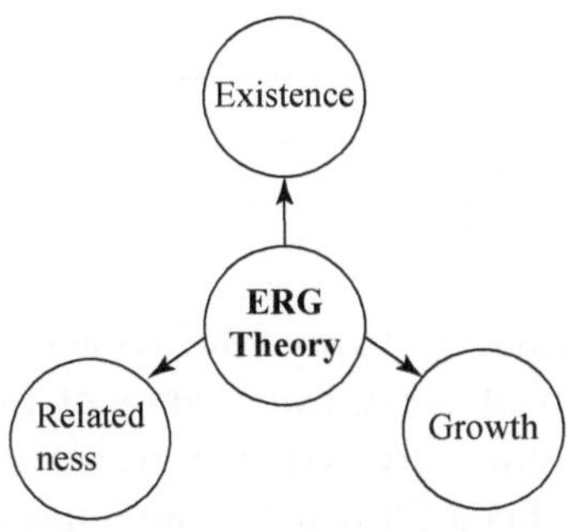

ERG theory's main contribution to the literature is its relaxation of Maslow's assumptions. For example, ERG theory does not rank needs in any particular order and explicitly recognizes that more than one need may operate at a given time. Moreover, the theory has a "frustration-regression" hypothesis, suggesting that individuals who are frustrated in their attempts to satisfy one need may regress to another one. For example, someone who is frustrated by the lack of growth opportunities in his job and slow progress toward career goals may regress to relatedness needs and start spending more time socializing with one's co-workers. The implication of this theory is that we need to recognize the multiple needs that may be driving an individual at a given point to understand his behaviour and to motivate him.

3. Two-Factor Theory

Frederick Herzberg approached the question of motivation in a different way. By asking individuals what satisfies them on the job and what dissatisfies them, Herzberg came to the conclusion that aspects of the work environment that satisfy employees are very different from aspects that dissatisfy them. Herzberg labeled factors causing dissatisfaction of workers as "hygiene" factors because these factors were part of the context in which the job was performed, as opposed to the job itself. Hygiene factors included company policies, supervision, working conditions, salary, safety, and security on the job.

In contrast, motivators are factors that are intrinsic to the job, such as achievement, recognition, interesting work, increased responsibilities, advancement, and growth opportunities. According to Herzberg's research, motivators are the conditions that truly encourage employees to try harder.

Two-factor theory of motivation

Hygiene factors	**Motivators**
Company Policy	Achievement
Supervision and Relationship	Recognition
Working conditions	Interesting work
Salary	Increased responsibility
Security	Advancement and growth

4. Acquired Needs Theory

Among the need-based approaches to motivation, Douglas McClelland's acquired needs theory is the one that has received the greatest amount of support. According to this theory, individuals acquire three types of needs as a result of their life experiences. These needs are need for achievement, need for affiliation, and need for power. All individuals possess a combination of these needs.

Those who have high need for achievement have a strong need to be successful. A worker who derives great satisfaction from meeting deadlines, coming up with brilliant ideas, and planning his or her next career move may be high in need for achievement. Individuals high on need for achievement are well suited to positions such as sales where there are explicit goals, feedback is immediately available, and their effort often leads to success. Because of their success in lower-level jobs, those in high need for achievement are often promoted to higher-level positions. However, a high need for achievement has important disadvantages in management. Management involves getting work done by motivating others. When a sales person is promoted to be a sales manager, the job description changes from actively selling to recruiting, motivating, and training sales people. Those who are high in need for achievement may view managerial activities such as coaching, communicating, and meeting with subordinates as a waste of time. Moreover, they enjoy doing things themselves and may find it difficult to delegate authority. They may become overbearing or micromanaging bosses, expecting everyone to be as dedicated to work as they are, and expecting subordinates to do things exactly the way they are used to doing.

Individuals who have a high need for affiliation want to be liked and accepted by others. When given a choice, they prefer to interact with others and be with friends. Their emphasis on harmonious interpersonal relationships may be an advantage in jobs and occupations requiring frequent interpersonal interaction, such as social worker or teacher. In managerial positions, a high need for affiliation may again serve as a disadvantage because these individuals tend to be overly concerned about how they are perceived by others. Thus, they may find it difficult to perform some aspects of a manager's job such as giving employees critical feedback or disciplining poor performers.

Finally, those with high need for power want to influence others and control their environment. Need for power may be destructive of one's relationships if it takes the form of seeking and using power for one's own good and prestige. However, when it manifests itself in more altruistic forms, such as changing the way things are done so that the work environment is more positive or negotiating more resources for one's department, it tends to lead to positive outcomes. In fact, need for power is viewed as important for effectiveness in managerial and leadership positions.

McClelland's theory of acquired needs has important implications for motivating employees. While someone who has high need for achievement may respond to goals, those with high need for affiliation may be motivated to gain the approval of their peers and supervisors, whereas those who have high need for power may value gaining influence over the supervisor or acquiring a position that has decision-making authority. And, when it comes to succeeding in managerial positions, individuals who are aware of the drawbacks of their need orientation can take steps to overcome these drawbacks.

McClelland identified three types of manifest needs, namely, Need for Achievement (N-Ach.), Need for Power (N-Pow) and Need for Affiliation (N-Aff.) as follows.

Need for Power (N-pow.): If a man "speculates about who is boss", he has a concern for power. Need for power, in effect, is the "concern for influencing people" or the behavior of others for moving in the chosen direction and attaining the envisioned objectives. In common perception, politicians, social-religious leaders Chief Executive Officers (CEOs), Government Bureaucrats/ Civil Servants typify the need for power.

Need for Affiliation (N-aff): If a man "readily thinks about interpersonal relationships", he has a concern for affiliation, wrote Mc-Clleland. It implies, among other things, "a tendency of the people to conform to the wishes and norms of those whom they value." Apparently, social activists, environmentalists, teachers, and doctors and nurses may seem as predominantly driven by these needs.

Need for Achievement: (N-ach) Concerns issues of excellence, competition, challenging goals and overcoming difficulties. A complete achievement sequence would comprise, "... defining the problem, wanting to solve it, thinking of means to solving it, thinking of difficulties that get in the way of solving it (either in one's self or in the environment), thinking of people who might help in solving it, and anticipating what would happen if one succeeded or failed."

Accordingly, a person with need for achievement would want to take personal responsibility for solving problem. One is goal oriented, that is, one sets moderate, realistic, attainable goals. One also seeks challenge, excellence, and individuality, one takes calculated/ moderate risk and is willing to work hard for that. One is always keen to find out how well one is doing and likes concrete feedback on performance.

Need for Autonomy: The need for autonomy is a desire for independence which, in effect, becomes a desire to do work of one's choice and at one's pace, defining one's own rules of the game, taking initiative, making independent and innovative choices and being responsible and accountable to oneself rather than some external authority for performance.

Four theories address

- Explain how employees are motivated according to Maslow's hierarchy of needs.
- Explain how ERG theory addresses the limitations of Maslow's hierarchy.
- Describe the difference between factors contributing to employee motivation and how these differ from factors contributing to dissatisfaction.
- Describe the needs for achievement, power, and affiliation, and how these needs affect work behaviour.

Why motivating livestock farmers

Investments into livestock farming have resulted in increased production. The negative environmental externalities from the practices have reoriented the focus to the sustainability aspects of intensification (Jhamtani, 2010). It involves application of multiple inputs, technologies and practices in an integrated way to increase agricultural productivity while simultaneously increasing the contribution to natural capital and environmental services (Pretty, 1997; Godfray*el al.*, 2010). Determinants of acceptance and use of technologies have been highlighted by literature on adoption of practices. These studies focus on socio-economic factor to explain the adoption decision.

However the socio-psychological farmer features have received less attention in these studies. Hence, it is essential to work on such socio-psychological factors to improve adoption, decision-making on technologies and practices to be adopted on the farm context or system. Considering its importance farmers need to be motivated for increased farm productivity for a satisfied and sustained farming.

Conclusion

Rewards must be based on individual performance. Identical rewards for all employees are ineffective in motivating employees. Employees should be treated equally. The employee should not feel that merit was ignored in selecting staff in recruitment or further training which may lead to frustration and lowered motivation. Staff performance need to be assessed accurately based on standards that employee perceive to be fair, achievable and equal for all. For better motivation, the motivation factors include uniform evaluation, dependable supervisors, work incentives, pay, praise and work location, housing, transportation, job security and unbiased administration and supervision.

With respect to motivating farmer, it is important to adopt sustainable practices that promote personal satisfaction, eco – diversity and eco –

efficiency. Also farmers prefer to have social support and resources for which extension service need to provide solutions to their critical issues that help to enhance their income and level of satisfaction. This in a long run motivate farmers adoption decision towards improved practices / innovations for increased productivity based on their socio-economic conditions and external drivers on introducing on-farm innovation process and policies that support their well-being. Each of the theories discussed in this section explains factors that promote work environment of veterinarians and farmers which may be utilized to maintain a higher level of energy for improved performance.

20

Extension-Plus New Dimension of Future Extension

Arunasis Goswami and Sukanta Biswas

Veterinary and Animal Husbandry Extension Education
West Bengal University of Animal and Fishery Sciences
Kolkata-700037, West Bengal, India

Emerging Paradigm of Extension Plus:

This is now widely recognized that Animal Husbandry extension needs to reform in ways that allow it to fulfill a diverse set of objectives in worldwide. This ranges from better linking of farmers to input and output markets, to reducing the vulnerability and enhancing voice of the rural poor, development of micro-enterprises, poverty reduction and environmental conservation and strengthening and support of farmer organizations'. So while technology transfer is important, what is also required is the strengthening of locally relevant innovation processes and knowledge systems. Extension is being forced to embrace a broadened mandate that while in reality has always existed, has rarely been addressed. The limitations of a single model of extension for all kinds of situations are now well recognized and there is an increasing realization that new extension approaches need to emerge locally, based on experimentation, learning and adaptation to prevailing circumstances. The need for this new and expanded view of extension is clearly emerging in the case of Indian agriculture, which is characterized by declining land and water availability, degradation of natural resources, an unfavorable price regime, low value addition, particularly in rural areas and increasing competition from import of agricultural commodities. Farmers thus find themselves in an ever more complex production and market environment, with an expanding need for information and services.

Extension Plus in Action

A range of experiences of extension initiatives from the public & private sectors that display the expanded agenda embodied in the concept of extension-plus. The four (04) cases of KHDP, MSSL, BASIX & BAIF's are illustrative of a number of points, concerning both content and process of extension innovations. All the four cases illustrate the need for extension type organizations' to act as a nodal point for linking farmers to both technology & non-technology services.

As instance, for *Kerala Horticultural Development Programme (KHDP), extension-plus* meant development and strengthening farmer organizations; improving farmers' ability to find solutions to technical, credit related and marketing problems; assisting sourcing better technical knowledge available with other organizations; and strengthening the capability of farmer organizations' to negotiate with the state, traders and banks for changes in terms, policy and practice.

In *Mahindra ShubhLabh Services Limited (MSSL), extension-plus* includes the delivery of a wide range of services, namely, making available quality inputs at the right time, provision of field based advice on technology use, reduction of number of intermediaries, and getting better prices. The central innovation of MSSL is that, it has evolved an integrated system that delivers all these services to farmers at one point, and delivering it as a viable business.

Similarly for BASIX, extension-plus means, linking primary producers to processors, promoting value addition at the local level and linking producer groups to other agencies, in addition to providing technical support and credit.

In BAIF Development Foundation (BAIF), setting up producer co-operatives, helping farmers acquire production, processing, managerial and marketing skills, and linking their produce to new and existing markets are all part of extension-plus.

All these cases reveal the importance of experimenting with new strategies and learning from them as a way of developing optimal arrangements. For instance, KHDP's farmer markets and new credit package for lease land farmers evolved through a series of failures *(eg: reluctance of banks to provide credit to lease-land farmers, resistance from traders to procure goods from farmer markets, etc)*, but these failures provided KHDP with lessons on how to go forward and try better arrangements each time. Similarly for MSSL, the failures from its first Mahindra Krishi Vihar (MKV) established at Madurai and its subsequent closure and the series of innovations made by its own franchisee "Bhuvi-care" to the MSSL approach helped it to evolve new location specific approaches while expanding MKVs to new locations. BASIX's interventions are based on system diagnosis in each location to identify critical interventions and potential partners. The key operational strategy is learning through small experimental interventions. Similarly BAIF's interventions were experimental.

Learning from each of these experiments led to the development of subsequent interventions. All the above cases thus reveal the *processes adopted, viz, experimentation, reflection and learning to evolve successful arrangements.* Moreover, these new institutional arrangements evolved through *partnership with other organizations'*, networks and schemes already in place. For instance, KHDP partnered with research organizations', banks and traders to make the whole arrangement work. MSSL has evolved this new business venture in partnership with input companies, agro-processors and financial institutions. BAIF and Dhruva are working in partnership with people's organizations', producer co-operatives and a rural development bank. Similarly, BASIX has been building its interventions around existing organizations' and is working in collaboration with *NGOs, such as Association of Sarva Seva Farms in Virudhnagar, Gram Abhyudaya Mandal in Nizamabad, and Rural Development Trust in Anantapur and with producer co-operatives like Andhra Pradesh Diary Development Co-operative Federation in Mahabubnagar and vegetable producer groups in Virudhanagar.*

From Policy To Practice-Key Constraints in Extension Plus

The National Agricultural Policy of India and the Policy Framework for Agricultural Extension (PFAE) acknowledges the need for extension to engage with issues beyond technology dissemination. The PFAE affirms that the "policy environment will promote private and community driven extension to operate competitively, in roles that complement, supplement, work in partnerships and even substitute for public extension. However, to fulfill this expanded role, extension organizations' need to change considerably both in scope and mode of operation. While the need to provide a wide range of services as envisaged in extension-plus is all too apparent, a clear roadmap on reforming extension is not evident. States face a number of dilemmas: how much of past arrangements should be retained and which innovations in extension provision are desirable, affordable and politically possible given opposition from staff unions, and declining enthusiasm from donors and political patrons for a stand-alone extension that deals with only technology dissemination. The learning from the past does not seem to have made any difference to the way extension reform is approached. For instance, although the limitations of a single model of extension are well known (for example T&V), the merits are being considered of ATMA (Agricultural Technology Management Agency) as a model for extension that can be replicated across all states and districts.

Moreover, the planning and implementation of extension programs still rests only on extending technologies to farmers. Public sector extension is yet to make any experimentation with perfecting new marketing arrangements that reduce the number of intermediaries, eliminate exploitative weighing and payment methods, and help farmers to get better prices. Current efforts that provide information on prices and market arrivals in major markets alone have limited operational merit. But policy can't seem to get beyond this impasse of prescription without subsequent analysis and refinement. The cases described above suggest a number of broad principles: the need to build on existing structures and strengths in different locations; the need to establish new programs in ways that explicitly recognize the experimental nature of the reform and change process; and the need to recognize the value of diversity of approaches and arrangements. Those involved in the reform process will need to build skills that allow them to reflect on progress (both successes and failures) and change course accordingly. It will require approaches that are less target-driven and more concerned with learning and the development of new capacities to deal with local circumstances. However, the current organizational culture in general restrict the ability of public sector extension to realize the vision of extension-plus precisely because the principles outlined above are counter to deeply held norms in the public sector. *Table-1 illustrates the key shifts required for operationalizing extension-plus.*

The following features need to be the focus of measures to reform the existing extension arrangements.

- Rigid professional hierarchies and patterns of control, with highly centralized modes of planning. This tends to stifle deviation from prescribed procedures, restricting innovation, particularly by middle and lower level staff.
- A tradition of assessing performance in terms of technology adoption and hence a focus on improved technology transfer mechanisms at the expense of other activities that may have a perfectly legitimate role in supporting farmers.
- A history of only rewarding successes and thus a reluctance to report and analyze the reasons of failure of a technology or a new approach.
- A tradition of working independently and a mistrust of other agencies. This is particularly so with regard to external agencies, NGO's and private sector, but also with other public agencies including research organizations.
- A tradition of up-ward accountability for resource utilization rather than output achievement and client satisfaction.

Rules and conventions related to recruitment, qualifications, transfer, contractual appointments and performance assessment further prevent accessing a wider range of expertise. The combined effect of these professional and administrative traditions is a prevailing culture in public sector extension that views its operational mandate-technology transfer-in very narrow terms, but also a culture in which the incentives and capabilities to learn and innovate are highly restricted. It is perhaps this weakness in the current culture of extension agencies and associated planning bodies that need to be addressed as one of the key issues by the reform process.

Way Forward In Extension Plus

The underlying principles of extension-plus include a broad scope of service provision; the extensive use of partnerships to fulfill an expanded mandate; a learning-based approach that includes negotiations with a wide range of stakeholders in order to develop workable and effective arrangements in line with specific local circumstances and objectives; and a larger degree of accountability to client groups.

To operationalize extension plus, there is a need for a broad agreement on the need to reinvent extension as a nodal agency that provides technological and non-technological services to farmers. Extension needs to play a facilitating role enabling access to services by acting as a bridge connecting farmers, the poor and vulnerable groups with different service providers.

Table 1 Key Shifts In Operationalizing Extension-Plus

Items	From	To
Form/Content	Technology dissemination Improving farm productivity Forming farmer groups Providing services Market information	Supporting rural livelihoods Improving farm and non-farm income Building independent farmer operated organizations Enabling farmers to access services from other agencies; Market development
Monitoring & Evaluation	Input and output targets	Learning
Planning & Implementation Strategy	Doing it alone	Partnerships
Sources of innovation in Extension	Centrally generated	Locally evolved (through local experimentation)
Approaches	Fixed/uniform	Evolving/diverse
Capacity Development of staff	Training	Learning by doing, facilitated experimentation
Capacity development of Extension system	Personnel and infrastructure	Development of linkages and networks
Policy Approach	Prescriptive/blue prints	Facilitating evolution of locally relevant approaches

Items	From	To
Introducing new working practices	Staff training	Changing organizational culture through action learning
Underpinning paradigm	Transfer of Technology	Innovation system

Operationalizing extension-plus requires a new organizational culture. Next steps to developing this new culture might include:

a. Capacity Development: Shifting from training to a "learning by doing" approach whereby staff are encouraged and enabled to initiate small experimental projects that address broad livelihood needs and use partnership as a central approach. By treating small projects experimentally and facilitating staff to reflect on their meaning and outcomes, this would build skills related to experimentation, learning and evaluating innovative extension approaches.

b. New skills: Constituting a core group of specialists at the district level with non-traditional extension skills such as: market development; institutional development; post-harvest; enterprise development and agribusiness management.

c. Organizational & Monitoring Review: An organizational & management review of existing extension system, primarily to explore possibilities of recruiting limited number of better qualified field staff, creating new incentive structures and to provide more administrative and financial freedom at the lower levels.

d. Better informed policy process: As part of the reform and planning process, resources should be used for systematic institutional analysis of promising extension innovations so that generalizable principles can be drawn and new strategies suitably informed.

Only if extension takes learning-based approach to changing its role and improving its performance, will reforms succeed. But if this cultural change is to flourish, it needs to be supported and legitimized wholeheartedly and unambiguously at the most senior levels of the extension services and in other allied organizations. Challenging as this may be, without a new organizational culture, the far-reaching reforms needed to operationalize extension-plus will not succeed.

Extension-Plus-Examples From The Field:

Government initiative: *Kerala Horticultural Development Programme (KHDP)* was conceived in 1992 as a project to improve the overall situation of fruit and vegetable farmers in Kerala; by increasing and stabilizing their income; reducing cost of production and improving the marketing system. KHDP used SHGs as its key concept for promoting the development of farmers and experimented with different approaches to provide better access by farmers to technology markets and credit. Every SHG selects three master farmers; one each for production, marketing and credit related activities and each one of them are trained by KHDP. KHDP has so far constituted 2312 SHGs, involving 41913 registered farmers. KHDP has encouraged group marketing where farmers now form their own market and got traders to come and buy. In the year 2002-03, about 31 thousand tons of produce worth around Rs.29 crore was traded through 112 marketing centers. KHDP developed a unique credit package that could be availed by lease-land farmers and at the same time acceptable to the banks. Loans totaling Rs. 52 crore has been disbursed to farmers. To generate and access needed technologies for its farmers, KHDP contracted the state agricultural university for research and also undertook participatory technology development with farmers. With the end of funding support from European Union in 2001, the organization was registered as a company and it currently provide support to growers in 11 districts. An impact study reported a significant increase in area under fruit and vegetables in 86% of the SHGs and an increase in income in 75% of the SHGs7. The same study also reported that the number of farmers availing credit increased from 21% in the pre-KHDP period to 41% by 1999 and an increase in the efficiency of loan disbursal and increase in size of loans.

Agri-business initiative: *Mahindra Shubh Labh Services Limited (MSSL)* was formed in 2001 as a subsidiary by Mahindra and Mahindra, one of the leading tractor manufacturing firms in India. The objective was to provide what the company describes as “integrated yield and profit solutions”. The company has established through its franchises “Mahindra Krishi Vihar” (MKV), a one stop shop for farmers (who registers with them on a fee), that provide access to quality inputs and machinery, credit, access to advisory and field supervision services, buy back and better prices. MSSL initiated this service in paddy in Tamil Nadu and currently this service is being expanded to more crops and districts. In Tirunelveli, the Mahindra franchise, Bhuvi Care Private Ltd has successfully established this scheme in paddy and maize. In 2003-04 II season (October -February), 105 farmers have registered 305 acres of paddy at Rs.500/ per acre/season and 314 farmers have registered 1392 acres of maize at Rs.150/per acre/per season. In paddy, the participant farmers realized 12% increase in yield and 27% increases in net returns per acre and for maize, 10% and 40% respectively.

Financial institution initiative: *BASIX is a group of financial services* and technical assistance companies, established for the promotion of sustainable livelihoods. It is currently operating in five states, namely, Andhra Pradesh, Karnataka, Maharashtra, Orissa and Jharkhand. According to BASIX, credit is necessary, but not a sufficient condition for generating sustainable livelihoods. In Andhra Pradesh, BASIX has identified a few sub-sectors in its area of operation (districts) such as groundnut in Anantpur, cotton in Adilabad and milk in Mahabubnagar. In Tamil Nadu (Virudhanagar) and Jharkhand (Ranchi), BASIX has initiated activities in vegetables9. Besides intervening in areas, which leads to direct increase in productivity or output, BASIX has been involved in finding out alternate market channels (eg: directly linking of cotton growers to spinning mills and groundnut growers to oil millers or wholesale traders) or value addition possibilities in these subsectors (eg; contracting with decorticating unit to decorticate groundnut by farmers) with an objective of raising the income of the primary producers. BASIX in all these cases worked in collaboration with local NGOs, or producer groups.

NGO initiative: *BAIF Development Foundation, an NGO* has been implementing the Wadi programme in three states, Gujarat, Maharashtra and Karnataka covering more than 50,000 families. In South Gujarat, Dhruva, an NGO promoted by BAIF has facilitated establishment of fruit orchard (wadi) on the land belonging to adivasis. When the trees (mango and cashew) started yielding, the project realized the need to intervene in value addition and marketing if the tribal producers have to benefit from the intervention. At Vansda, BAIF facilitated the establishment of a producer co-operative "Vasundhara VrixVanwadiJalsinchan Vikas Sahkari Mandal Samiti" with an objective to help the member producers to increase income through post-harvest processing of fruits into marketable products and establish marketing linkages. By 2002-03, 13,000 adivasis have been assisted and an area of 11,897 acres of private land has been covered. Dhruva assisted the Vasunadhara Co-operative in designing appropriate systems (technical and organizational) to preserve fruits, process them (eg: cashew nuts, and as mango pickles, jams, and jellies) and access local and urban markets under the brand name "Vrindavan". This project funded by KFW, (a German donor) is implemented by Dhruva in partnership with "Village Ayojan Samities" and the National Bank for Agriculture and Rural Development (NABARD).

Acknowledgement

The authors are thankful & acknowledge the great contribution in the research Paper of Sulaiman, R.V. and Hall A.J. of 2017 & 2004 published in https://www.researchget.net.

21

Emotional Intelligence in Extension Education

P. Ramesh

ICAR-National Academy of Agricultural Research Management, Hyderabad Telangana, India

Our emotions play quite a significant role in guiding and directing our behavior. Many a times they are seen to dominate our behavior in such a way that we have no solution other than behaving as per their wish. On the other hand, if a person has no emotional current then he becomes crippled in terms of living his life in a normal way. Hence, emotions play a key role in providing a particular direction to our behavior and thus shaping our personality according to their development.

Etymologically, the word emotion is derived from the Latin word '*emovere*' which means 'to stir up' or 'to excite'. Emotion implies a state of being stirred up or aroused in one way or another. Therefore, emotion may be understood as an agitated or excited state of our mind and body. It involves extensive visual disturbance and includes many feeling tones or varying degrees of satisfaction or annoyance. Feeling may be a simple degree of emotional experience. Psychologists and physiologists are in agreement that emotion involves feelings, impulses and physiological reactions.

Thus, whatever may be the terminology used by different psychologists, their definition tends to describe "*emotions as some sort of feelings or affective experiences which are characterized by some physiological changes that generally lead them to perform some or the other type of behavioral act*".

To sum up, the following are the important characteristics of emotions:

Emotional experiences are associated with instincts or biological drives. When the basic need is satisfied or challenged (the satisfaction is in danger), the emotion plays their part.

Emotions are the product of perception. The perception of a proper stimulus (object or situation) is needed to start an emotional experience. Organic changes within the body (favorable or unfavorable) may then intensify the emotional experience.

The core of an emotion is feeling. Actually every emotional experience, whatever it maybe, involves feelings – matter of the heart. Feelings and emotions both are affective experiences. There is only the difference of degrees. After perceiving a thing or a situation, feelings like pleasure or displeasure can be aroused. There may be some intensity or degree of strength in these feelings. When the feelings are so strong that they are able to disturb the mind and excite an individual to act immediately they are turned into emotions. Therefore, the urge to do or act is the most important emotional experience.

Emotions bring physiological changes. Every emotional experience involves many physical and physiological changes in an organism. These changes become so specific and distinguishable in human beings that a simple glimpse can enable us to detect a particular emotional experience in an individual and we can see whether he is in anger or scared.

Working environment in any organization poses a variety of challenges. These challenges may be self-created or experienced from others. If a person wants to succeed one must have the ability to respond positively to such challenges. Otherwise, it may lead to emotional disturbances in the form of frustration, anger, anxiety etc., which in turn affect individual productivity. There is increasing interest in how people process emotionally relevant information and the ability to process it efficiently and accurately can have an effect on an individual's life outcomes such as achieving success at work and their general well-being (Salovey and Grewal, 2005; Brackett *et al.,* 2011).

Emotional intelligence (EI) is "the ability to monitor one's own and others' feelings and emotions, to discriminate among them and to use information to guide one's thinking and actions" (Salovey and Mayer, 1990). The concept of EI was popularized by Goleman (1995) in his book, "Emotional Intelligence: Why it can Matter More than IQ". He described a connection between emotional competencies and pro-social behavior and declared EI is more powerful than intelligence quotient (IQ) in predicting success in life.

Emotional intelligence is hypothesized to influence the success with which employees interact with colleagues, the strategies they use to manage conflict and stress, and overall job performance (Ashkanasy and Daus, 2005; Lopes *et al.,* 2006a; Martins *et al*., 2010). Employees with higher EI also received better peer and supervisor ratings of interpersonal facilitation, stress tolerance and leadership potential than those with lower EI (Lopes *et al*, 2006b).

Robert Sternberg (1985) more recently proposed a 'Triarchic' theory of intelligence, in which he argued that intelligence, is comprised of three separate facets; analytic, practical and creative. Sternberg's work is significant, as it was one of the first major theories of intelligence to include both cognitive and non-cognitive variables. It is also, therefore, one of the most comprehensive theories of intelligence. Sternberg's work helped to widen the scope of intelligence, as he argued that IQ tests only measure specific aspects of intelligence and do not assess social and emotional factors that impact everyday functioning. Over time, as theorists such as wschler and Sternberg began to question the efficacy of the psychometric approach and as a more substantial body of research was undertaken in this respect, researchers began to realize that intelligence was far from easy to quantify, or even to define. For example, Sternberg and Detterman, in 1987 asked 24 leading experts in the field to provide a definition of the word 'intelligence' and received twenty-four different definitions! Accordingly, Bar-On (1997) claimed that it is obviously easier to measure intelligence than it is to define it, since researchers clearly encounter difficulties defining intelligence, yet still prodigiously use intelligence testing in varied settings. In addition, several theorists have argued that rather than being a unitary construct, intelligence is in fact comprised of a number of separate but related constructs and that we should speak not of intelligence in the singular, but of multiple intelligences.

For example, **Howard Gardner** (1983) suggested that intelligence is multi-dimensional and comprises both cognitive and emotional aspects. In his seminal text 'Frames of Mind', he argues in favour of multiple intelligences and proposed that there are eight distinct forms of human intelligence as follows:

- **Linguistic intelligence** – This area pertains to verbal abilities, both spoken and written, including oration, debating, reading, writing and memory for names and dates.
- **Logico-mathematical intelligence** – This area pertains to numerical and reasoning abilities, including pattern recognition, scientific investigation and numeracy.
- **Spatial intelligence** – This area pertains to abilities to visualize and mentally manipulate objects and includes hand-eye coordination, visual memory and sense of direction.
- **Bodily-kinesthetic intelligence** – This area pertains to physical abilities, including sport, dance and building or making objects.
- **Musical intelligence** – This area pertains to auditory and musical abilities, including rhythm, composing and musical performance.
- **Interpersonal intelligence** – This area pertains to the ability to interact with other people and includes empathy, leadership skills and communicative abilities.

- **Intrapersonal intelligence**-This area pertains to self-awareness and includes introspection, emotional self-awareness and self-reflection.
- **Naturalist intelligence**-This area pertains to awareness of natural phenomena, including weather patterns, the ability to nurture animals and crops and classifying objects.

Emotional Intelligence (EI) or **Emotional Quotient (EQ)** is the ability of individuals to recognize their own and other people's emotions to discriminate between different feelings and label them appropriately, and to use emotional information to guide thinking and behaviour. Emotional intelligence, like general intelligence, is the product of one's heredity and its interaction with his environment. Until recently, we have been led to believe that a person's general intelligence measure as I.Q. or intelligence quotient is the greatest predictor of success in any walk of life- academic, social, vocational or professional. However, researchers and experiments conducted in the 90's onwards have tried to challenge such over-dominance of intelligence and its measure I.Q. by replacing it with the concept of emotional intelligence and its measure emotional quotient (E.Q.). Studies reveled that a person's emotional intelligence measured through his EQ may be a greater predictor of success than his IQ.

The term emotional intelligence was introduced by Mayer and Salovey (1990) in their attempt to develop a scientific measure for knowing the differences between people's ability in the area of emotions. However, the credit for popularizing the concept of emotional intelligence goes to Daniel Goleman (1995).

"Emotional Intelligence may be defined as the capacity to reason with emotions in four areas: to perceive emotion, to integrate it in thought, to understand it and to manage it" (Mayer & Salovey, 1997).

According to this definition, every one of us may be found to have varying capacities and ability with regard to one's dealing with emotions. Depending upon the nature of this ability, he or she may be said to be more or less emotionally intelligent in comparison to others in the group.

A person will be termed emotionally intelligent in proportion to his ability to:

- Identify and perceive the various types of emotions in others (through face reading, body language and voice tone etc.).
- Being aware of his own feelings and emotions.
- Incorporate or integrate the perceived emotions in his thought (such as using his emotions, feeling in analyzing, problem solving, decision making etc.).

- Have proper understanding about the nature, intensity and outcomes of the emotions.
- Exercise proper control and regulation over the expression and use of emotions in dealing with his self and others in view of promoting harmony, prosperity and peace.

Dimensions of Emotional Intelligence

1. *Self-Awareness*: Knowing what we are feeling at the moment, and using those preferences to guide our decision making; having a realistic assessment of our own abilities and a well-grounded sense of self confidence.
2. *Managing Emotions*: Handling our emotions so that they facilitate rather than interfere with the task at hand; being conscientious and delaying gratification to pursue goals; recovering well from emotional distress.
3. *Self-Motivation*: Using our deepest preferences to move and guide us towards our goals, to help us take initiatives and strive to improve, and to persevere in the face of setbacks and frustrations.
4. *Empathy*: Sensing what people are feeling, being able to take their perspective, and cultivating rapport and attunement with a broad diversity of people.
5. *Handling Relationships*: Handling emotions in relationships well and accurately reading social situations and networks; interacting smoothly; using these skills to persuade and lead, negotiate and settle disputes, for cooperation and teamwork.

The Importance of Emotional Intelligence in Leadership

Emotional intelligence has recently become one of the key talking points when it comes to leadership. One thing we know for sure is that it is a trait that can be measured and developed. But what exactly is it and how does it influence the concept of leadership as we know it today?

Emotional intelligence has to do with one's ability to both recognize and control their own emotions, while harnessing said emotions appropriately to have the most optimum reaction as situations dictate. It also has to do with one's awareness of and sensitivity towards others' emotions.

Emotional intelligence is therefore an important characteristic for anyone at any level of an organization but it is particularly important for those who occupy positions of leadership. A leader's emotional intelligence can have sweeping influence over their relationships, how they manage their teams, and all in all how they interact with individuals in the workplace.

What happens when leaders are emotionally intelligent?

Leaders who are emotionally intelligent foster safe environments, where employees feel comfortable to take calculated risks, suggest ideas and to voice their opinions. In such safe environments, working collaboratively isn't just an objective, but it gets woven into the organizational culture as whole. When a leader is emotionally intelligent, they can use emotions to drive the organization forward. Leaders often have the responsibility of effecting any necessary changes in the organization, and if they are aware of others' possible emotional reactions to these changes they are able to plan and prepare the most optimal ways to make them. Furthermore, emotionally intelligent leaders don't take things personally and are able to forge ahead with plans without worrying about the impact on their egos. Personal vendettas between leaders and employees are one of the commonest hindrances to productivity in many workplaces.

What happens when leaders aren't emotionally intelligent?

Leadership is a naturally stressful mandate, being responsible for the fate of hundreds or even thousands of other people can take its toll. Leaders who are low in emotional intelligence tend to unravel in stressful situations because they fail to handle their own emotions and this might manifest as verbal attacks on others and being passive aggressive.

This can create an even more stressful environment, where workers are always walking on eggshells trying to prevent the next outburst from happening. This often has disastrous effects on productivity and team cohesion because the employees stay too distracted by this fear to focus on work and bond.

Not being emotionally intelligent hinders collaboration within the organization. When a leader doesn't have a handle on their own emotions and reacts inappropriately, most of their employees tend to feel nervous about contributing their ideas and suggestions, for fear of how the leader will respond.

However, a leader who lacks emotional intelligence doesn't necessarily lash out at their employees. Not being emotionally intelligent can also mean an inability to address situations that could be fraught with emotion. Most leaders deal with conflict, and a leader who isn't clued into others' emotions will often have a difficult time recognizing conflict in the first place let alone dealing effectively resolving it.

How do leaders use Emotional Intelligence?

Successful leadership is about being effective in three ways: leading self, leading others, and leading the organization.

Leading self

Successful leaders know that they are not perfect. They are aware of their strengths and weaknesses, and strive for continuous improvement. A Chief Executive that does not acknowledge their own flaws or blind spots, who tries to do everything by him- or herself, doesn't learn from mistakes and is unable to delegate, will soon be derailed. If you're self-aware as a leader you can work to overcome your weaknesses either through personal development and learning new skills, or by empowering others and using their skills. Motivation is equally important here. Having goals to work towards, and setting high standards for yourself, means acknowledging that there will be obstacles along the way. As a leader, this means constantly challenging yourself, finding ways round the obstacles, and picking yourself up when things go wrong. And you need self-regulation to manage your emotions as a leader. Leadership is tough. So having the ability to keep calm, deal well with pressure and stay optimistic is vital. Mastering leadership of self requires admitting you're not perfect and striving for improvement.

Leading others

Leaders know that they need other people-after all, leadership doesn't mean a lot without followership. Being personally motivated isn't enough-leaders need to unlock the potential of others. This means understanding what matters to people, what their motivations are and how these motivations relate to the purpose of the organization. Not everyone is the same which makes social skills are important. Successful leaders understand that they need to be flexible and adaptable, as well as able to read and understand others. You need to spend time with different teams, and not just your direct reports. As a leader you don't have to be the master of all trades, but you do need to be willing to listen, to respect the expertise of others and to change your mind, if it's appropriate. And in this time of change, you need to be able to demonstrate real empathy to undertake the most difficult workplace conversations with tact and sensitivity.

Leading organizations

Successful leaders know how to inspire others. Leadership means being visionary, keeping in mind at all times the bigger picture. Leaders can articulate that big picture to others – and the best leaders help people to see their role in that big picture. They also hold themselves and their organization accountable to that goal. The goal is what is important, not personal gain or success. Leaders need to build strong relationships with boards, partners, stakeholders and even competitors to reach organizational goals. They demonstrate political astuteness, recognizing that power and influence in organizations does not work in neat hierarchical lines. They ensure success through influencing and by networking. Mastering leadership of organizations requires inspiration, accountability and relationship building.

Tips and Ways to increase your Emotional Intelligence

Self-Awareness: Knowing and understanding your own emotions is essential to knowing what you really want and understanding the impact you have on other people.

1. Accept your emotions

Whatever your feelings are, accept them as yours. Realize that your inner self is doing the best it can right now. Giving yourself a hard time because you "shouldn't" be feeling a certain way is not going to help you. If you don't like the way you're feeling, there are ways you can change it.

2. Get in touch with your emotions

Notice how you feel right now. Now let your eyes stray down towards your dominant hand (the one you write with). Notice how you feel now - are you more intensely aware of it?

3. Take the labels off your feelings

If you don't like the way you're feeling, ask yourself: "How do you know you are feeling that?" Forget the label that you've given the emotion - sadness, anxiety or whatever - what are the physical sensations and where in your body are they? How intense are they? Are they constant or do they change? After doing this for a couple of minutes, you may feel different.

4. Keep an emotional journal

Take ten minutes at the start and end of each day to write down your feelings, without judging or censoring yourself. Notice what you learn.

5. Meditate

When you meditate, it's easier to be aware of your feelings without being distracted by the busyness and noise of everyday life. Often creative ideas will come to you as well.

6. Listening to emotional messages

What if that troublesome emotion is trying to tell you something? No wonder it won't go away - you've not listened to its message yet. So ask yourself: "If this feeling has a message for me, what is it trying to tell me?"

7. Feelings about feelings

We can have feelings about the way we feel. For example, we might feel guilty about getting angry. So if you catch yourself feeling bad, ask yourself "How do I feel about that emotion?"

8. See yourself as a friend sees you

Other people may see aspects of us that we are unaware of. Put yourself in the shoes of a friend or someone who loves you - stand like them, breathe like them, 'be' them. Notice how you look through their eyes and how they feel about you. You may be pleasantly surprised by how different you seem from the outside.

9. Listen to your heart (and gut)

The heart is traditionally the source of love, acceptance and self-in-relation to-others. For problems that you can't solve with logic alone, put your hand over your heart, close your eyes and imagine you are breathing into this area. When you have identified with your heart area, ask your heart what to do. Notice what new insights come to you, and how you feel differently about the problem and life in general from this perspective. Repeat the exercise using the area just below your navel; notice what extra perspectives you get from this viewpoint.

10. Other people as mirrors

Sometimes we can deny unpleasant feelings within ourselves and 'project' them onto other people. So if you find that, for example, other people are often angry with you and you don't know why, ask yourself, "When am I like that?"

Self-Regulation: Being able to control your own emotional state is essential for taking responsibility for your actions, and can save you from hasty actions that you later regret.

11. Take responsibility for your feelings

Once you accept that these are your emotions and you are responsible for them, your attitude can change from the powerless "Why am I feeling this way?" (or even worse, "Why are they 'making' me feel this way?") to the more empowering "What do I need to do to change the way I feel?"

12. Be kind to your body

The biggest single difference you can make to your emotional stability is to cut down on coffee. Caffeine (also present in smaller doses in tea, cola and chocolate) mimics the effect of adrenaline to give you an energy surge followed by a dip. This can have a roller coaster effect on your emotions. Sugary foods have a similar effect.

13. Respect your body's natural cycle

We have a natural cycle of rest and activity. Left to ourselves, we would have an hour and a half of activity followed by 20 minutes' rest. The further we get from that natural cycle; the more stress we experience. So take a break in the middle of the morning and the middle of the afternoon, and leave work at a reasonable time.

14. Stand tall

Your physical posture can have a big effect on how you feel. Try it now: first, slump over and hang your head while trying to remember a good time. It's not easy, is it? Now stand up straight, look up, and spread your arms wide, and notice how much easier it is to feel good!

15. Calm yourself instantly

Focusing on your breathing (tip 5) is one quick way to calm yourself. Here's another that instantly activates the body's relaxation response and works for both fear and anger:

16. Monitor your body for tension

Every so often, check your body for tension. If any areas are tense, relax them by imagining that you are breathing into them.

17. Centre yourself

Pay attention to the centre of your body, a few inches below your navel and half way between your stomach and your lower back. Relax your body and imagine your feet are firmly rooted to the ground. Notice how physically strong and centered you feel, and how paying attention to your centre also makes you feel stronger and calmer.

18. Project an energy bubble

Imagine you're protected by bubble of energy projected from your central point, so that anything stressful just bounces off and away.

19. Anchor your good feelings

Remember a time when you felt really good and in control. Choose a word, an image, and a physical gesture that sum those feelings up. As you relive that time and the good feelings are coming to a peak, repeat the word to yourself, see the image and physically make the gesture. Practice getting into those good feelings until they are 'anchored' in, and you can access them any time you need them just by using the word, the image or the gesture.

20. Rise above uncomfortable emotions

If you are feeling overwhelmed, imagine you are floating above the situation looking down at yourself. Float up until you reach a height at which you are completely comfortable. Ask your inner self, "What do I need to learn from this?"

21. Challenge negative self-talk

Another way of dealing with an 'inner critic' is to train it out of negativity by challenging it. Every time you catch yourself saying or thinking "I can't do that" ask yourself "What would happen if I did?" If you find you are saying, "I mustn't do that", ask yourself "Who says I mustn't? And what would happen if I did?"

Motivation: We can use our deepest emotions to move and guide us towards our goals, helping us to take the initiative and to persevere in the face of setbacks.

22. Discover what you really want

If it's not easy to motivate yourself now, maybe you're not doing what you really want to do. What do you love doing so much you'd do it for free? What are you interested in? What excites you? What gives you energy?

23. Clarify your values

Values are what's important to us. They motivate us and are our criteria for knowing if we are doing the right thing. To clarify your values for a given area of your life - e.g. career, health and fitness, relationships - make a list of what's important to you about that area. Better still, get someone else to ask you: "What's important about <area>?" Get them to keep asking you that even past the point where you think you've run out of answers - this is when your deepest motivations often surface. Are these values being satisfied in your life now?

24. Prioritize your values

What's the most important value on that list (if you could only have one?) What's the next most important? Values determine how we spend our time, so in practice only the top six or seven values get significant time devoted to their fulfillment.

25. Resolve values conflicts

If you're not achieving your goals, it can be because two values are in conflict. If you find this, for each value keep asking "What's important about that?" until you reach a higher-level purpose that can satisfy both.

26. Establish if your motivation is 'towards' or 'away from'

For each value, ask yourself "Why is that important?" You may get a 'towards' answer - "Because I love the things it gives me"-or an 'away from' answer - "Because I hate not having it". There can also be 'concealed away forms' - "Because it's better to have it". Better than what? Better than not having it - which is an 'away from'.

27. Focus on what you want, not what you don't want

You tend to get what you focus on, so focus on what you want. 'Away from' motivation can be very powerful and great for getting you out of trouble, but it is directionless ('away' can be any direction) and runs out once you get far enough away from what you don't want. 'Towards' motivation gives you more direction and gets stronger the closer you get to your goal.

28. Make sure your goal is right for you

Does your goal raise your interest and renew your energy levels when you think about it? Will it be good for every area of your life? If not, do you really want it? Is it really your goal?

29. Make what you want more compelling

See yourself achieving your goal. How will you know when you have it? Notice how you feel in response to that picture. If it feels good, make that picture big, bright, colorful and moving, so your good feeling gets stronger. Add some sound. Step into the picture so you are there, and notice how good that feels. Turn those good feelings up even higher - then step back out of it so your goal is ahead of you. This will motivate you to get there.

30. Set your goal for a specific date

Set a date by which you can achieve your goal. This is very important - if you leave the date unspecified, the goal will always be at some vague time in the future and will never happen.

31. Install the goal in your future timeline

Imagine your future stretching out like a line that you could walk along. Take your goal and actually walk out along this imagined line until you get to the date you want it by. Let go of your goal, and let it float down and bed firmly into the timeline. Step into your goal and be there at the achievement of it. Notice how good that feels. Now step beyond your goal, turn around, and looking back down the past timeline, notice the steps you took to get there. Walk back along the line to now, only as quickly as you learn what you need to learn from each step along the way.

32. Set smaller, achievable milestone goals

If you feel overwhelmed by how much you have to do to achieve a task, break it down into smaller, achievable steps (maybe the steps from tip 34).

33. Plan a reward for each step achieved

Decide in advance how you will reward yourself for each milestone you achieve. This will give you additional motivation and prevent you getting disheartened before you achieve your main goal.

34. For things you don't feel like doing, focus on the end result

When people want something done but they don't enjoy the process of doing it - paying bills, doing the washing up they often make it harder for themselves by focusing on how tedious or hard it will be to do it. Instead, focus on how great it will be when you've done it. Imagine those dishes all clean and put away. Tell yourself how good you'll feel. Then just do it!

35. Set up a 'motivation anchor'

Remember a time when you really wanted something. Anchor that process (as in tip 20) and fire off that anchor whenever you need a little boost to get yourself motivated.

Empathy: Being able to sense and respond to emotions in others.

36. Notice visual clues

You already have the unconscious ability to read another person's emotional state from subtle changes in their expression, their movements, their posture, their breathing, and changes in skin colour and muscle tension. You can improve this ability by consciously paying attention to these changes.

37. Notice voice changes

In the same way, people's voice tone, pitch, volume and tempo can tell you a lot about their emotional state. The more you practice listening not just to the words that people say but to the tonal qualities of their voices, the more information about their emotions you will pick up.

38. Notice indicator words

The types of words that people use (as distinct from the content of what they are saying) give a lot of information about what they are feeling. For example, if a person uses words like "ought, must, have to, need to" that suggests they feel compelled to do things that they don't want to. If they use "can't" a lot, they may feel powerless.

39. Clues showing absence of emotion

If a person uses a lot of dry, abstract language, if they speak in a flat monotone, and if their habitual posture tends to lean back, they are probably not very in touch with their feelings and distrust emotions as a source of information.

40. Notice the images their words evoke

What kinds of pictures are conjured up in your mind by the words another person chooses? What kind of metaphors do they use? Are they positive and empowering or upsetting and draining? Their words are clues to their emotional state and what's really on their mind.

41. Put yourself in the other person's shoes

Briefly imagine that you are the other person. See things as they see them, stand as they stand, talk as they would talk, breathe as they breathe. Imagine how things look from their point of view and how the situation would feel from their perspective.

42. Notice your emotional responses

Sometimes we may seem to get a feeling from someone. If this is not 'projection' (tip 10), it could be something that we have unconsciously picked up about how they are feeling.

Social Skills: Being able to deal with other people's emotions and being able to influence and inspire others are essential foundation skills for successful teamwork and leadership.

43. Know what you want from your interaction

Every time you communicate with someone, have a desired outcome even if it's just to establish or maintain contact. That way, you can know when you've achieved what you want.

44. Allow other people to have their emotions

If you accept your own feelings and know you can control them, you will feel much more comfortable with strong emotions in other people. Remember, just like you, they are doing the best they can.

45. Match other people to achieve rapport

You can subtly match some of the aspects of voice, posture and movement that you noticed in tips 40 and 41. As long as it's unobtrusive, it will make the other person feel more comfortable.

46. Rapport the easy way

If the features in tips 40 and 41 seem too many to keep track of and follow the content of what the person is saying, just imagine the person has a motor driving them. Ask yourself "What speed are they running at?" and just match that speed.

47. Talk their language

People who use mainly visual expressions will get the picture more clearly if you also use visual expressions to shed some light for them. If they use mainly feeling or touch-based words, they'll feel more comfortable if you use words they can get a handle on. And if you hear them using sound-related words, it will be music to their ears if you use words which will resonate for them. To make your written communication richer, use a mix of words that appeal to different senses.

48. Dealing with 'difficult' people

If you find a particular person difficult to deal with, adapt tip 8 to guess at how they feel and how you appear to them. Also rise above the situation (tip 21) and look objectively at the interaction between the two of you. These different perspectives will give you extra information and change how you feel about the person (and they will adapt their behavior to reflect that change).

49. In meetings and negotiations, aim for a win/win outcome

Don't get drawn into nitpicking disagreements. Keep yourself and the 'other side' focused on what's really important about your negotiation.

50. Key tip: stay true to yourself. As long as you maintain rapport, others will respond to your passion and commitment.

Summary

All the great leaders know there is a lot of power in their emotions so they make sure to learn how to identify, understand and manage them, and also go ahead to teach those they lead how to do the same. This is referred to as having emotional intelligence and is one of the most important traits for any leader in any modern day organization to have.

22

Occupational Health Hazards and Risks in Livestock Rearing Among Rural Women

Hema Tripathi

(IG and M&E)
Indian Council of Agricultural Research (ICAR), NAHEP, New Delhi

The ICAR / Agriculture Universities are playing key role in addressing the gender issues in agriculture as a whole through development of women friendly technologies, efficient extension system and technical backstopping because of the fact that women are the backbone of as nearly contribute 33% of agriculture workforce and silently adorning myriad roles in agriculture sector from home maker to cultivator and even entrepreneur. Traditionally, managing the home, nurturing and grooming children have been considered to be the primary responsibility of women. Besides attending the household chores, they attend to arduous agricultural operations like sowing, transplanting, weeding, harvesting, threshing, agro processing in crop production and cutting and transportation of fodder, milking, cleaning of cattle shed and making of cow dung cakes in livestock rearing. The role of Indian rural women is increasing evidently due to migration of males to urban areas which is having profound and far-reaching effects.

According to National safety and health law, agriculture is one of the most hazardous occupations worldwide, which includes livestock rearing, breeding of poultry, apiculture and fish farming, manufacture of animal husbandry products besides the tillage of soil, cultivation and harvesting, seed and plant production, forestry work and forest conservation and primary processing of agricultural products. World statistics shows that some 2.3 million women and men around the world succumb to work-related accidents or diseases every year; this corresponds to over 6000 deaths every single day. Worldwide, there are around 340 million occupational accidents and 160 million victims of work-related illnesses annually. The ILO updates these estimates at intervals, and the updates indicate an increase of accidents and ill health. (https://www.ilo.org). In several countries, the fatal accident rate in Agriculture is double the average of all the industries.

Gender inequality

The role of livestock sector in generating employment especially for rural women needs no emphasis. In spite of their immense contribution, she does not receive due recognition. Due to gender stereotypes, they are not treated as equal partners in the family. The major concerns of women are lack of education and technical skills, marriage at an early age, neglect of their health and little or no control over resources. Hence, they are many a times denied opportunities for their development and active participation in society.

Hardships and potential health hazards in livestock rearing

Livestock production and consumption can lead to human health risks which include the diseases transmitted from livestock to humans; environmental pollution; food borne diseases and risks and diet-related chronic diseases etc. Over 150 zoonotic diseases that can be transmitted between animals and humans have been identified worldwide, with approximately 40 significant for human health (Donham 1985). The hotspots for emerging zoonotic diseases exist throughout the world, the high burdens of zoonotic diseases are associated with poor livestock keepers and many of the hotspots are indeed in the developing world. (Ahuja, 2013).

Animal husbandry-the rearing and use of animals-involves a wide variety of activities, including breeding, feeding, moving animals from one location to another, basic care, care for injured animals and activities associated with particular animals (e.g., milking of cows, shearing of sheep, working with draught animals). Such handling of livestock is associated with a variety of injuries and illnesses among humans. These injuries and illnesses may be due to direct exposure or may be due to environmental contamination from animals.

The risk of injury and illness is dependent largely on the type of livestock and on the particulars of animal behaviour. Finally, the specific hazards depend on methods of handling livestock, which have emerged from geographical and social factors that vary across human society. Close association between the worker and the animal, often has unpredictable behaviour, puts the livestock worker at risk. Many livestock have superior size and strength. Injuries are often due to direct trauma from kicking, biting or crushing against a structure and often involve the worker's lower extremity.

The tools, implements and techniques are either defective in design or are not suiting to stature of women invariably leads to various health hazards like injury, fatigue, exhaustion etc The most disturbing aspect of the farm task is excessive spinal loading due to awkward work posture maintained over extended period of time, cardio respiratory strains, skin irritation, allergies, eczema due to use of chemicals and pesticides due to husk and dust particles, cuts, wounds, injuries, congestion, swollen and sore hands and feet, sun stroke, body ache, physical tiredness, psychological fatigue, eye irritation, brucellosis, leptospirosis, animal tuberculosis, pesticide intoxification etc.

The women adopt long static postures for some of the activities which increase the static muscular effort resulting in high physiological cost and low productivity. They perform the activities in their own convenient postures like sitting, standing, bending, and squatting without realizing harmful effects on the body.

Majority of these activities are full of drudgery and have not supported by the mechanical advantages of tools and appliances. Many of these operations involve a lot of physical strain, which do in long run, create health problems particularly those who are above the middle age group. The behavior of workers may also contribute to risk of injury. These constitute important areas not only for further research but also for health promotion programs.

Classification of potential health hazards

Potential health hazards are often classified as physical, chemical, biological, or psychological. Types of human health problems associated with livestock production includes health problems from direct physical contact (Allergic contact dermatitis, allergic rhinitis, bites, kicks, crushing, envenomation and possible hypersensitivity, asthma, scratches, traumatic injury); **Health problems from organic agents** (agrochemical poisoning, antibiotic resistance, chronic bronchitis, contact dermatitis, food-borne illnesses, "Farmer's lung", hypersensitivity pneumonitis, mucous membrane irritation, occupational asthma, organic dust toxic syndrome (ODTS), allergies from pharmaceutical exposures, zoonotic diseases); **Health problems from physical agents** (hearing loss, machinery-related trauma, methane emission and greenhouse effect, musculoskeletal disorders, stress, allergies from drug residue food exposures).

The most frequent hazards related to agriculture are due to machinery (such as tractors, harvesters, use of piercing tools), hazardous chemicals fertilizers and other veterinary products, toxic or allergenic agents (plants, flowers, animal waste etc), carcinogenic substances, transmissible animal diseases (Brucelloses, Bovine tuberculosis, Rabies, Listeriosis), other parasitic diseases (faciolosis, malaria, noise, contact with wild and poisonous animals and ergonomic hazards (use of inadequate equipment's, and tools, unnatural body positions, prolonged static postures, carrying of heavy loads, repetitive work, excessive loading), extreme weather conditions.

Research Base Evidences

To ensure better health and safety and to improve work efficiency and to reduce the health hazards, drudgery, accidents and injuries among rural women, it is important to have an understanding through an empirical data in a gender perspective. Although a number of research work has been carried out and commonly found that women had lack of knowledge and awareness regarding occupational health hazards and risks in livestock rearing activities. They also had lack of knowledge of various diseases associated with their work and implications of being infected with zoonotic diseases and other biological hazards. Females who work in dairy farming had greater self-reported stress and risks of developing hand, wrist, shoulder and low back pain whereas male workers reported more risks in shoulder, upper leg, ankle, feet etc after performing the operations related to breeding, management, health related work and marketing etc. Although both male and female workers were found to be at risk of hazards in livestock farming, females reported greater risk and hazards. Specific interventions to prevent animal-associated hazards should target the women farmers first with intense educational efforts. (Tripathi, 2010; Tripathi, 2015, Tripathi,et al 2017) These constitute important areas not only for further research but also for health promotion programs.

Livestock handlers are at risk for developing respiratory illness from exposure to inhaled dusts. Hair cutters and sheep shearers face several hazards. Cuts and abrasions may result during the shearing operation. Animal hoofs and horns also present potential hazards. Slips and falls are an ever- present hazard while handling the animals. The control of insects on cattle, sheep and goats with pesticide spray or powder can expose workers to the pesticide. Field experiments were conducted on rural women in twelve different villages of Uttar Pradesh and determined their occupational workload and muscular stress based on physiological responses in selected drudgery prone and strenuous activities revealed high physiological workload.

The drudgery index showed highest drudgery in transplanting of paddy followed by chaffing fodder. Introduction of improved tools and techniques saved the cardiac cost to the extent of 16.03% for harvesting, 26.05% for milking, 66.03% for dibbling, 82.88% for hoeing, 29.43% for cleaning of shed and 34% on maize shelling (Tripathi, 2010) & (Kumari et al 2017). Agarwal (2000) emphasized that psychological hazards play very important role and affect the health. Various psychological and behavioural changes like depression, hostility, anxiety and alcoholism may result from frustration, lack of job satisfaction, insecurity, poor human relationship; tension etc. Occupational studies of stress have repeatedly identified farmers as a high-risk group. Meenakshi and Panneer revealed that occupational health hazards have a direct impact on the physical and mental health of women workers and suggested that implementation of social security and welfare measures by the Government for the agricultural women could enhance the health of women workers.

A cross-sectional survey was carried out to determine the hazard exposures of workers of animal related occupations in Abeokuta Southwestern, Nigeria. A total of 230 workers consisting of animal health workers, veterinarians, abattoir workers, livestock keepers, poultry attendants, animal handlers and fish farm workers were randomly surveyed using a well- structured questionnaire. A prevalence of 69.6% occupational hazard exposures was discovered and workers were at risk of myriad of occupational specific and non-specific hazards. 6.5% work related hospitalization was observed among the workers, Thirty-three (14.3%) of the respondents have experienced occupational related diseases/sickness. Workers have average to adequate knowledge of zoonoses but poor knowledge of preventive measures. Employers' responsibilities towards prevention and control of occupational hazards were inadequate. The findings in this study have provided a baseline list of hazards from different occupations in this study area for future researches and also the findings may be useful for developing policies for preventing occupationally-related hazards in animal related establishments (Awosile *et al.*, 2013). A study on knowledge, attitude and practices about zoonosis was done in a rural area of West Bengal by Chattopadhyay and Rashid (1980), revealed that 68.2% of 500 families interviewed did not have knowledge about zoonotic diseases in rural Bengal.

Extension Strategy/intervention/implications to improve the working conditions for minimizing the occupational health hazards and risks while performing various livestock related activities:

Based on the experiences during the field work and available literature, the following specific interventions have been developed that may help in preventing animal-associated injuries which includes intense educational efforts, selecting animals that are more compatible with humans, selecting workers who are less likely to agitate animals and engineering approaches that may decrease the risk of exposure of humans to animals.

- There is need to increase public awareness through creation of public health initiatives for preventive measures and safety precautions to minimize the hazards.

- A plan can be developed based on the identified self-reported hazards and risks to use available resources to address the greatest need first. Here education of farmers, farm women and other stakeholders on possible reasons and risks in livestock rearing - including closer interaction with extension workers may pave a way for better provision to researchers and policy makers of information on farming activities.
- Guidelines may be developed on the safety measures for handling and rearing of livestock in framing effective and holistic messages for the various stakeholders.
- Continued collaboration is essentially required between researchers, policy makers, farmers, non-governmental organizations, and other stakeholders in the promotion of safe rearing of livestock in rural areas.
- Waste management is one of the key challenges faced by livestock farmers. If not properly managed, animal waste can be a significant source of human health hazards, and is one of the major public health concerns. Therefore, appropriate technologies are required in treatment and recycling of animal waste as manure, or feed utilizing best practices in the region.
- Infected animals often shed infectious agents in their faeces, urine and other bodily fluids. The agents may contaminate feed, water and housing. To reduce the risk of spreading disease, a manure plan is needed to install to prevent environmental contamination, removal of manure frequently from animal tying area/shed and holding areas to prevent completion of life cycles by parasites and flies to control the fly population by removing manure, using insecticides, using biological predators (wasps) or combinations as control measures.
- Most of the men and women in rural areas had inadequate knowledge regarding transmission of disease from domestic animals. However, these diseases can be prevented if they have adequate knowledge regarding these diseases. Hence there is a need to disseminate the knowledge up gradation programs for them where domestic animals are more prevalent particularly in the rural areas.
- To bring change, the livestock and human health sectors is needed to work together more closely. The livestock sector should develop and build clear guidelines in local languages on ways/methods of rearing the domestic animals that promote healthier production practices for reducing exposure to hazards.
- Improper disposal of dead animal /carcasses can be a hazard to people and other animals. To minimize the contamination and risk of spreading disease, owners need to be educated the proper method of disposal, immediately after

death, including all contaminated bedding, milk, manure or feed to prevent scavenging by dogs, cats, birds, foxes, including cleaning of protective cloths and disinfecting the area that was occupied by the dead cattle.

- Demonstration and training awareness camps may be organized to improve livestock practices/ technologies on minimizing the health hazards along with precautionary measures should be available in the villages.
- Posters specifying the clear messages may be displayed on the public places in the villages to minimize the risks of health hazards
- Educate on washing of hands before milking and after working with sick animals, wearing of protective plastic or rubber gloves for calving cows, control / minimize the movement of stray animals in animal shed, timely vaccinating the animals against contagious diseases including the dogs and diseases common in the area may help in decrease in spread of contaminants
- Solutions to reduce ergonomic risk include intensified educational efforts focused upon appropriate handling of animals, as well as engineering efforts to redesign the work environment is needed.
- Women need to be educationally empowered regarding the availability and proper handling of appropriate Labor-saving technologies (LSTs) technologies which can enhance their productivity and income through livestock farming.
- It is recommended to institute a comprehensive programme on appropriate interventions including the capacity building programs for the women with respect to age to educate them at doorstep about the severity of effects of these hazards and the safety precautions and the appropriate measures to reduce the burden of injury, risks and hazards. Training programmes should be formulated by considering some important aspects like duration, time (season), place, month and interval of training as per the responses recorded by the farmers.

Conclusion

Occupational safety and health in livestock rearing is needed to be addressed multifaceted with well-defined strategy/interventions and must be integrated in the rural development policy with special reference to small scale livestock farming.

Theme-02

Applied Extension and Communication Strategies for Sustainable Livelihood Through Animal Husbandry and Allied Farming System

23

Mass Communication Through Community Radio Station in Agriculture

Debabrata Basu

Department of Agricultural Extension
Bidhan Chandra Krishi Viswavidyalaya, Nadia, West Bengal

Introduction

A community radio station is characterized by its ownership and programming and the community it is authorized to serve. It is owned and controlled by anon-profit organization whose structure provides for membership, management, operation and programming primarily by members of the community at large. Its programming should be based on community access and participation and should reflect the special interests and needs of the listenership it is licensed to serve.

While community radio is a form of public-service broadcasting, it has an approach that is different from conventional broadcasting. Its specific focus is to make its audience the main protagonists, by their involvement in all aspects of its management and programme production, and by providing them with programming that will help them in the development and social advancement of their community.

Background

The success of agricultural development programmes in developing countries largely depends on the nature and extent of use of mass media in mobilization of people for agricultural development. The planners in developing countries realize that the development of agriculture could be hastened with the effective use of mass media. Radio and television have been acclaimed to be the most effective media for diffusing the scientific knowledge to the masses. In a country like India, where literacy level among the farm population is low, the choice of communication media is of vital importance. In this regard the television and radio are significant, as they transfer modern agricultural and information technology to literate and illiterate farmers alike even in interior or rural areas within short time.

Among the several mass media, newspaper and farm magazine are still commonly used. They have a vital role to play in the communication of agricultural information among the literate farmers. Increasing rate of literacy in the country offers new promises and prospects for utilizing print medium as a means of mass communication. The print media widened the scope of communication. It is cheap and people can afford to buy and read them at their convenience. It is a permanent medium in that the message are imprinted permanently with high storage value which makes them suitable for reference and research.

The Evolution of Community Radio

The pioneering experiences from which today's community radio has evolved began some 50 years ago in Latin America. Poverty and social injustice were the stimulus for those first experiences, one beginning in Bolivia in 1947 and known as the Miners' radios and another in Colombia in the same year, known as Radio Sutatenza/ accióncultural Popular. These experiences in Bolivia and Colombia set a trend, even if today's concept of community radio has evolved considerably. For example, the Miners' radios in Bolivia were working in the decades of ideological clash between Marxism and capitalism. Thus, their principal focus was to unite the community of miners to battle for better and fairer working conditions. They were generally considered to be trade union radios, even if the miners provided much of the finance for the purchase of equipment and running costs. Radio Sutatenza/ACPO in Colombia, although inspired by the aim of supporting the community of peasants, was not owned or directly managed by them. There was much feedback from peasants – some 50,000 letters a year – and these certainly ensured the integration of the peasants' desires and needs into the radio's programming. But it was not truly 'radio by the people for the people', which is today's aim. Even so, this first systematic effort by Radio Sutatenza to educate by radio created a movement that "...spread and was later consolidated through ALER, the Latin American Educational Radio Broadcasting Association. This inter-linkage of radio and education is basic to the idea of public service and marked the birth of community media in Latin America.".

However, even if the groundbreaking work was in Latin America, it was in Europe that community radio first became a vital phenomenon, an alternative to – or a critique of – mainstream broadcast media. The first challenges to state public service broadcasting were in the 1960s-70s when "swashbuckling entrepreneurs boarded the airwaves illegally and seized as much of the audience as they could carry away from the treasure chest monopoly controlled by the state." In the West, these pirate stations proved a catalyst in motivating governments and national broadcasting systems to introduce legitimate local radio. In Africa, the establishment of community radio became, in a broad sense, a social movement after the demise of the apartheid regime in South Africa. This was followed by democratization, decentralization, and to some extent structural adjustment, elsewhere in that continent. The pressure groups that have instigated community radio in many parts of the world (e.g. Miners, pirate radio operators, missionaries and democracy movements) have been less present in Asia. In their place, international agencies such as UNESCO and other external donors have often taken initiatives to help get community radio off the ground. And in some cases, it has been the national broadcasting organization that has itself started community radio services. Community radio arguably demystifies the broadcaster's profession by taking community members as message producers. It is also a school for fledgling broadcasters, where they, of course, acquire valuable technical skills. But there is another factor that makes people trained in community radio particularly valuable. They are podcasters who live among their listeners, share many of the same problems and get constant feedback-positive and negative - on the formats of their programmes and on their interest and usefulness this gives them unique insights into the broadcaster /audience relationship and into radio as a tool for change and development. It is not uncommon; therefore, for community broadcasters go on to join the staff of mainstream broadcasting.

Principles of public access and participation

Citizens have a democratic right to reliable, accurate, and timely information. Based on this right, it is a public interest of broadcasting that it should incorporate the principles of access and participation. Access implies the availability of broadcasting services to all citizens; participation implies that the public is actively involved in planning and management, and also provides producers and performers. In concrete terms, for community radio these concepts mean that:

- A community radio's broadcast pattern reaches all members of the community it aims to serve;
- The community participates in formulating plans and policies for the radio service and in defining its objectives, its principles of management, and its programming;
- The community participates in decisions concerning programme content, duration and schedules People select the types of programmes they want, rather than having them prescribed by the producers;
- The community is free to comment and criticize;

- There is continuous interaction between producers and receivers of messages. The radio itself acts as a principal channel for this interaction, but there are also mechanisms that allow easy contact between the community the programme producers, and the management of the radio station;
- There are unrestricted opportunities for members of the community, as individuals or groups, to produce programmes, and be helped by the radio station staff, using the technical production facilities available;
- The community participates in the establishment, management, administration and financing of the radio station.

Essential Features of Community Radio

- **The Audience as Protagonists**

While community radio is a form of public-service broadcasting, it has an approach that is different from conventional broadcasting. Its specific focus is to make its audience the main protagonists, by their involvement in all aspects of its management and programme production, and by providing them with programming that will help them in the development

And social advancement of their community.

- **A special slant on news, entertainment and education**

Entertainment is provided in a form that is a collective cultural expression, rather than a featuring of refined performers. It is more like singing Karaoke than listening to a professional artist. Education is more the sharing of experiences and learning from others in the community than listening to an expert or teacher talking.

- **Ownership**

The facilities of community radio are almost invariably owned by the community through a trust, foundation, cooperative, or some similar vehicle. However, there could be cases where formal ownership was in the hands of a body external to the community, but which has passed the facility to the community for its independent and exclusive use.

- **Management**

Irrespective of formal ownership, the station's policies, management, and programming must be the responsibility of the community in order for it to be considered a true community radio. There will usually be a representative community committee, or Board of Directors, to set overall policies.

- **Inclusion of minority and marginalized groups**

Community radio includes minority and marginalized groups on equal terms, rather than giving them an equal opportunity to participate.

- **Representation of different groups and interests in the community**

Communities are inevitably made up of different groups and interests. Community radio broadcasts programmes that cater to these and also encourages them to express themselves on air. Clearly, however, programme and time allocation are approximately proportional to the size of any particular group or interest in the community, taking into account any special circumstances or needs.

- **Principles of public access and participation**

Citizens have a democratic right to reliable, accurate, and timely information. Based on this right, it is a public interest of broadcasting that it should incorporate the principles of access and participation

- **Funding**

A community radio service is set up and run as a non-profit organization. It relies on financial support from a diversity of sources, which may include donations, grants, membership fees, sponsorship or advertising. A combination of these is the most desirable in order to ensure independence. Many community radios also organize fund-raising events among their audience. The overall aim is always to reach a state of financial self-sufficiency.

Functions of community radio in general

- Reflect and Promote Local Identity, Character, and Culture
- Create a Diversity of Voices and Opinions on the Air
- Culture is also Language:
- Encourage Open Dialogue and Democratic Process
- Promote Development and Social Change
- People in poor communities
- Encourage Participation, Sharing of Information and Innovation
- Promote Good Governance
- Promote Civil Society
- Give voices to voiceless

Relevance of community radio in Indian agriculture

- Can target local indigenous and grassroots technologies and networking the community

- Create and sustain networks between researcher and field
- Help in conservation and protection of biodiversity
- Providing appropriate markets to farmers
- Catering solutions to problems related to production, processing, markets, livelihoods etc.

Some examples of Indian community radio

- Krishi Community Radio Station 90.4 FM of Dharwad (UAU)
- AID in Jharkand
- Kutch Mahila Vikas Sangathan in Bhuj, Pastapur (Decacan Development Society in A.P)
- NammaDhwani Community Radio in Kolar district of Karnataka

There are many community radio stations serving the needs of Indian farmers. Among them the Sangham Radio, a community radio was launched in Telangana (earlier in Andhra Pradesh), India, on World Rural Women's Day that is on October 15, 2008 by the Deccan Development Society, a non-governmental organization (NGO) that works with 100 groups of the economically poorest Dalit women. This CR radio is owned, managed, and operated exclusively by women from rural marginalized communities (the "Dalit" caste). The radio broadcasts covers 25 kms that includes 100 villages. The programme content of broadcast includes news and views of local people, tips on herbal medicines, news and reports on farming tools of agriculture, folk songs, stories etc.

The themes include seed sovereignty and women; food sovereignty and women; women and biodiversity; women and land, ownership; women and ecological agriculture; ecological enterprises for women, healthcare and plant medicines; creating awareness about child education and its importance, legal education for women etc. DDS helps the farming communities and women specially in many ways including-getting credit and linking women to banks, conducting participatory natural resource documentation and planning exercises, overcoming resistance from men and upper castes, trying to get women ownership over or rights to lands they are cultivating (Kothari, 2015). The community radio provides a lot of information on the dangers of chemicals, fertilizers, hybrid and genetically modified seeds. It also helps the women and other farmers in marketing of their organic produce through a cooperative called Sangham Organics. Krishi Community Radio is established on May 17th, 2007 by the University of Agricultural Sciences, Dharwad in Karnataka. It covers in 15-20 km area in and around the University.

The CR is completely dedicated to the service of agriculture and the rural community, keeping in mind the largest economic growth sector and broad in the rural community. The community radio station is engaged in active involvement of farmers in production of programmes. It creates a platform for the farmers and also looks at preserving local culture of the farmers. A study was conducted by Madhu et al in 2009-10 to analyze the impact of the Krishi Community radio on its listeners. According to them the CR-gives useful information on agriculture as the major reason followed by-information on pesticides, helps to adopt new agricultural technologies, information about new varieties and increases knowledge (Madhu et al 2012).

The community radio also helping the listeners in gaining knowledge about-improvised varieties of seeds, seed treatment, seed selection, storage, better methods of agricultural practices, control of pesticides and diseases and harvesting technique (Madhu et al 2012). Another community radio Sharada Krishi Vahini launched on January 18, 2011. It was launched by Krishi Vigyan Kendra, in Pune, This CR is funded by the Agriculture Technology Management Agency (ATMA) scheme of the Government of India and the station also receives funding by broadcasting local advertisements. It provides latest information in the field of agriculture to the farming community in and around 25 km from Krishi Vigyan Kendra, Baramati. It provides a platform for the farmers, farm women to share their experiences, skills, art, problems and needs to their other farmers and farm communities. Farmers, Self Help Groups (SHG), students, doctors, local artists, agriculture businesspersons, teachers, experts in agriculture participate in programme production.

The programme producers of the stations goes around the farmers in villages in collecting information about their problems of livelihood, their farming techniques and experiences and record them and broadcasted on the CRS. The CRS also records local folk songs from the members of the community and they were played in the CRS. The CRS airs information by agriculture scientists and experts to help the farmers to improve their farming. The CR also broadcast programmes on human health, market prices and weather forecasts. A study of Sharada Krishi Vahini revealed that-a majority of the farmers (67%) preferred agricultural success story programme followed by live interactive program (62%) and phone in programme (57.50%). A majority of the farmers were interested in programme like rainfall prediction, agricultural news, disease and pest predictions and inputs availability (Indian Agricultural Research Institute). Vasundhara Krishi Vahini community radio station was launched on April 2004 by Vidya Pratishthan Institute of Information Technology (VIIT), Baramati, Maharashtra. It focuses on the socio, economic development of the farming community in its region. It was launched to bridge the gap existing in terms of information needs of the farmers.

A study was conducted by Mahekhka (2007-08) for her dissertation to Mudra Institute of Communication, Ahmadabad to analyze the communication gap if any that exists between the providers of the initiative and the beneficiaries and the role of Vasudhara Krishi Vahini CR in it. It caters the farmers by providing a lot of information relating to agriculture like new varieties of seeds, updated commodity rates, weather forecasts, various pesticides and medicines, animal diseases and information on research done by the scientists from various agricultural universities. It airs Bhumiputra a programme on success stories of farmers, Shashandarbarprogramme on governmental schemes, Pashudhan-Dairy and animal husbandry, krushisandesh –weather report and agricultural advices for the benefit of farmers. According the study the CR-can leverage and empower the community with a platform to address their issues. It can not only be used for addressing the issues and information needs of the farming community but also for providing social development to the entire community (Mahekhka,2007-08). It is providing -social, economic and cultural development (Mahekhka, 2007-08). There is a few more community radio stations established for the purpose of promoting agriculture in the country. They are Allahabad Agricultural Institute Deemed University, Uttar Pradesh launched a community radio station called Radio Adanto promote agriculture. It engages villagers and farmers in programme production to increase their knowledge in various fields of agricultural crops/ produces.

The themes of the programming include agriculture, health care, hygiene and social issues as they are relevant to for the community members. The programmes are produced with the help of agriculture experts with an aim to inform and educate the farmers. The primary aim of the Radio Adan is to empower its listeners with skills and capacities to enhance their agricultural incomes and strengthen their livelihoods and other security opportunities. Another community radio station Pantnagar Janvani was launched on August 15, 2011 by Govind Ballabh (G.B.) Pant University of Agriculture & Technology in Uttarakhand. It reaches more than 80 villages in the radius. The community radio station was launched to create a platform for the rural people and to use the radio as a tool of participatory development at grassroots level. Along with that the community radio disseminates agricultural information to promote sustainable development.

The radio as part of extension and communication efforts by the university disseminates the relevant need based research and technological information to the farmers and allied beneficiaries. The programming of the radio station includes agriculture, animal husbandry, fishery, health and other issues. One more community radio Chaudhary Charan Singh (CCS) Haryana Agricultural University in Haryana called CCS Radio. The CR was launched to disseminate technology related to agriculture and its allied sciences among the farmers, farm women and rural youth. The programmes of the station not only interest them but also benefit them with the information which they acquire from the station broadcast. The station was launched with the infrastructure and other support provided by the Ministry of Information and Broadcasting. The station broadcasts success stories of farmers to motivate them. These stories help the listeners (farmers) in knowing the problems faced and helps them in finding out the ways for solving them. Along with that, the radio broadcasts agricultural information on day-to-day, monthly basis and seasonal basis. The broadcasting programmes includes _do‘ and _don‘t‘ of agriculture, knowledge of new seeds, fertilizers and pesticides, rabi and kharif crops, remedies for various plant diseases. It also includes veterinary and animal husbandry information, dairying and animal products. The —farmers, farm women, scientists of university and people residing in the coverage area participate in programme production.

TANU e-Community radio (Tamil Nadu Agricultural University) launched in October 2009. It covers 15 to 20 kms radius. It was established with the help of World Development Foundation (WDF) (a NGO based in Delhi) and Media Lab Asia (MLA) (it has been promoted by The Department of Electronics and Information Technology, MCIT, Government of India as a non-profit company). Both WEF and MLA joined together through a Memorandum of Association and started community radio stations for enhancing the life of poor and marginalized sections. The e-community radio was launched to provide information for farmers which benefit them. It uploads information on TNA Agri Portal for wider coverage and to effectively reach its audience. The TNAU e-radio is integrated into the University e-extension network and it aims to compile, record, edit and fine tune the content of the technologies for the benefit of farmers, farm women, youth and other stakeholders in the broad domain of agriculture and rural development. Kisanvani, a community radio station established as an extension tool by the Indian Society of Agribusiness Professionals (ISAP) a Delhi based NGO established for community development. The CR reaches surrounding 350 villages. The ISAP also runs a Kisan Call Centre which is located in Bhopal. The CR was launched on September 30, 2009 in Madhya Pradesh. The CR station covers entirely farm specific useful information, social issues of the community, important announcement from the government departments along with information on various schemes of government departments and banks. It covers agricultural information, market information (market prices), weather, health programmes, government schemes and subsidies etc. The programme formats include Drama, Folk Songs, Farmers choice (includes phone-in, farmer talk, farmer goshtietc), interview with personality (include persons from agriculture, medical, administration, public figure, health, food etc), live play, special features on various occasion like festivals, world literacy day, women's day, children's day, tuberculosis day, independence day, republic day and so on. The community radio also broadcasts farmers and community benefit schemes and programmes in the state and central supported by the government in the state (i.e Madhya Pradesh) and around the country. The local community is benefiting with the CR services as it covers a wide range of topics that are required by farmers. It acts as advisory instrument on plat protection, irrigation, market prices of commodities, credit and finance for farmers, bank schemes along with some programmes mend for promoting health and education.

Conclusion

Community radio which are established specifically for the promotion of agriculture in the country pays special attention to rural development and agriculture. As a radio set is an affordable and accessible medium for many in rural India and it also can run with the battery as many of the farmers can carry the radio set with them to their fields and listen to the station. It is proved as an effective medium in conveying farm/ agricultural messages to its listeners. CR stations have started with a motive to promote agriculture have become very popular among the agricultural community as it provides them information about weather, new technologies, pesticides, agricultural inputs, information on seed varieties, market rates and new farming techniques etc. Kakade (2013) concludes that a large percentage of farmers opined that the information which broadcast through agricultural radio programmes as practically applicable and reliable. Kujur et al (2009) concludes that most of the farmers felt that the information provided in Kisanvani (community radio) could be actually practices/ adopted but the degree of adoption varied from year to year. Kothari, (2015) says that Sangham Radio (community radio) provides a lot of information on the dangers of chemicals, fertilizers, hybrid and genetically modified seeds. It also helps the women and other farmer members in marketing of their organic produce. Madhu et al (2012) concludes that Krishi Community Radio provides useful information on agriculture and pesticides helps in adopting new agricultural technologies by farmers and create awareness about new varieties and increases knowledge. It also helps the listeners in gaining knowledge about —improved varieties of seeds, seed treatment, seed selection, storage, and better methods of agricultural practices, control of pesticides and diseases and harvesting techniques (Madhu *et. al.,* 2012). The study of Sharada Krishi Vahini revealed that-a majority of the farmers (67%) preferred agricultural success story programme followed by live interactive program (62%) and phone in programme (57.50%). A majority of the farmers were interested in programme like rainfall prediction, agricultural news, disease and pest predictions and inputs availability (Indian Agricultural Research Institute). The study on Vasundhara Krishi Vahini community radio concludes that the CR is providing-social, economic and cultural development (Mahekhka, 2007-08).Community radio (agricultural) impact studies proved that the CR is an essential medium in conveying the farm related information to farm community.

24

Approaches for Impact Evaluation of Extension Programmes

Souvik Ghosh

Department of Agricultural Extension, PalliSiksha Bhavana (Institute of Agriculture), Visva-Bharati University, Sriniketan Birbhum-731236, West Bengal

Monitoring and Evaluation are the two management tools that help in keeping a control on the extension programmes as well as raising the level of performance. Monitoring refers to an organized process of overseeing and checking the activities undertaken in a project, to ascertain whether it is capable of achieving the planned results or not. Conversely, evaluation is a scientific process that gauges the success of the projector programme in meeting the objectives. The primary difference between monitoring and evaluation is that while monitoring is a continuous activity, performed at the functional level of management, evaluation is a periodic activity, performed at the business level.

Evaluation in a broad sense is concerned with the effectiveness of a programme. Evaluation has been defined in many ways, although the central focus in all the definitions is the same. UNDP in 2002 has defined evaluation as a selective exercise that attempts to systematically and objectively assess progress towards and the achievement of an outcome. World Bank has defined evaluation as systematic and objective assessment of an ongoing or completed project or programme, and its design, implementation and results. The aim is to determine the relevance and fulfillment of objectives, development efficiency, effectiveness, impact, and sustainability (ICAR, 2020).

Impact evaluation is done to find out causal effect/relationship between a programme and a set of outcomes. An impact evaluation tries to find out whether a programme is responsible for changes in outcomes. The outcomes of agricultural development programme, for example, are to improve farm livelihood, raise farm income, improve farmer's knowledge, attitude and skills, reduce input cost, etc. The programme managers and policy makers focus only on measuring the inputs and outputs of a programme, for example, against the budgetary allotment how much money has been spent, how many frontline demonstrations have been laid, how many training programmes or farmers field schools have been organized, instead of finding whether agricultural development programmes have achieved their goals and improving farmers wellbeing and livelihoods (ICAR, 2020).

Myths About Evaluation

Several evaluation myths have often discouraged extension managers from engaging in useful evaluation (Deshler, 1997).

Myth 1: Evaluate only when mandated. Many funded programmes require evaluation as a form of accountability. However, it is a myth that evaluation should occur only if it is mandated. On the contrary, evaluations that are self-initiated are more likely to be taken seriously for immediate programme improvement. Programmes become responsible and excellent just as often through self-initiated evaluation.

Myth 2: Evaluation is an add-on. It is a myth that evaluation is an add-on activity or at most a pre-test with a post-test. It is most meaningful when it is integrated with decision making at every stage of programme planning and operation (Patton, 1991).

Myth 3: Evaluation is an activity for experts. It is a myth that evaluation should be undertaken only by technical experts. However, systematic evaluation can be undertaken by inexperienced managers, and specialists and educators themselves can be helped to critique their own work.

Myth 4: Outside evaluators are best. It is a myth that evaluation should be done only by external evaluators. Yes, external evaluators are often useful in challenging insiders to address what they have overlooked because of their near-sightedness. However, internal, self-initiated, and subjectively oriented evaluations also can be rigorous and valuable. In fact, because they often are participatory in generating, analyzing, and interpreting data, they may result in greater acceptability of the findings and recommendations.

Myth 5: There is one best evaluation approach. Another myth is that there is one best way to conduct an extension programme evaluation. Some approaches are probably better than others for addressing particular types of questions or concerns. However, various types of evaluation approaches have their own strengths and limitations. Some situations require quantification and measurement, while others require qualitative, descriptive, and subjective data.

Myth 6: Quantitative data are best. A mixed-methods approach combining qualitative and quantitative methods can lead to better understanding and appreciation of phenomena under evaluation and provide triangulation, convergence, and corroboration of results from different methods. Qualitative methods are best for understanding the nature of something, while quantitative methods help in appreciating its extent.

Major Elements in Evaluation

There are at least five major elements in most evaluations:

1. Focused questions
2. Objects or events to be evaluated
3. Data or evidence
4. Analysis and interpretation using judgment perspectives
5. Judgments, conclusions, or findings.
6. Purposes and approaches or models may vary, but these elements will be present in one form or another.

Process of Evaluation

Evaluation is usually focused to judge the effectiveness, efficiency and sustainability of a programme. It is intended to provide feedback in order to modify and improve future programmes. The procedures for conducting evaluation are:

(a) Analysis of situation

(b) Planning the study

(c) Collection of data

(d) Analysis of data

(e) Presentation of results

The steps in evaluation process are as under

(a) Defining the purpose for which evaluation efforts are being made that may be programme improvement, accountability and knowledge generation.

(b) Defining the issue in form of structure of the programme, its design and intended results.

(c) Selecting a model to be followed for taking up the evaluation. The models can be classified in three categories: effectiveness models, economic models and professional models. The models have to be decided based on the purpose of evaluation and specific issue to address.

(d) Choosing the right method for evaluation amongst different qualitative and quantitative methods.

Types of Evaluation

Based upon the object under evaluation and its purpose, evaluation can be classified into various types:

Every day evaluation: It happens every day. The observation and drawing inference are everyday evaluation. These may happen by individual contacts, meetings, discussions etc. Simple observation or inference is a casual type of evaluation.

Informal evaluation: It is also known as informal studies. It involves review and analysis of information from secondary sources like annual reports, survey and PRA studies. Informal studies are conducted to simply compare the present with past performance of any programme. It is the most common of evaluation in social work and community activities.

Formal studies: It is scientific in plan and carried out to provide objective information as a basis for achieving the objective or the effectiveness of the methods used. The formal studies follow the scientific procedure for data collection, analysis, use of statistical methods to draw conclusions.

Formative evaluation: Formative evaluations are conducted during programme development and implementation. These are useful when directions are sought on bow to achieve goals or Improvement in programme. Formative evaluations thus strengthen and improve the object being evaluated (ICAR, 2020). Formative evaluation includes need assessment, evaluability assessment, structured conceptualization, implementation evaluation and process evaluation.

Summative evaluation: Summative evaluations examine the effects or outcomes of some object. They summarize it by explaining the consequences of the programme or technology delivery. They are meant to assess the causal effect of an object to lead to the outcome. Summative evaluation further aids-in determining the overall impact of the causal factor beyond only the immediate target outcomes; and estimating the relative costs associated with the object (ICAR, 2020). Summative evaluation includes outcome evaluation, impact evaluation, cost-effectiveness and cost-benefit analysis, secondary analysis and meta-analysis.

There are different models of evaluation which can be used for evaluating extension programme.

Logsdon (1975) suggested three models of evaluation:

Experimental method: It is characterized by random selection from a large pool of population to their assigned group and their control group. In other words, to have this type of evaluation, we have to take two groups (i) programme group and (ii) control group. When we compare the difference between these two groups, the impact is determined.

Survey of subjective opinions and skills learned: In this model, objective tests of the skills learned can be given before and after the programme. The difference between after and before programme reveals the effect of the programme.

Group process model: In this model, a series of group discussions are made at all levels of hierarchy. Out of discussion the inference is drawn. Brack(1975) listed four models for evaluation of extension programme:

Controlled field experiment: In this model, variables are manipulated and their effects on other variables are observed. Here, we need the knowledge of research design. It is a difficult method but gives more accuracy.

Goal-free evaluation: According to this model, the evaluation is made not only for the objective but anything emerges as a result of programme completion.

Transactional evaluation: In this case, a transact of the population involving in programme are drawn and information collected from them to draw the inference. The evaluator must be familiar with, and skilled at inter-personal relations.

Adversary model: In this case, the decision maker listens the positive and negative effects and draws the conclusion. Stuffle beam (1971) suggested four models (CIPP model) on which evaluation can be made:

Context evaluation: This model of evaluation is concerned with social structure and power structure related to programme action to draw the conclusion. It mainly emphasizes on surrounding environment as contributing factors in programme outcomes. Context assesses needs, problems and opportunities within a defined environment.

Input evaluation: This evaluation makes analysis of resource use and output obtained. The resource input may be human resource, programme activities, facilities, equipment and needed training. Input evaluation assesses competing strategies, work plans and budgets of approaches chosen for implementation.

Process evaluation: In this type of evaluation, the process and procedure followed in planning and execution of the programme are examined. Process evaluation monitors, documents and assesses activities, and also helps in carrying out improvement efforts to maintain accountability records of their execution of action plans.

Product evaluation: Product evaluation is concerned with outcome of total programme. It may be physical power or internal resources. The product evaluation assesses the programme may be in terms of production and productivity or knowledge, skills and attitude. Product evaluation identifies and assesses short-term, long-term, intended, and unintended outcomes.

Clark (1960) proposed Objective-based Evaluation. This model is simple and involves five steps as follows:

(a) Selecting the objective

(b) Selecting the critical properties of the objective

(c) Making critical properties as operational as possible

(d) Using critical properties to prescribe materials and instruction

(e) Using critical properties to prescribe evaluation

Kirkpatrick /Phillips model (1996) is used in analyzing and evaluating the results of training and educational programmes. This model can be implemented before, throughout, and following training to show the value of training programmes. The five levels followed in the model are as follows:

Level I: Reaction - At this level, trainees' reaction to the training programme is measured. It is important to measure reaction of trainees because it helps in understanding how well the training was received by the participants.

Level 2: Learning - At this level, the extent of increase in trainees' knowledge as a result of the training is measured.

Level 3: Behaviour - At this level, change in trainees' behaviour as a result of the training programme is measured. Specifically, it looks at how trainees apply the acquired knowledge.

Level 4: Results - At this level, final results of the training programme are analysed. It includes outcomes that the organization determines to be good for its objectives and employees.

Level 5: Return on investment - ROI is the ultimate level of evaluation. It compares the monetary benefits from the programme with the programme costs. Although the ROI can be expressed in several ways, it is usually presented as a percentage or cost/benefit ratio.

The formula for ROI is:

(Total programme benefits - Total programme costs) × 100% / Total programme costs (ICAR, 2020)

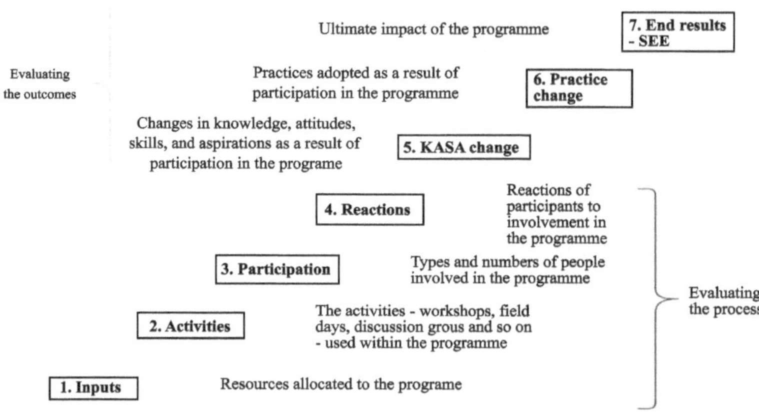

Fig. 1. Hierarchy of Programme Evaluations (Bennett, 1975)

Evaluation hierarchy of Claude Bennett (1975) is a useful evaluation model consisting of seven categories for planning and evaluating extension programmes. According to it, chain of events begins with (i) inputs followed by (ii) programme and activities (iii) programme delivery and client participation (iv) clients' reactions/satisfactions (v) changes in knowledge, attitudes, skills and aspirations (vi) changes in practices and (vii) end results (improved social, economic and environmental condition) with which chain of events ends. As the hierarchy is ascended, evidence of programme impact becomes stronger. Although change in knowledge, attitudes, skills and aspiration (KASA) is a key category in the hierarchy, the major emphasis of the model is laid upon practice change and end results (ICAR, 2020).

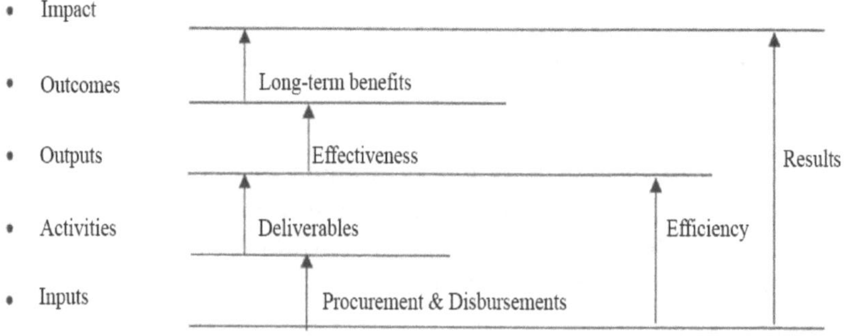

Fig. 2a Result Hierarchy in the casual chain

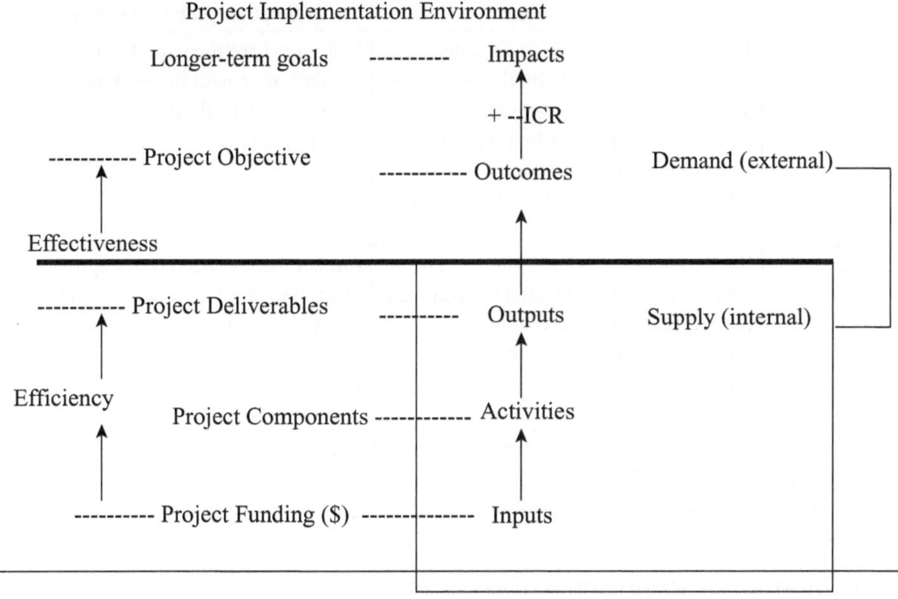

Fig. 2b Demand and supply side effects in the result chain

Source: Alex and Byeriee, Monitoring and Evaluation for AKIS Projects, World Bank, 2000

The terminology used in the results frame work is defined in the following Table.

Table 1. Results Framework Terminology Defined

Terms	Explanation	Relevance to causal chain*
Inputs	Financial, human, and other resources mobilized to support activities undertaken by a project	Inputs are converted into activities by the implementing agency
Activities	Action taken or work performed by which inputs are converted into specific outputs.	Activities are designed to deliver outputs. Through intermediate deliverables each activity will have a deliverable at the end of a specified time interval
Outputs	Project deliverables (on the supply-side) that are expected to add value for potential users and are designed to stimulate development out comes (on the demand-side) based on the causal chain.	Outputs are designed to stimulate outcomes. One output may result from more than one activity & even more than one objective.

(Contd.)

Terms	Explanation	Relevance to causal chain*
Outcomes	Expected or actual demand-side behavioral responses by the end users and other stakeholders outside the control of the project that demonstrate uptake, adoption and use of project outputs—thus validating the causal chain	Outcomes are measured before the end of project implementation which will fulfill one or more of clients demands
IImpact	Positive and negative, primary and secondary long-term effects produced by a development intervention, directly or indirectly, intended or unintended.	Impacts' are expected to begin after the end of implementation as an extension of the project's causal chain (and are typically measured 5 years after the end of implementation).

* The causal chain refers to inputs to activities to outputs (Supply side)and outcomes producing impacts(Demand side) in Fig.2.

Source: Adapted from Alex & Byeriee, Monitoring & Evaluation for AKIS Projects, World Bank, 2000

Major Models for Programme Evaluation

Several models are suggested for extension programme evaluation (Deshler, 1997):

Expert Model: This approach relies on expert judgment (Eisner, 1983). Usually, documentation is prepared in advance of experts' visits. The experts then interview, analyze documents, and make judgments using their own judgment perspectives or those set as standards by the outside organizations or stakeholders.

Goal-Free Model: This approach assumes that outside evaluators do not know, or need to know, what the programme has intended to accomplish, but that it is the task of the evaluators to uncover what is actually happening relative to farmers' interests regardless of stated goals and intentions. The focus point is to identify environmental and farming conditions and then to compare these needs with what people are actually experiencing as a result of the extension programme. The gap is then viewed as a starting point for making changes in the programme. This approach relies heavily on open-ended interviewing and observation by persons who do not have a vested interest in the programme (Scriven, 1972).

Attainment of Objectives Model: This approach assumes that the success of a programme can be determined by measuring a programme's outcomes against its own goals and objectives. This type of evaluation begins with clarifying measurable objectives and then gathering data that validate the extent to which these objectives have been met. For this model to be credible, an essential feature should be added, namely, the evaluation of the appropriateness of goals and objectives, given the circumstances and needs of farmers. This model also has a "black box" limitation in that it tends to ignore the extension process, thereby failing to provide explanations for outcomes (Provus, 1971).

Management Decision Model: The purpose of this model is to provide relevant information as a management tool to decision makers. It assumes that evaluation should be geared to decisions during programme initiation and operation stages to make results more relevant at each particular stage. Participation of stakeholders is central to the process because evaluation should serve their decisions. One limitation of this model is the tendency for the decisions of major stakeholders to be viewed as more important than those of various types of farmers, especially women in agriculture who may not benefit directly from such an evaluation unless care is taken.

Naturalistic Model: This model assumes that a programme is a natural experiment and that the purpose of evaluation is to understand how the programme is operating in its natural environment. There is an assumption that programmes are negotiated realities among the significant stakeholders and that evaluation serves this value-laden negotiation (Cronbach, 1981; Guba & Lincoln, 1989).

Experimental Model: The purpose of this approach is to determine whether changes in programme outcomes (learning accomplishments) were due to the contributions of the programme and not just to life's experiences or from other influences (Goldstein, 1986). This model asks the question, "Were differences in sustainable agriculture practice attributable to the programme?" The simplest way to determine causality between the programme inputs and comparable groups, a group that received the educational treatment and a group that did not. It is recommended that this model be used only when major changes are expected or when a major failure is anticipated in pilot efforts where causal claims are central to making major programme investments (Rossi & Freeman, 1982).

Participatory Evaluation Model: The purpose of this model is for extension educators and farmers themselves to initiate a critical reflection process focused on their own activities. This is done through identifying a persistent major situation such as extension's neglect of women in agriculture; subject it to critical reflection, underlying assumptions, habits of mind, and cause and effect expectations; and then after creating new assumptions, change practices and validate or invalidate the results. The model assumes a democratic participatory process along with autonomy on the part of educators and learners at the local level (Brunner & Guzman, 1989; Greene, 1988).

Focusing the Evaluation Effort

According to Deshler (1997), there are eight major areas of focus for programme evaluation:

1. Inputs-resources
2. Activities
3. Participation
4. Reactions
5. Individual Change
6. Organizational Change
7. Community Change
8. National impacts (Political stability, economic fairness, agricultural environmental sustainability)

Evaluations rarely cover all and limit to a combination of items that pertains to selected evaluation model and focus of stakeholders. The focus of evaluation is narrowed during planning with the major stakeholders of a programme (farmers, extension personnel, etc). The key here is to determine the decisions that stakeholders intend to make based on the evaluation findings.

The expert model most often focuses on data from inputs, activities, and participation, while the goal-free model tends to focus on individual change, organization change, or community change, ignoring the inputs and activities. The attainment of objectives model usually compares the philosophy, goals, and objectives of inputs to the extent of individual or organizational change outcomes. The naturalistic model emphasizes understanding activities, participation, and reactions as processes that occur within cultural, economic, and political contexts. The experimental model emphasizes causal relationships between inputs and individual or organizational change. The participatory evaluation model emphasizes activities and their relationship to benefits and values to farmers. It also emphasizes participation of farmers themselves in planning the focus, data collection, interpretation, and implementation of action that emerges from the evaluation process (Deshler, 1997).

Conclusion

In the development projects, monitoring and evaluation play diverse roles, in the sense that monitoring is an ongoing process, where as evaluation is performed periodically. Further, the focus of the assessment also differentiates the two, i.e., monitoring is all about what is happening, evaluation is concerned with how well it happened. Impact evaluation can be short-term, mid-term and long-term. Short-term evaluation assesses changes in knowledge, skills, attitude and aspiration of programme beneficiaries. The mid-term impact may be in term of assessing adoption of practices disseminated through extension programmes, while long-term impacts can be economic benefits, social outcomes and environmental outcomes.

25

Conservation & Extension of Threatened Small Animals in Native Tract of West Bengal

Keshab Chandra Dhara

Directorate of Research, Extension and Farms
West Bengal University of Animal and Fishery Sciences
Kolkata, West Bengal

India is one of the few countries in the world, which has contributed richly to the international livestock gene pool. Small animal particularly sheep and goat biodiversity in India is characterized by high degree of endemism in different agro climatic regions , and has led to the development of various breeds/strains that are well adapted to specific set of environmental conditions. These breeds have generally been named after their place of origin and some based on their prominent characteristics. Indigenous sheep and goat contribute greatly to the agrarian economy, especially in areas where crop and dairy farming are not economical, and play an important role in the livelihood of a large proportion of small and marginal farmers and landless laborers. Sheep and Goat rearing and production has been the important source for sustainable livelihood of the rural people mainly in arid , semi-arid and temperate regions of India as it serves their various needs and provides an unceasing source of income round the year. Goat has been reared mainly for the mutton whereas sheep are reared for mutton as well as wool production since ages; however, recently the trend has shifted more towards the enhanced mutton productivity and profitability. Moreover, these small ruminant acts as source of instant income in the event of emergency situation. These sheep and goat can even thrive in draught and harsh conditions on minimal input thereby providing poor marginal and landless farmers livelihood and nutritional security. There is rich genetic diversity of sheep and goat in India. In India total well characterized and accredited breeds of sheep and goat are 44 and 32 respectively. In India, small animal are mainly being considered as sheep and goat as they predominant and thus the discussion related to Conservation & Extension of threatened Small Animals in native tract of West Bengal will be focused on sheep and goat. Sheep and Goats are integral part of agriculture and key component of global livestock genetic diversity. These animals are widely distributed across all agro-ecological zones and play an important role in the rural areas by providing income, nutrition, socio-cultural linkages, employment opportunities and insurance against risk in harsh environments (Devendra, 1991). Indigenous animals have evolved within the ecosystem by providing a sustainable and environmentally sound agriculture. The genetic potential of Sheep and Goats has not fully exploited. The diversity present in small ruminant species also reflects their wide range in production conditions. Sheep and Goats are associated with smallholder production systems in which they use by-product feeds, lowly productive common grazing lands or under-utilized forages along roadsides. Active conservation of the goat genetic resource means both the creative utilization of that genetic resource in sustainable production systems and the long-term preservation of key genetic types to meet unseen future needs. Further, it has an important role to play in meeting the animal protein requirement for huge human population comparatively at lower cost. FAO has defined population sizes at which breeds could be labeled endangered and at risk of extinction. Although, such numbers need not be taken literally, they provide useful guidelines. To prevent breeds from becoming extinct, various measures are recommended. *In-situ* conservation schemes involve support of live populations of such size that viable breeding programmes should be possible to maintain, while avoiding inbreeding problems. The aim of *ex situ* conservation schemes is twofold: maintaining gene banks by cryo-preservation (semen and embryos) and, if possible, maintaining the remaining small populations (see FAO, 2007a; FAO, 2011). As the effects of breeding programmes are determined on a long-term basis, it is quite important to continuously monitor changes in population sizes and immigration of genes between populations. The Global Strategy for the Management of Farm AnGR provides a technical and operational framework for assisting countries as laid out in chapter 3.4. Additionally, FAO has developed a communication and information tool, the Domestic Animal Diversity Information System [DAD-IS], to implement the Global Strategy [FAO, 2007b-GPA]. The objective of DAD-IS is to assist countries and country networks by providing extensive searchable databases, tools, guidelines, a library, links and contacts for the better management of all AnGR used in food and agriculture. That way, it would be possible to effectively apply certain measures to conserve threatened breeds. However, for the systems to work, the country-level participation must remain highly proactive and professional and use participatory approaches with livestock keepers, Otherwise, one may consistently get stuck with projects aimed at rescuing the remaining small number of animals of a breed, but at a stage when it is too late to develop the breed.

Extension: Extension is the science of making people innovative, it is deals with people's knowledge and resources, encompasses all aspects of life and emphasizes on behavioral change of target communities. The word 'extension' is derived from the Latin roots, 'ex'-meaning 'out' and 'tensio' meaning 'stretching'. Stretching out is the meaning of extension. The word 'extension' came to be used originally in USA during 1914 which means "a branch of a university for students who cannot attend the university proper. In other words, the word "extension" signifies an out-of school system of education.

The extension methodology to be applied for the purpose as **training and visit, demonstration farm projects, producers' meetings, educational materials, and use of mass media**. Extension activities must be multi-media to direct the process of technological change and development effectively.

Communication Channel	Step in the Extension Process
Traditional leaders	First contact with community
Village meeting	Introduction of sheep and goat farming
Slide show	Visualize small animal farming and discuss general issues concerning sheep and goat farming; create mutual background of information regarding opportunities and constraints of target group when adopting such farming.
Farm visits	Assist farmers to take decisions concerning use and management of their resources
Motivators	Provide contact between other farmers and the project and give advisory support to late adopters
Pamphlets	Give specific information about sheep and goat husbandry practices..

2. Sheep Population in India

The total population of sheep in India is 65.06 million (2012) which was 71.60 millions in 2007. There has been negative trend in population growth. According to the Livestock Census 2012, United Andhra Pradesh ranks first in sheep population with nearly 40.57% sheep population followed by Karnataka (14.73%) and Rajasthan (13.95%). The total contribution of mutton, wool, skin and manure from sheep rearing are 441, 47.09, 56.30 and 190 million Kg respectively. It provides employment to 6 million people and the revenue generated from export of wool and animal fiber is 178539 thousand USD.

2.1. Sheep Breeds

Based on the agro-climatic conditions and habitat of sheep it can be divided into four regions.

(a) **North Temperate Region**: North Temperate Region comprises of Jammu and Kashmir, Himachal Pradesh and Uttarakhand having medium wool type breeds. Sheep breeds found in this area are Gaddi, Rampur Bushair, Bhakarwal, Poonchi, Karnah, Gurenz, Kashmir Valley and Changthangi.

(b) North western arid and semi-arid region: North western arid and semi-arid region includes the States of Rajasthan, Punjab, Haryana, the plains of Uttar Pradesh, Gujarat and Madhya Pradesh having carpet wool type sheep breeds. Sheep breeds found in this area are-Chokla, Nali, Marwari, Magra, Jaisalmeri, Pugal, Malpura, Sonadi, Pattanwadi, Muzaffarnagri, Jalauni, Hissardale and Kheri. Marwari sheep has been numerically the most important and largest contributor to carpet wool production in the country (Acharya R M, 1982).

(c) Southern peninsular region: Southern peninsular region covers of the states of Maharashtra, Andhra Pradesh, Karnataka and Tamil Nadu having meat type breeds. Sheep breeds found in this area are Deccani, Nellore, Bellary, Hassan, Mandya, Mecheri, Kilakarsal, Vembur, Coimbatore, Nilgiri, Ramnad white, Madras Red, Trichi Black and Kenguri. Deccani sheep is numerically most important and is largest contributor to the meat production in the country.

(d) Eastern region: Eastern region comprises of the states of Bihar, West Bengal, Orissa, Assam and North Eastern states having hairy breeds. Sheep breeds found in this area are Chottanagpuri, Bolangir, Ganjam, Tibetan, Bonpala and Garole. Garole sheep in Sunderban areas of West Bengal are reputed for multiple births.

2.2. Sheep breeds and their unique characters*.

Breed	Unique characteristics
Magra	Lustrous wool, excellent for carpet manufacture
Changthangi	Alpine sheep of high altitude for fine wool
Chokla	Fine carpet quality fleece
Garole	High fecundity- twins and triplets common. Survival under saline conditions.
Mecheri, Madras Red	High quality skin and mutton
Mandya	Excellent meaty conformation, high quality and meat palatability.
Patanwadi	Carpet wool and good milk producer
Nellore	Tallest sheep breed of India.
Muzaffarnagari	Best mutton producing breed
Marwari, Deccani ,Jaisalmeri	Hardy and capable of walking long distances during migration.
Kendrapada	High fecundity- twins and triplets common.

**Source*: (Bhatia and Arora, 2005)

2.3. Sheep Breeds considered being at risk

In India, 21% of the total breeds (Ganjam, Bhakarwal, Gurez, Karnah, Nilgiri, Poonchi, Poogal and Magra) show declining trends in their population and demand conservation. Criteria of breeds at risk if breed able population is around 50,000 it is considered to be normal, once population is in the range of 30,000 –50,000 with constant decline it is called as insecure. If the population range is 15,000 – 30,000 this condition is defined as vulnerable. Endangered is a situation where population ranges from 8,000 – 15000. It becomes critical once it is less than 8000.

Breeds/strains of Indian sheep considered at risk*

Breed/strain	Location	Risk status	Main causes for decline
Bhakarwal, Gurej, Karnah, Poonchi	Jammu & Kashmir	Endangered	Indiscriminate crossbreeding with exotic fine wool breeds
Changthangi	Ladakh	Endangered	Smaller flocks scattered in large area of fragile ecology
Rampur Bushair	Himachal Pradesh	Endangered	Indiscriminate crossbreeding
Tibetan and Bonpala	Sikkim	Endangered	Smaller flocks scattered in large area of fragile ecology
Muzaffarnagari	Uttar Pradesh	Declining	Small grazing area
Malpura, Chokla	Rajasthan	Declining	Introduction of Marwari inheritance through migratory flocks
Magra	Rajasthan	Endangered	Crossing with Marwari\Kheri
Pugal	Rajasthan	Declining	Crossing with Marwari/Kheri
Jaisalmeri	Rajsthan	Declining	Intermixing with Chokla
Mandya	Karnataka	Endangered	High incidence of cryptorchidism
Nilgiri	Tamilnadu	Endangered	No demand of wool in Tamil Nadu and their indiscriminate slaughter
Kilakarsal	Tamilnadu	Endangered	Crossing with Vembur/Ramnad white.

**Source:* (Bhatia and Arora, 2005)

3. Goat Breeds

India has the largest goat population in the world. Their number has increased at the annual rate of approximately 3.2%, which appears to be the highest rate among all species of livestock in the country. India possesses 22 recognized breeds of goat apart from non-descript. India has been divided into four eco-zones for the purpose of description of goats depending upon their production and adaptability and has been evolved primarily through natural process relevant to diversified agro-climatic conditions.

(a) Temperate Himalayan region:	Changthangi, Chegu, Gaddi, Shingari.
(b) North-Western region:	Barbari, Beetal, Jamnapari, Jakhrana, Marwari, Sirohi, Surti, Zalawadi.
(c) Southern region:	Malabari, Osmanabadi, Sangamneri.
(d) Eastern region:	Assam hill, Black Bengal, Ganjam.

There is large variation among the breeds with respect to their production traits namely, milk, meat and fiber in the different eco-zones of the country. The goat breeds of temperate Himalayan region include Cheghu and Changthangi, which possess the finest natural fiber as under coat commonly known as Pashmina. All the milch breeds, Beetal, Jamunapari, Surti, Jakhrana are found in the hot dry belt of the **North-Western** India. In the **Southern and Western Zones** of India long legged dual-purpose breeds, Malabari, Marwari, Kutchi, Zalawadi, Mehsana and Sirohi are prevalent. Highly prolific dwarf breed, Black Bengal covers a major part of **Eastern** India. Assam Hill goats (Syn. Khasi) are a hairy well-built, short-legged animal adapted to hilly climate of undivided Assam. Wild goats of Andaman have drawn the attention of Scientists recently as they survive on seawater, leaves and fruits. Most of the goat breeds of **Western** region are suitable for meat production under intensive grazing; **Southern and Eastern** region goat breeds attain early maturity and are more prolific. In **Southern region** most of the goats are non-descript and only two breeds i.e. Malabari and Osmanabadi have been recognized. Recently, some local types have been identified (e.g. Salem Black in Tamil Nadu and Attappady Black in Kerala).

3.1. Unique characteristics of Indian Goat Breeds

1	Milch type	Jamunapari, Beetal, Surti and Jakhrana
2	Meat type	Bengal, Barbari, Sirohi, Kutchi, Marwari, Zalawadi, Sangamneri, Mehesana and Osmanabadi.
3.	Fibre type	Gaddi and Khasi (long hairy), Changthangi and Cheghu (Fine undercoat - Pashmina)

3.2. Threatened Goat Breeds of India

Due to constant decline in population of some goat breeds of India they have been listed under threatened breeds viz; Jamunapari, Beetal, Jakhrana,

Surti, Sangamneri, Osmanabadi, Ganjam, Malabari, Changthangi, Chegu and Attappady Black goat. There is dire need to conserve these breeds in order to meet the future requirements.

4. Importance of conservation of Sheep and Goat Breeds

Pastoralists and small and marginal farmers are somehow or other are dependent on the livestock those have been their companions since ages. They symbolize their culture, knowledge systems and societies. These animals are unique with respect to tolerance to biotic and abiotic stresses. These animals and breeds continue to produce meat, wool and other produce without much input on feeding, care and veterinary assistance. In spite of this, these breeds are in danger of extinction, pushed out by modern production techniques and diluted by experiments such as inheritance of exotic germ-plasm. Today, in the time of competition, the focus of farmer as well as government is diverted towards the high producing breeds those can meet the demand and in turn the diversity of the sheep and goats breeds faces challenges for existence. This small number of high producing breeds leads to narrowing the genetic base, as native breeds are neglected in response to market forces. The diversity of animal genetic resources is essential to satisfy basic human needs for food and livelihood security. Genetic diversity defines not only animals' production and functional traits, but also their ability to adapt to different environments, including food and water availability, climate, pests and diseases. It has also been found that the Indian sheep breeds are more resistant to the gastrointestinal parasites as compared to the crossbreds or exotic sheep. There are many sheep genetic resources which are unique and therefore popular among the local population (Bhatia and Arora, 2005). Thus, we need to preserve this trait which is possible only if we can save these breeds form extinction.

4.1. Different Methods of Conservations of Sheep and Goat in India

(A) *In situ* conservation: It is the method of conservation where animals are bred in their home tract with the purpose of increasing their breed able population. Different ways of *In situ* conservation are:

(a) Genetic Improvement and Sustainable management.

(b) Institutional flock.

(c) In farmers' flock

 i. Creation of breed societies.

 ii. Financial assistance to farmers.

iii. Increased extension services.

iv. Provision of improved breeding rams.

v. Creation of public awareness and mass movement.

vi. Incentives and awards.

(B) ***Ex Situ*** **conservation:** It is the method of conservation where animals are reared away from the home tract and production system. It includes the different biotechnology tools to save the population for future use.

(a) Cryopreservation: It is used for future use, when probably the breeds shall be extinct, or a specific desired character goes missing

- Semen, ova, embryos, tissue, *etc.* for potential future use are cryo-preserved.
- National Animal Gene Bank where genome of the animals are preserved. In India, it has been established at NBAGR and frozen semen of different sheep and goats are maintained.

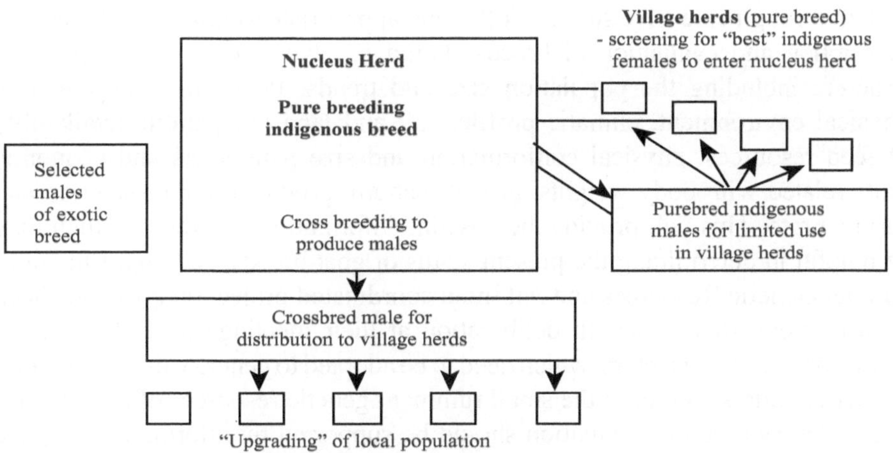

5. Evaluation, Conservation and Management

No serious attempts for description, evaluation, conservation and genetic improvement of Sheep and Goats have been made. Perhaps Sheep and Goats are the most neglected species with respect to their evaluation and genetic improvement. In the recent past, considerable emphasis was given on crossbreeding of indigenous breeds with exotic as well as with indigenous improver breeds in order to enhance their productivity. The resultant outcome was very inconsistent due to many shortfalls including inadequate infrastructure.

However, there is now growing realization for the importance of indigenous breeds because of their suitability and adaptation to diversified agro-climatic and socio-economic situations. With this view, the breeding strategies and improvement programmes were, therefore devised considering the efficiency of production in relation to physical environment, feed and fodder resource availability, management and health aspects. The information on small ruminant genetic resources is not adequate and whatever information available is based on limited number of animals under organized and institutional sector, which is not representing their production status and performance under their natural habitat. Efforts made in the direction to identify and evaluate the breeds and to bring them on record are also restricted making it difficult to decide as what to conserve. It is therefore necessary to view this process in an integrated manner comprising to establish the identification of the breeds at the first instance, their evaluation and documentation of the data, conservation and management.

5.1. Evaluation

It is necessary to evaluate the breeds in their home tract under native management system through extensive surveys following appropriate sampling methods. The description and evaluation of breeds should involve studying the population structure including the population size and trends, flock size and structure, physical environment, climatic profile, soil and land use pattern, availability of feed resources, physical conformation and size parameters and economic traits related with body weights, growth pattern, production, reproduction and survival rate. This will provide the baseline information on breeds, which may be helpful in determining the present status of goat breeds. National Bureau of Animal Genetic Resources and All India coordinated project on goat and sheep Improvement after in length deliberation at their meetings have devised the format on breed descriptors, which need to be adopted to generate the information for better understanding of the small ruminant genetic resources of the country. Breed description and evaluation should be supported by information on gene markers, karyotypes, blood groups and other variable of protein types in order to utilize such information for identification of breeds/ breed types.

5.2. Need for conservation

The planned conservation programme of goat breeds in India is neglected one and more importantly, the adapted goat breeds at high altitude, harsh environment and marginal agricultural regions have neither adequately maintained in their habitat nor tried for improving the productivity. No attention has been made for valuable traits like fecundity, disease resistance, grazing habit, cheese quality, meat quality, skin characteristics, though crucial for the development programme of Sheep and Goats The goat breeds should be conserved for these specialties in their home tract for future use. However, India is facing major environmental problem due to increase in agricultural land, human population, rangeland management and forests protected for wild life etc. The livestock sector is facing problem due to shortage of grazing land, availability of feed and fodder and loss of habitat etc. The pure Jamunapari population has declined seriously and it is less than 10,000 in its habitat due to different reasons. Beetal is drawing attention for conservation as the number is declining because of changing agricultural patterns in the Punjab. Barbari is facing dilution in breed characteristics due to cross breeding with Sirohi and Jamunapari in its home tract. Due to decrease in natural browse and geographical restriction Surti and Jakhrana are decreasing in number. There is also danger in India that attention to the improvement of breeds such as Beetal, Barbari and Jamunapari could result in these breeds becoming dominant nationally and eliminating other distinctive breeds by cross breeding. Means for the conservation, multiplication and improvement of these breeds in the pattern of ONBS have been suggested by Acharya et al., (1982). Moreover Epstein (1974), Acharya et al (1982) and Devendra and Burns (1983) have drawn attention for the conservation programme for specific goat populations in developing countries.

5.3. Identification of Conservation

If the breeds are disappearing in its natural habitat, then action to conserve the breed should be taken immediately. The range of information is needed in order to identify the populations, which is in danger of extinction and should be considered as candidate for conservation. *The following information should be gathered and to be used in planning conservation strategy.*

1. Descriptive information on breeds, geographical location and information on production characteristics.
2. Estimating the availability of total number of animals in relation to sex and the population trend including selling pattern.
3. The proportion of the female population being used in cross breeding. By estimating the number of purebred males and females along with the number of young stocks with evidence of cross breeding it is possible to estimate the rate of breed dilution. Even a 20% per year decrease in purebred young stock will result in a very dramatic crash in population size over a relatively short space of time.

4. The number of herds or breeding units available in natural habitat as large size herds may be more vulnerable to decreases and affected more seriously due to economic or political changes than the smaller herds.
5. Estimate the health risk, whether the population in owns where lethal epidemics are endemic may be at greater risk than those in regions where such diseases are not present.
6. Estimate the other risks, political, climatic or economic. In particular the risk of drought, storms, flooding, war or rapid socio-economic change, this could result in the disappearance of indigenous populations.
7. Characterization of the breed which includes the measurement and description of external appearance, production characteristics, climatic adaptation, disease resistance, parasite tolerance, management and any other special feature, it may also involve the collection of biochemical information from blood types, milk proteins and the comparative analysis of DNA fragments, All of this information is useful in determining the long term conservation strategy with respect to a breed but is not essential in establishing an initial programme to prevent the early loss of a breed or population.

5.4. Mechanism of Conservation

The mechanism for the conservation of individual genes within populations is closely linked to the conservation of species and breeds. The most important feature of a small population conservation programme is the rate of genetic loss and the increase in homo-zygosity. The increase in homo-zygosity within a small population causes the loss of ability to adapt, inbreeding depression and extinction. Viable population size must be therefore linked to the ability to conserve genetic diversity within any conservation population. The maintenance of diversity in a population depends on founder population and effective population size. The population size, birth and survival rates, sex ratio and levels of variation must be taken into account before deciding the manner the breeds will be conserved.

Mechanism for conserving genetic resources conservation is not an end itself, but rather a means of ensuring that animal genetic resources are better understood and available and more effectively used and eloped. Generally, two approaches Ex-situ and In-situ have been used for conserving the goat population in India.

In situ: The generation and loss of alleles is a dynamic process that should be maintained at close equilibrium through sound management. The maintaining animal in its natural habitat or in their adaptive environment as close as possible is called in-situ conservation.

Ex Situ: It is the storage of animal genetic resources, which farmers are not currently using in field condition. It includes cryogenic preservation and maintenance of breeds of domesticated animals in farms, zoos and other location away from its home tract. It is the preservation of semen, ova or embryos, DNA segments in frozen blood or other tissue. As technologies for conserving semen, embryo has been standardized at CSWRI, Avikanagar and CIRG, Makhdoom. Both In-situ and Ex-situ methods are equally feasible for conserving small ruminant genetic resources. Technological means are available for conserving the germ plasm in the form of gametes and embryos with liquid nitrogen, thereby creating a gene bank to face the problems of extinction.

5.5. Conservation in research organization

Mostly selective breeding has been practiced in research Institutes and Universities for increasing the efficiency in productivity. In India crossbreeding in goat has been practiced for more than a decade that resulted into very inconsistent results due to many shortfalls and inadequate. Infrastructure. Now a day there is growing realization for the importance of indigenous genetic resources because they are more relevant to meet out the nutritional needs under their natural habitat.

5.6. Breeding policy for sheep and goat (National Livestock Policy-2013, DADHF)

1. This aims to improve growth, body weight, reproductive efficiency, meat and wool quality and quantity, and to reduce mortality.
2. An area specific approach would be adopted to improve quality and quantity of coarse wool and fine wool.
3. Main focus will be to produce and distribute good quality rams/bucks of quality indigenous breeds which can thrive in different agro-climatic conditions.
4. Artificial insemination would also be encouraged.
5. Cross-breeding with high yielding exotic and other native breeds of goats will also be considered.

Future thrust

India is very rich in goat and sheep genetic resources and number of breeds with great diversity is available having good potential for production of meat, milk and fiber. Very little work has been done for breed characterization and their proper evaluation. It is necessary and recommended that concerted efforts should be made to characterize and evaluate the indigenous breeds including genetic characterization. Further it is suggested that regional programme for sustainable development and purposeful use of goat and sheep genetic resources need to be developed and put to function. The programme should be designed in such a manner so as to contribute both immediate production needs and long-term improvement programmes in order to take up breed characterization, evaluation and utilization. It is necessary that each State Govt. should establish an appropriate infrastructure at provincial level with adequate allocation of funds. National Bureau of Animal Genetic Resources as nodal agency on Animal Genetic Resources from time to time encourage research Institutes/SAUS, State Governments to give adequate priority to management and development of small ruminant genetic resources for food security, poverty alleviation and rural development. The experts and technicians may be trained in the area of management of animal genetic resources conservation. Adequate support including funding should be provided by the Government to carry out the National small ruminant Genetic Resources Conservation work plan.

Following areas may need attention:

- Breed characterization and evaluation.
- Recording system and data management.
- Development of suitable breeding strategies including ONBS, Gene, markers and Genetic Identification.
- Management and utilization of small ruminant genetic resources.
- Monitoring the population those are identified at risk.
- A national information network should be established to provide an opportunity for the exchange of information on Animal Genetic Resources including goats and sheep within country as well as to other countries.

Recommendations

1. Livestock census gives information on sex ratio, population of different age groups and production status. However, it should be conducted on breed basis so that the population of sheep breeds showing declining trend can be monitored and conservation programs are undertaken.

2. An expert panel should be appointed at National level to determine the basic norms for a breed registration.
3. Breed societies be created and should get patronage, funding and scientific support for the conservation and sustainable utilization of goat genetic resources.
4. A National Watch List of endangered breeds of livestock should be established like that of wild life and plants supported by strict legislation.
5. The financial aid given to the breeders through Government programs may be given strictly for raising animals of recognized breed of the area.
6. The facilities available in the Government farms should be improved to keep the recognized indigenous breeds of livestock for in-situ conservation.
7. Genetic improvement programs with high intensity of selection should be adopted for each breed. These selected elite animals would thus be economically viable and would be preserved / conserved by the farmers due to their utility.
8. Wherever feasible, live animal reserves for keeping to limited number of animals of a rare breed should be encouraged.

A large infrastructure is available in the country for the semen/ embryo collection, storage and deep freezing. In should be mandatory for them to keep sample of semen doses/embryos in addition to their development needs.

26

Climate Resilient Agriculture for Sustainable Production of Agriculture and Allied Sectors in Eastern India

F.H. Rahman and R. Bhattacharya

ICAR- Agricultural Technology Application Research Institute Kolkata Bhumi Vihar Complex, Salt Lake, Kolkata- 700097

Climate change refers to a change of climate that is attributed directly or indirectly to human activity that alters the composition of the global atmosphere and that is in addition to natural climate variability observed over comparable time periods (FCCC).

Overall, climate change could result in a variety of impacts on agriculture. Some of these effects are biophysical, some are ecological, and some are economic, including:

- A shift in climate and agricultural zones towards the poles
- Changes in production patterns due to higher temperatures
- A boost in agricultural productivity due to increased carbon dioxide in the atmosphere
- Changing precipitation patterns
- Increased vulnerability of the landless and the poor

Evidences of Climate Change

Physical evidences: Rise in atmospheric temp and CO_2 level; Depletion in rainfall; Shifting and shrinking of cooling period; changing pattern of monsoon; Occurrence of natural disaster

Biological evidences: Early blossoming of trees; Appearance of grasses in Antarctica; Changing cropping pattern.

It has been reported that due to climate change there is raise in sea level of 1-3 mm/year in coastal areas of Asia and which projected to 5 mm/year over the next century and thereby increase from 13 million to 94 million people would be flooded annually in South Asia under very conservative scenario 40 cm by 2100 (Cruz *et al.* 2007; Wassmann *et al.* 2004)

Abundance and lifetime of greenhouse gases in the atmosphere

Gases	Pre-1750 tropospheric conc.	Recent tropospheric conc.	GWP- (100 yr time horizon)	Atmospheric Lifetime (years)
CO_2 (ppm)	280	399.5	1	~100-300
CH_4 (ppb)	722	1834	28	12.4
N_2O (ppb)	270	328	265	121

(*Source*: *US Department of Energy-CDIAC-2016)*

Climate Variability during the Recent Past

- 2002- Drought
- 2003- 20 day heat wave during May in AP & extreme cold winter in the year 2002-03
- 2004- Drought like situation in India in July
- 2005- Abnormal temp. in March 2004 and Jan 2005; Floods and Cold wave 2005 - 06
- 2006- Floods in arid Rajasthan & AP and drought in NE regions
- 2007- Abnormal temp in 3rd week of Jan to 1st week of Feb
- 2009 - All India Severe drought , Severe Cyclone Aila in WB
- 2010 - One of warmest years
- 2011 - Failure of September rains in AP
- 2012 - Drought in Punjab, Haryana, Gujarat and Karnataka. Neelam cyclone, AP floods
- 2014-Hailstorms, Early season dry spells, Kashmir floods and Hudhud cyclone
- 2015 - Drought, floods
- 2016 - Drought, floods
- 2017 - Floods, cyclone, drought
- 2018- Drought, floods
- 2019 - Floods, cyclone
- 2020 - Cyclone , floods
- 2021 - Cyclone, floods

Future impacts of climate change in India

- Decreased snow cover
- Erratic monsoon with serious effects on rain-fed agriculture
- Drop in wheat production by 4-5 mt with 1^{0}C raise in temperature
- Raising sea level
- Increased frequency and intensity of floods

Impact of climate change by 2050

- > 25m children will be malnourished
- Irrigated wheat yield will decreased by 30%
- Irrigated rice yield 15%
- Climate change will increase prices in 2050 by 90% for wheat, 12% for rice and 35% for maize
- It is reported that at least US$7 billion a year are necessary to improve agricultural productivity to
- Prevent adverse effects on children (IFPRI 2010).

Impact of climate change on Rice production

- An increase of 2 - 4°C results to 15% reduction in yields
- Rain fed and drought prone areas 17 to 40%
- Water scarcity affects 23mha in Asia
- Additional CO_2 can benefit crops but this effect was nullified by an increase of temperature

Critical temperatures for the development of rice plant at different growth stages

Growth stages	Critical temperature (^{0}C)		
	Low	High	Optimum
Germination	16-19	45	18-40
Seedling emergence	12	35	25-30
Rooting	16	35	25-28
Leaf elongation	7-12	45	31
Tillering	9-16	33	25-31
Initiation of panicle	15	-	-
Panicle differentiation	15-20	30	-
Anthesis	22	35-36	30-33
Ripening	12-18	>30	20-29

(Source: Nguyen, 2006)

Symptoms of heat stress in rice

Growth stage	Symptoms
Vegetative	White leaf tip, chlorotic & white bands and specks
Reproductive stage	Reduce spikelet number and sterility
Ripening	Reduced grain filling

Rice crop response to variations in temperature

Yield and yield attributes							
Climate scenarios	**Temp. change**	**Crop duration (days)**	**Grain yield (kg ha^{-1})**	**Grains (m^{-2})**	**Grains (ear^{-1})**	**Biomass (kg ha^{-1})**	**Straw (kg ha $^{-1}$)**
(% deviation over normal scenario)							
Extreme warm	+2.0 °C	-3.3	-8.4	-8.4	-12.4	-7.4	-6.4
Greater warm	+1.5 °C	-2.6	-8.2	-8.2	-8.3	-6.5	-4.7
Moderate warm	+1.0 °C	-2.0	-4.9	-4.9	-6.1	-3.6	-2.2
Slight warm	+0.5 °C	-1.3	-3.2	-3.2	-2.4	-1.3	-0.7
Normal warm	Normal	153	6136	18846	494	10220	4943

(*Source*: Mathauda*et al.*,2000)

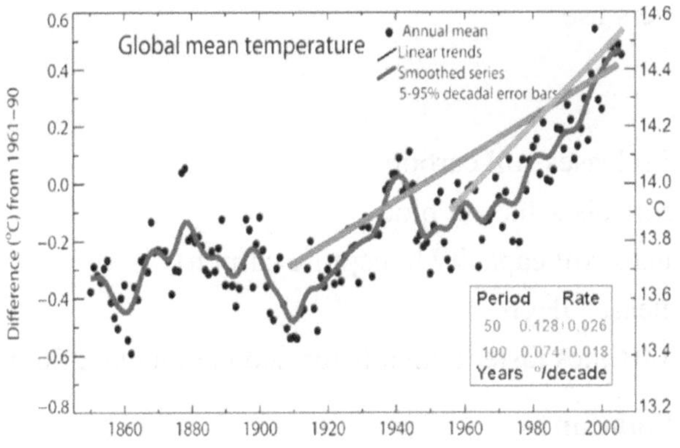

Fig.4: Trends in global temperature over the years (IPCC, 2007)

The global *mean annual temperature* at the end of the 20th century, as a result of GHG accumulation in the atmosphere, has increased by 0.4 - 0.7 ºC above that recorded at the end of the 19th century. The past 50 years have shown an increasing trend in temperature @ 0.13 °C/decade.

The Inter-Governmental Panel on Climate Change has projected the Temperature increase to be between 1.1 °C and 6.4 °C by the end of the 21st Century (IPCC, 2007).

Impact of climate change on pest and diseases

- Hymenopteran parasitoids and small predators
- Brown plant hopper is 17 times more tolerant at 40 ^{0}C than its predator *Cyrtor rhynu slividi pennis*
- Rise in winter temperature may help to continue the life cycle of pests
- High temperature and RH is very much conducive for rapid proliferation of sheath blight disease
- Bacterial leaf streak emerged as an alarming proportion in South and SW parts of country might be due environmental factor
- Minimum temperature In winter may rise in further increased severity of sheath blight and stem rot

Agriculture contributes to Climate Change

- While agriculture produces food, it also produces GHGs (methane, nitrous oxide, carbon dioxide) - about 17 % nationally, after energy 57% and industry 22%.
- Methane emissions from paddy fields and livestock
- Nitrous oxide from fertilizers use
- Carbon dioxide from
- Crop residue burning
- Ploughing and tilling land releases soil carbon
- Excessive use of agro-chemicals kills soil biota,
- Depleted soil fertility reduces soil capacity to capture carbon
- Slash and burn systems release GHGs
- Soil erosion - soil is lost 100 times faster than it is formed in ploughed fields

Agriculture as part of the Solution

- Agriculture can reduce global CO_2 emissions by 10-15%
- Well-maintained soils sequester carbon
- Conservation tillage prevents further loss of soil erosion and soil fertility; enhances carbon capture
- Agro-forestry : trees on farm sequester carbon
- Homestead gardens - fruit trees - contribute to nutrition & capture carbon
- Rotations with cover crops, legumes, green manure enhance soil fertility

Climate Smart Agriculture

- Holistically addresses food security & Climate Change
- Primary objective is to sustainably increase productivity and income of farmers
- Develop Adaptation/ Coping strategies in times of depleting soil fertility and increasing water stress
- Strengthen resilience of smallholder farmers and reduce their vulnerabilities to extreme events
- Reduce agriculture GHG emissions by CSA practices
- Mitigation through carbon sequestration as co-benefit of the primary objective

Key issues in crop production under climate change scenario in India

Climate Change	Possible Effects on Agriculture
Deviation in temperature	Quick break down of soil organic matter. Quick loss of water from soil resulting low WUE. Higher transpiration loss of water Quick loss of applied N from soil resulting low NUE Creating heat stress condition for rabi crops
Deviation in rainfall	Unpredictable rainfall pattern called for contingency measure Adverse effect of seasonal variation on cropping sequence Changed SW monsoon behavior may hamper crop production Increased soil and nutrient loss due to higher no of extreme rainfall Lowering of ground water table due to lifting during dry spell and insufficient recharge
Occurrence of extreme events	Higher possibility of occurrence of drought during kharif season will greatly hamper rice production Increased possibility of flood will also adversely affect production kharif paddy as well as cropping pattern Untimely occurrence of heavy cyclone will badly affect kharif rice and pre-kharif crop like jute, maize etc.
Changes in sea level	1 m rise in sea level will result in loss of 5764 sq km land area squeezing per capita land availability More intrusion of saline water into agriculture land resulting conversion to waste land

National Innovations on Climate Resilient Agriculture (NICRA)

National Innovations on Climate Resilient Agriculture (NICRA) is a network project of ICAR launched in February, 2011.The project aims - at enhancing resilience of Indian agriculture to climate change and climate vulnerability through strategic research and technology demonstration.

The objectives of this network project are:

- To enhance the resilience of Indian agriculture covering crops, livestock and fisheries to climatic variability & climate change through development and application of improved production & risk management technologies
- To demonstrate site specific technology packages on farmers' fields for adapting to current climate risks
- To enhance the capacity building of scientists and other stakeholders in climate resilient agricultural research and its application

NICRA is a step towards climate-smart agriculture that includes application of proven practical techniques in major areas of water management, crop husbandry, livestock management, farm implements and others. Getting existing technologies into the hands of small and marginal farmers and developing new technologies like drought or flood tolerant crops to meet the demands of a changing climate also come under the purview of NICRA programme

The project is comprised of four components-

- Strategic research on adaptation and mitigation
- Technology demonstration on farmers' fields to cope up with current climate variability
- Sponsored and competitive research grants to fill critical research gaps
- Capacity building of different stakeholders

100 KVKs all over India were selected for implementation of the project (TDC) in the first phase. Simultaneously the project was spreaded over **121 KVKs** of the country during 2015-16. The research on adaptation and mitigation covers crops, livestock, fisheries and natural resource management. Technology Demonstration Component programme are carried out in 22 KVKs from different states of eastern part of the Country based on different climatic vulnerabilities like drought, flood, cyclone, heat wave which are as:

- Seven districts of Bihar: Aurangabad, Buxar, Jehanabad, Nawada, Saran and Supaul
- Six of Jharkhand: Chatra, East Singhbhum, Gumla,Koderma and Palamu
- Five of Odisha: Kendrapara, Ganjam, Kalahandi, Jharsuguda and Sonepur
- Three of West Bengal: Coochbehar, Malda and S 24 Parganas
- One of A & N Islands: Port Blair

The interventions covered with the following modules:

Module I: Natural Resource Management

In-situ moisture conservation, construction/renovation of new water harvesting and recycling structures/farm ponds/ checks dams/tank roof water harvesting tank, land shaping & RWH improved drainage in flood prone areas, conservation tillage where appropriate, artificial ground water recharge and water saving irrigation methods, green manuring, 5% model of irrigation, crop residue management, bunding of field, Broad Bed Furrow, soil test based nutrient application, micro irrigation techniques, compost pits

Module II: Crop Production

Introducing drought, salt and flood tolerant/ resistant varieties, advancement of planting dates of rabi crops in areas with terminal heat stress, water saving paddy cultivation methods (SRI, aerobic, direct seedling), community nurseries for delayed monsoon, location specific intercropping systems with high sustainable yield index, introduction of new crops/ crop diversification, custom hiring centers for timely planting, low temperature tolerance, promotion of pulses utilizing post-monsoon rainfall, integrated crop/pest/ disease management, growing vegetables as contingency crop

Module III: Livestock and Fisheries

Use of community lands for fodder production during drought/flood, improved fodder/feed storage methods, improved shelters for reducing heat stress in livestock, management of fish ponds/tanks during water scarcity and excess water, breed up-gradation, balanced feed & fodder management through mineral mixture, feed blocks & silage making, azolla feeding, breed animal health management through deworming and vaccination, fish pond cleaning and fish farming, pig farming, clean milk & fodder production

Module IV: Institutional Interventions

Strengthening the existing or initiating new ones relating to Seed bank, fodder bank, commodity groups, custom hiring centre, collective marketing group, introduction of weather index based insurance and climate literacy through a village weather station are part of this module

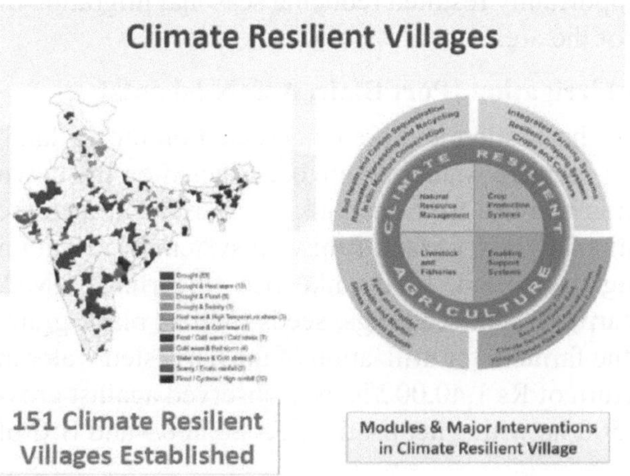

Cases of Successful and scalable interventions

- **Sand Bag Check dam (*Bora Bandi*)[Gumla, Jharkhand]**

Earlier pakka check dam was constructed on river but damaged after one year and the dams became purpose less. No water storage at this slope. After creation of low cost temporary structure through sand bag was made on river of 50 meter length huge quantity of water was reserved for supplemental and drinking (Animal) purpose. Recharging of well in nearby of the village was also done. Water table has risen by 44% followed by area expansion under off-season vegetable cultivation in 40.0 ha, summer paddy cultivation in 50.0 ha, wheat cultivation in 50.0 ha and safe harvesting of standing paddy from 30.0 ha during acute scarcity of rainwater. Mono-cropping has turned into double and in some cases multiple cropping in the village. All together more than 100 numbers of check dam created during ten years. Seeing the success of the intervention Govt. of Jharkhand has declared to replicate the technology in each district of the state.

- **Land shaping and rain water harvesting [S 24 pgs, WB]**

1600 ha mono-cropped land converted to multiple cropping (220 % Cropping Intensity), Net income Rs. 1.39 lakh/ha, 1774 man days per ha per year, Migration to city for other job reduced, Soil salinity significantly reduced, Carbon sequestration increased, 1500 ha × Rs. 1.39 = Rs. 22.2 crore net profit per annum, 10 million cu m. rain water harvested every year, 28.3 lakh man days of farm work created every year. Rs. 25 crore mobilized from other Department for up-scaling the technology in the entire Sundarbans Islands. Vegetables cultivation in land embankment during *kharif*and*rabi* season which fetched an additional income of Rs. 11000/- to 15000/- per acre. Pisci-culture opportunity along with paddy compounded by this technology which created handsome income and job opportunity resulted reducing seasonal migration of the farmers and rural youth of the area

- **Tank cum well system of irrigation [Port Blair, A & N Islands]**

Tanks are used for rain water harvesting and are constructed on the up land. Wells are used for harvesting seepage water and are constructed on the down slope of the pond. Irrigation is allowed from the tank till March and then the well water is used for irrigation. 40 nos. of tank cum well system of irrigation has been popularized during the period. Inputs like fish fingerlings (IMC, freshwater prawn & grass carp), brinjal seedlings, seeds (maize, black gram, pumpkin) were supplied to the farmers for utilization of the harvested water in cultivating crops. A gross return of Rs 1,40,000/ha was observed against gross cost of cultivation of Rs 59,500/ha with a net profit of Rs 80,500/- and B:C of 2.35 in one demonstration.

- **Improving the Resilience of Poor Farmers by Reclaiming Cultivable Wastelands [Nawada, Bihar]**

The cluster of villages Vidyasagar & Gadimajhila, Nawada is predominantly inhabited by Rajvanshi and Ravidas communities. The undulated lands are located in the fringe areas of forests and not cultivated despite being fertile. These were completely unprotected from grazing animals and rainwater harvesting and storage structures (*ahars*) could not convey water due to their higher elevation. The cultivable fallow was brought back into crop production by motivating the community to participate in reclaiming the lands by bunding and leveling. About 15 ha was planted with pigeon pea during *kharif* leading to a harvest of 10,000 kg of pigeon pea worth Rs.3,50,000/-. For the first time, the farmers of these villages could realize such a harvest and this helped them to appreciate the worth of their land.

- **De-silting of irrigation channels for coping with water [Saran, Bihar]**

The time required for irrigating one ha was brought down to 4.8 hr from 8 hr. This resulted in bringing 4 ha additionally under paddy. This generated an additional 600 man days of work. It also saved enough water to provide one supplementary irrigation of 5 cm over 15 ha. The additional 4 ha brought under paddy could yield about 10 t worth Rs. 1.0 lakh.

- **Renovation of Wells [Bihar and Jharkhand]**

So far, 125 wells have been renovated in this cluster of villages. The villagers are very happy with this intervention, as it has ensured them drinking water availability even in the midst of summer. The drainage line has also been developed leading to safe disposal of water. This has improved hygiene around the wells. In all, the well renovation intervention has been very well accepted by the villagers.

- **Renovation of *Ahar*[Aurangabad, Saran in Bihar]**
- Around 400 ha area was brought back into cultivation through the renovation of defunct *ahar.*
- **Rain water harvesting structures created in the zone**

Total Number	Storage capacity (mill cu m)	Protective irrigation potential (ha)
995	3.98	5535 ha of land

- **In-situ moisture conservation [in the zone]**

Technology Demonstrated	Area (ha)	No. of Beneficiaries	BC ratio
Summer Ploughing- Paddy (Var. Lalat)	412	1331	2.14
Green Manuring-Paddy (Var. Lalat)	505	1231	1.99

Technology Demonstrated	Area (ha)	No. of Beneficiaries	BC ratio
Brown Manuring in Paddy (Var. Anjali)	503	1305	2.54
Azolla application in Paddy (Var. Lalat)	501	1403	1.98

- **Rain water harvesting structure - 5% model [Chatra, Palamu, E Singhbhum in Jharkhand]**

5% models are created on medium upland rice field. In medium upland rice field the water retention capacity is low. Especially in late monsoon or insufficient rainfall transplanting of seedling are not done in time. By creating 5% model ditches in each plot to harvest and collect the rain water. Stored water increases the moisture level and helps in transplanting. Water stored in 5% model provides moisture during moisture stress later on. In this region mid land paddy suffer moisture stress at the time flowering and grain filling in case of early cessation of monsoon. Stored water in this structure provides moisture and life saving irrigation

- **In-situ moisture conservation through ridge & furrow method in cowpea (Jharsuguda, Odisha)**

It is used as contingent crop to protect from drought condition which improved water use efficiency up to 50%, increased in yield 28% more, maintain the gap of pulse and increase in net profit up to Rs. 78000 /- per ha.

- **Vegetables based Multi-tier Horticulture System (Malda, WB)**

Increased cropping intensity 197 %, Net income Rs. 1.08 lakh/ha, 368 man days per ha per year, Migration to city for other job reduced, Increase in diet diversity, Effective utilization of space, land and moisture

5520 man days of farm work created every year. All growing space is used as crop fit together vertically or horizontally (tall, medium & short) and underground (deep-rooted and shallow-rooted plants). Crops can be grown according to market preference and seasons

- **Post flood potato cultivation (Kendrapara, Odisha)**

Cropping Intensity increased up to 200%, 80 ha of river bank area converted to potato cultivation in post flood situation, Net income Rs.80.000/- per ha, 215 man days per ha per year, Increase in family income, increase in soil fertility, Farm biodiversity, Efficient use of silt in post flood situation, total 17,200 man days of farm work created every year

- **Soil Health Improvement through Azolla& Green Manuring [Sonepur, Odisha]**

	No. of demo	Bio-mass addition (q/ha)	C sequestration (kg/ha)	N addition (kg/ha)	% more in crop yield (q/ha)
Azolla	110	18-20	390	40-42	15-25
Dhaincha	60 3	28-30	820	50-60	15-28

- **Zero Tillage in Wheat [Bihar & Jharkhand]**

	Area	Grain Yield (q/ha)	Fuel for (L/ ha) land prepn	Fuel for (L/ ha) irrign	Man day (Nos/ha)
Demonstration	**> 500 ha**	**30.48(24.6)**	**20.19(36.1)**	**12.98(18.0)**	**84(118)**

Figures in parentheses for conventional practices

Technology demonstration under Crop Production [in the Zone]

Technology demonstrated	Area covered	No. of farmers covered	% increase
Drought tolerant vars (Sahbhagi, Anjali, A 404, Naveen, Abhishek)	2414.0	14499	16.8 – 150.5
Salt tolerant varsCARIDhan 5, User dhan 3, SR 268, Jarava, Geetanjali	2105.5	14184	16.7 – 35.5
Flood tolerant vars.Swarna Sub 1, Sabita	2184.0	13235	22 – 33.5
Advancement of planting datesfor wheat, lentil, mustard	2153.4	12046	31 – 231.5
Staggered community nurseries for paddy, brinjal, cauliflower, tomato	2119.3	1385	11.3 – 24.3
Location sp. intercropping	2158.3	6321	55.5 – 134.6
Crop diversification	1198.4	9534	26.0 - 68.8

- **Community Nursery for Paddy [Saran, Jehanabad in Bihar and Chatra, palamu in Jharkhand]**

One of the important interventions has been the promotion of community nursery for paddy as an approach to contingent availability of seedlings during drought or flood in the NICRA adopted village(s). Seedlings were raised by sowing of seeds at 15 days interval in three stages and farmers were allowed to take the seedlings as much as they could transplant depending upon rainfall conditions.

- **Organic mulching in vegetables [Coochbehar, WB]**

In situ moisture conservation through application of organic mulching (straw) in vegetable cultivation and use of zero tillage machine in wheat cultivation as resource conservation means with reduced cost of cultivation ensured timely sowing of wheat in NICRA adopted villages followed by production of off season vegetables

- **Advancement of planting dates [in the Zone]**

Advancement of planting dates of rabi crops to overcome terminal heat stress also recorded as much as 97.3, 75.6 and 68.8 percent higher yield in case of okra (Bhendi No. 64), bitter gourd (DEB-512) and french bean (*Arkakomal*) respectively than existing farmers practice

Technology demonstrate	Crop	Area (ha)	Yield		% increase
			Demo (t/ha)	Local (t/ha)	
Advancement of planting dates of rabi crops in areas with terminal heat stress	Okra (*Bhendi No- 64*),	1.0	7.5	3.8	97.3
	Bitter gourd (*DEB-512*)	0.5	7.2	4.1	75.6
	French bean (*Arkakomal*)	0.4	8.1	-	100

- **Crop diversification** through introducing crops like ori (vars. *Pusatarak, Pusavijay, Pusa 28*) as less water requiring crop as contingent crop planning during deficit rainfall in kharif
- **Breed Improvement through Improved Buck [Saran, Jehanabad in Bihar]**
  - Ensuring Descript services among 10 no. of goat.
  - For 14 no of kids in F1 generation.
  - Rs 45000/- more income was recover from 14 no of kids
  - Body weight increased by 40%.
- **Cultivation of sudan grass – a low water requiring fodder crop [in the Zone]**

Sudan grass, a fodder crop is suitable for drought affected areas. In general 2-3 cuttings at 60, 100, 140 days could be made from this crop. The crop required low water and the growth is very fast compared to other fodder crops. It has been recorded fodder yield of 503 q/ha in 2 months from cultivation of sudan grass.

- **Livelihood security through Pig Farming: Introduces T&D breed of Pig [Jehanabad, Saran in Bihar and Gumla, Chatra in Jharkhand]**

More Feed Conversion ratio that's why better growth, very low skin disease occurrence, high income, Benefit cost ratio is better than Local breed, Body weight enhanced by 120%

- **Preventive vaccination [in the Zone]**

Various vaccination camps were organized against FMD of Cattle; PPR against goat, Ranikhet of poultry, BQ vaccine, deworming etc. in all different NICRA adopted villages regularly. Mortality rate reduce up to the extent of 100% and average increase in cattle milk yield up to 20% have been recorded after the vaccination camps organized

- **Improved cross ventilated Poultry, Dairy and Goatary shed[in the Zone]**
  - Improved Poultry shed with well-ventilated system reduced mortality rate
  - Improved sheds in shady area reduced heat stress, mortality of calves & increased milk yield
  - Recommended spacing in improved shed resulted into better performance in poultry, dairy animals and goat
- **Roof Top Rain Water Harvesting for Asian Catfish Hatchery[S 24 pgs, WB]**

Roof Top Rain Water Harvesting in Bongheri, Sunderbans was developed to start Asian Catfish Hatchery cultivation. Fresh groundwater is required for breeding and larval rearing of Asian catfish but the village doesn't have a single bore well to serve the purpose. The roof top rainwater was collected in a 1500L capacity storage tank and used for larval rearing of Asian Catfish and Koi. The harvested rainwater was portable and measured 6.85 of pH and 0.05 of EC suitable for breeding and larval rearing. The storage tank was filled for three times during the rainy season that supported 3 breeding cycles of Asian catfish and Koi. Around produced 12000 Asian catfish and 12000 *Koi* fry were produced and earned a net profit of Rs. One lakh in 1st year and more in subsequent years. The technology is now up-scaled in nearby villages of Sunderbans

Institutional Intervention

Institutional interventions including seed bank, fodder bank, commodity groups, custom hiring for timely operations, community nursery raising, irrigation, collective marketing climate literacy through a village level weather station and awareness developed 1221 units covering of 1365.8 ha area of 8351 number of farmers in the Zone. Custom Hiring Centre has the provision of various farm implements like Power tiller, Thresher, Reaper, Water pump, Zero- till Drill, Raised bed planter, Sprayer, Weeder etc. There is a provision of Mini Automatic Weather Station through which farmers are provided weather forecasting data.

Village Climate Risk Management Committee (VCRMC)

Village Climate Risk Management Committee (VCRMC) was constituted after in-depth discussion with the villagers about the mitigation of the climatic vulnerabilities of the villages and the strategies to be adopted under NICRA. The members of the committee were selected by the villagers under the facilitation of KVKs where NICRA was being implemented. VCRMC became operational with opening of a bank account in their name being jointly handled by the President of VCRMC and the Programme Coordinator of the KVK concerned. The custom hiring of various farm tools and implements was being supervised by VCRMC apart from taking important decisions on the technological interventions to be implemented at the village in consultation with the KVK. Jay Prakash VCRMC constituted at KVK Nawada, Bihar generated highest amount (approx. Rs. 3.0 lakh) in the bank account of VCRMC and got National Award of best performing VCRMC in 2014.

Custom Hiring of Farm Implements and machinery at NICRA Villages

The custom hiring of various farm tools and implements was being supervised by VCRMC apart from taking important decisions on the technological interventions to be implemented at the village in consultation with the KVK have now become immensely popular among the farmers and substantial amount has also been generated. Timeliness of agricultural operations is crucial to cope with climate variability, especially in case of sowing and intercultural operations. Access to implements for planting in ridge-furrow, broad bed furrow and raised beds is essential for widespread adoption of resilient practices for *in situ* soil moisture conservation and drainage of excess water in heavy soils. In rain fed areas, availability of such farm implements to small and marginal farmers is important. Similarly in irrigated areas, residue management of *kharif* crops through zero till cultivation of *rabi* crops reduces the problem of burning of residues and adds to the improvement of soil health and increases water use efficiency. The rates for hiring the machines /implements are decided by the members of VCRMC. This committee also uses the revenue generated from hiring charges and deposits in a bank account opened in the name of VCRMC. The revenue is used for repair and maintenance of the implements and 25% share is earmarked as a sustainability fund. Different types of farm machinery are stocked in the CHCs, the most popular being Zero till drill, Happy seeder, BBF planter, drum seeder, multi crop planter, power weeder, mechanical weeder, chaff cutter, cono weeder, duster, sprayer, leveler, FIRB planter, sub-soiler, zero-till frti-seed, disc harrow, bucket leveler, reaper, thresher, cultivator, rotavator, pump set *etc.*

Resource Generated through Convergence by NICRA with Ongoing Other Development Schemes

Huge number of convergence programmes was carried out by each of the NICRA implementing KVK with ongoing development schemes. The prominent development schemes: NAIP, MGNREGA, National Micro and Minor Irrigation Scheme, Pradhan Mantri Gram SadakYojana, Chief Minister SadakYojna, Backward Rural Grant Fund, Silk Board, Sunderban Development Board, NFSM, IWMP, IVRI, Forest Department, MESO (Marine Environmental Support Office), IAP (Integrated action plan) Yojana*etc.* NICRA implementing KVKs being part of the different convergence programmes generated an amount of Rs. 52.87 crore during last 10 years in WB, Odisha, Bihar and Jharkhand.

27

Extension Strategies for Popularization of Livestock Based Entrepreneurship Models

Prabhat Kumar Pal

Extension Education
Uttar Banga Krishi Viswavidyalaya, West Bengal-736165

Over the time, the concept of extension education transformed from an educational system to an empowerment tool. It is a programme and a process of helping village people to help themselves in view to increase production and raise their general standard of living. As a science, Extension education deals with the creation, transmission and application of knowledge designed to bring about planned changes in the behaviour-complex of people. This particular branch of agricultural science is devoted to bring changes in perception and attitude towards scientific farming techniques, adoption of hi-tech horticulture, precision farming, improved machineries of pre and post-harvest management etc. through vocational training, capacity building, participatory approaches and through many other approaches. A proper planning of extension strategy will help to popularize livestock-based system of production, processing and economics associated with it.

Extension Approaches Followed In India Till Date

From the pre-independence period, different extension approaches were adopted in our country. In pre-independence era, extension services started with micro-level attempts under individual leadership of eminent personalities. Programmes like Gurgaon experiment, Sriniketan experiment, Etowah pilot project etc. were some of such attempts initiated to mobilize rural people. Although these efforts could not impact extensively, but we could learn how to initiate rural development programmes. Based on the experiences of individual approaches extensive development approaches like Community Development Programme, National Extension Service or *Panchayeti Raj* system were adopted focusing on all round development with nationwide network of delivery system, facilitated grass-root participation. Subsequently another extension approach that was Intensive extension approach followed which was highly input intensive in terms of requirement of seeds, fertilizers, pesticides, irrigation, credit etc and food production increases (cereals and wheat).Programmes under this approach were Intensive Agricultural District Programme, Intensive Agricultural Area Programme, High Yielding Variety Programme etc. In this way, with the experiences in each approach, other approached like target group/area specific approach, mono-purpose extension approach or group approach came in different phases. All these approaches were having various limitations like having too narrow focus limiting to crop production technologies only, low ratio of skilled experts in relation to no. of serving households under each expert, uncoordinated and duplication of efforts etc. (Swanson, 2006; Reddy and Swanson, 2006; Birner and Anderson, 2007; Singh et al.,2014).

A critical review of working of extension systems prevailing in India with respect to livestock development and promotion

The extension system described in foregoing section helped India to achieve3.7 times increase in food production with 45% increase in per capita production against 2.55 times increase in population taking 1965 as the base year. This transformed India not only to a food self-sufficient country, but also to a food exporting country. So far livestock sector is concerned, it plays an important role in Indian economy and about 20.5 million people depend upon livestock for their livelihood. Livestock contributed 16% to the income of small farm households as against an average of 14% for all rural households. Livestock provides livelihood to two-third of rural community. It also provides employment to about 8.8 % of the population in India. India has vast livestock resources. Livestock sector contributes 4.11% GDP and 25.6% of total Agriculture GDP (accessed from www.vikaspedia.in). Although public extension system has adopted a range of extension programmes but the emphasis was predominantly given on increasing the production and productivity of popular and conventional crops, emphasis on livestock sector is still meagre. In private sector also, efforts are comparatively less than crop-based interventions. It may be due to the fact that trained manpower in livestock sector is extremely shorter than crop sector. Moreover, livestock being the member of animal kingdom is associated with more risks due to health and nutritional aspects than that of crop production sector. It also requires more intensive and higher skills for day to day management of livestock resources.

Exploring new extension approaches for promotion of farming and entrepreneurship in livestock sector

New approaches are initiated in extension service delivery which can be explored for promotion of farming and entrepreneurship in livestock sector. These approaches are:

- Pluralism and convergence of extension activities of different extension actors.
- Formation and utilization of Grass root extension organizations like Farmer Producer Organizations, Commodity Groups or Farmer Interest Groups etc.
- Use of ICT tools for database management, knowledge management and skill development
- Development of Agri-Start-ups by youth empowerment.
- Exploring public-private partnership in enhancing livestock based entrepreneurship.

Community-oriented models should be developed integrating the foregoing approaches in these models. A model is proposed which works on the principle of pluralistic and convergence approach engaging public-private-corporate-community organizations at various stages of supply chain.

Steps to be followed for establishment of such models

- Conducting a community oriented situational analysis to explore the gap and scope of integrating livestock resources in existing model of livelihood.
- Exploring the technological option for cultivation and processing of livestock products and making institutional back-stopping linkage for this.
- Organizing producers into Farmer Interest Group/Farmer organizations.
- Training and skill development of farmers for scientific cultivation or processing.
- Supply-chain management and marketing of produce.

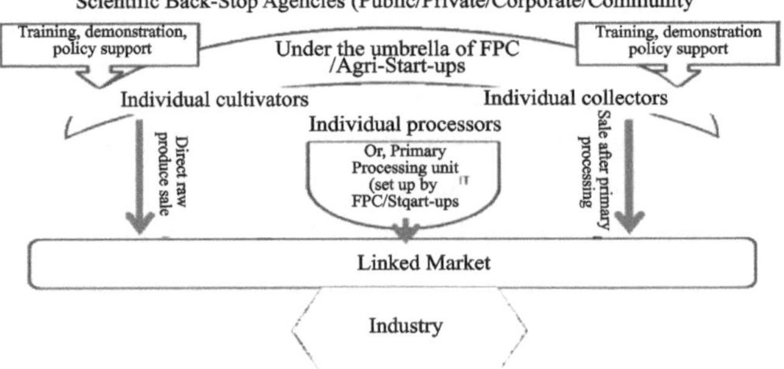

Production and processing oriented model

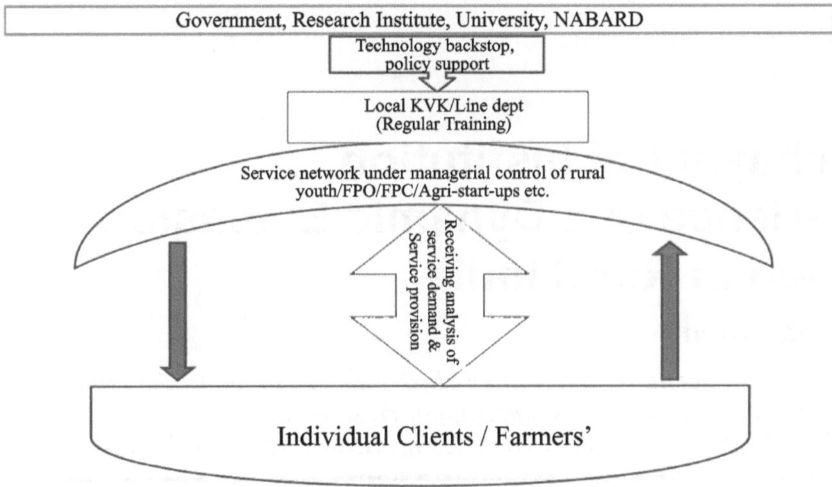

Service oriented model

Factors making farmers ready to be an actor of such models

With above illustration can easily understand different factors responsible to encourage individual farmers/community/group to take part into entrepreneurship model based on livestock. These factors are individual factors (behavioural aspects, education level, economic condition, managerial capability, marginality, needs and innovativeness of the farmer); community & socio-political factors (available institutional structures, norms & sanctions, group dynamic, political situation of farming community); technological factors (relative advantages, compatibility, complexity, observability and trialability of farm technologies); extension & policy factors (competence & dedication & communication behaviour of extension agent, Govt. policy premises).

Organizations can establish such type of Model

The different agencies like Agri-Start-ups, Farmer Producer Company (FPCs), Local KVKs, Agri-Innovative Projects, Science Technology and Innovation Hub andNGOs can establish community-oriented models for popularizing medicinal plant.

28

Panchayat Raj Institution Experience of a Dynamic Extension System in Rural India

Saidur Rahman

Department of Veterinary and Animal Husbandry Extension Education
College of Veterinary Sciences and Animal Husbandry
Central Agricultural University (I), Selesih, Aizawl, Mizoram-796014

Panchayati Raj is the oldest system of local government in the Indian subcontinent. Panchayati Raj Institutions have been in existence in India for a long time. In the old Sanskrit scriptures, word 'Panchayatan' has been mentioned which means a group of five persons, including a spiritual man. In the Rigveda, there is a mention of Sabha, Samiti and Vidatha as local self-units. These were the democratic bodies at the local level. The king used to get the approval of these bodies regarding certain functions and decisions.

After independence, as a development initiative, India had implemented the Community Development Programmes (CDP) on the eve of Gandhi Jayanti, the 2nd October, 1952.The National Extension Service followed the Community Development Programme as the vehicle through which idea of Community Development would be worked and to build up an administrative system which can tackle the welfare problems of growth at the local level. The Balvantray Mehta Study Team was appointed in January 1957 to study and to make report on the Community Development Projects and National Extension Service .The Team brought to focus the areas mentioned below:

- First, it argued that there should be administrative decentralization for the effective implementation of the development programme and that the decentralized administrative system should be under the control of elected bodies.
- Recommended an early establishment of statutory elective local bodies and devolution to them of the necessary resources, power and authority".
- This, according to the report, was the meaning of democratic decentralization

in operational terms. Secondly, the basic unit of democratic decentralization should be located at the block/samiti level.

- The National Development Council affirmed the objective in introducing democratic institutions at the district and block levels and suggested that each State should work out the structure which suited its conditions best.

The word "Democracy" is used the Greek roots 'demos' meaning the people and 'Kratos' meaning authority i.e. in democracy all authority originates from the people. Decentralization means distribution of functions and power from a central authority to regional and local authorities. Democratic Decentralization in the present context means that the government which has derived its authority from the people, redistributes it to some extent to the people for the decision and action at the local level. This is popularly known as 'Panchayat Raj'. The word "Panchayat" means assembly (ayat) of five (panch) and raj means "rule".

The recommendation of the Balwantray Mehta Committee came as a fresh breeze and gave a new lease to CD and extension service projects. It paved the way for new era of Panchayat Raj Institution (PRI), which was inaugurated by Jawahar Lal Nehru on 2nd October, 1959 at a national rally at Nagaur in Rajasthan..

Definition

- PRIis a system of **rural local self-government** in India.
- Local Self Government is the management of local affairs by such local bodies who have been **elected by the local people**.

Concept of Panchayat Raj (PR):

- Panchayat Raj is a means to achieve the end of Community development.
- It is an extension of democracy to the village
- It is an extension of administration up to the village level

Basic objective of PRI is to evolve:

- a system of democratic decentralization and devolution of power.
- Function and authority to the rural people with a view to ensure rapid socio-economic progress and speedier and inexpensive justice.

New Panchayat Raj System (Three -Tier System)

The 73rd and 74th Constitutional Amendments were passed by Parliament in December, 1992. Through these amendments local self-governance was introduced in rural and urban India. The Acts came into force as the Constitution (73rd Amendment) Act, 1992 on April 24, 1993 and the Constitution (74th Amendment) Act, 1992 on June 1, 1993.

Basic Features of 73rd Amendments of Constitution

- 3-tier system of Panchayat at the village, for all the states.
- All seats in Panchayat are filled by direct Election.
- Devolution of powers & responsibilities by the State Legislature.
- Constitution of finance commission in the state.
- Vest in the election commission, the super intendancy direction & control of election to the Panchayat at all three level.
- The Gram Sabha is a body consisting of all the people registered in the electoral rolls who belong to a village comprised within the area of the Panchayat at the village level. Gram Sabha is the smallest and the only permanent unit in the Panchayati Raj system. The powers and functions of Gram Sabha are fixed by state legislature according to the law on the subject.
- One-third of the total numbers of seats are to be reserved for women. One-third of the seats reserved for SCs and STs, are also reserved for women. This policy extends to the office of the chairperson at all levels as well (Article 243D). The reserved seats may be allotted by rotation to different constituencies in the Panchayat.
- There is a uniform policy with each term being five years. Fresh elections must be conducted before the expiry of the term. In the event of dissolution, elections compulsorily within six months (Article 243E).
- Panchayats have the responsibility to prepare plans for economic development and social justice with respect to the subjects as per the law put in place, which also extends to the various levels of Panchayat including the subjects as illustrated in the Eleventh Schedule (Article 243G).
- The Panchayati Raj Institution (PRI) consists of three levels:
- Gram Panchayat at the village level
- Block Panchayat or Panchayat Samiti at the intermediate level
- Zilla Panchayat at the district level

Subjects Transferred to the Panchayats- 29 subjects transferred to PRI

1. Agriculture, including agricultural extension
2. Land improvement, implementation of land reforms, land consolidation and soil conservation
3. Minor irrigation, water management and watershed development
4. Animal husbandry, dairying and poultry
5. Fisheries

6. Social forestry and farm forestry
7. Minor forest produce
8. Small scale industries, including food processing industries
9. Khadi, village and cottage industries
10. Rural housing
11. Drinking water
12. Fuel and fodder
13. Roads, culverts, bridges, ferries, waterways and other means of communication
14. Rural electrification, including distribution of electricity
15. Non-conventional energy sources
16. Poverty alleviation programme
17. Education including primary and secondary schools
18. Technical training and vocational education
19. Adult and non-formal education
20. Libraries
21. Cultural activities
22. Market and fairs
23. Health and sanitation, including hospitals, primary health centres and dispensaries
24. Family welfare
25. Women and child development
26. Social welfare, including welfare of the handicapped and mentally retarded
27. Welfare of the weaker sections, and in particular, of the Scheduled Castes and Scheduled Tribes.
28. Public distribution system
29. Maintenance of community assets

Reservation for women in PRI

- On August 27, 2009, the Union Cabinet of the Government of India approved 50% reservation for women in (PRI).
- The states of Andhra Pradesh, Assam, Bihar, Chhattisgarh, Gujarat, HimachalPradesh, Jharkhand, Kerala, Karnataka, MadhyaPradesh,Maharashtra, Odisha, Rajasthan, Sikkim, Tamil Nadu, Telangana,Tripura, West Bengal and Uttarakhand have implemented 50% reservation for women in PRIs.

Panchayat Raj Institutions Today

Sl. No.	Unit	No.
1.	Number of PRIs in the country.	2,62,617
2.	Number of Village Panchayats	255283
3.	Number of Intermediate Panchayats	6672
4.	Number of District Panchayats	662
5.	Number of Elected Members of PRIs	31.00 lakh (approx.)
6.	Number of Elected Women Representatives	13.75 lakh (approx.)

Achievements of Panchayat Raj Institutions

- The innovation has empowered the village community.
- Widened the democratic base of rural India resulting in inclusive and integrated growth.
- Resulted in amazing development – women empowerment and emergence of women as leaders.
- Large numbers of women are shouldering responsibilities with grace and competence, bringing enormous courage, enthusiasm and creativity.

Aberrations in the Effort

- Bureaucratic methods of the State Governments dilute the spirit of implementation.
- In some cases, Panchayats are becoming an institution to perpetuate cast inequalities that already exist.
- The power rooted in caste, gender and sometimes religion determines the functioning of Panchayat system.

Extension Education

"Agricultural Extension is an empowering system of sharing information, knowledge, technology, skills, risk & farm management practices, across agricultural sub-sectors and along all aspects of the agricultural supply chain, so as to enable the farmers to realize higher net income from their enterprise on a sustainable basis". (*DFI Volume X-2017*)

Objective of Extension

The fundamental objective of extension is to develop the rural people economically, socially and culturally by means of education.

1. To assist people to analyze problem
2. To develop leadership
3. To disseminate research information
4. To help in utilizing resources
5. To collect and feedback information

Scope of Extension

The scope of extension education includes all the activities directed towards the development of the rural people. The capacity of extension education to work for rural people is very wide.

Extensions appears to have unlimited scope in situations where there is need for creating awareness amongst the people and changing their behavior.

- Efficiency in agricultural production.
- Efficiency in marketing, distribution and utilization.
- Conservation, development, and use of natural resources.
- Management on the farm and in the home.
- Family living.
- Youth development.
- Leadership development.
- Community development and rural area development.
- Public affairs.

Role of PRI in Agri Extension

After the 73rd and 74th constitutional amendments, the PRI is the major driver in the development of rural areas. It acts as a single window for implementation of all developmental schemes. PRI is the main planning and executive agency for all kinds of development projects at the *Gram Panchayat* level.

- Participatory Planning and Development
- Technology Refinement
- Management of Agricultural Infrastructure
- Redefine Agenda of Research Institutions/Stations
- Implement Research - Extension Link Programmes

- Participatory Research and Refinement
- Programme Planning, Implementation and Disaster Management
- Input Distribution
- Institutional Co-ordination
- Agricultural Infrastructure and Resource Improvement
- Natural Resource Management
- Equal Sharing of Resources
- Conservation and Sustainable Use of Resources
- Environment Protection

Benefits of PRI

- Strong Grassroots level local democratic Institution-Local problems require local solutions. Problems arising in rural areas can be best attended and solved by members of the Panchayats, encouraging local leadership.
- The line departments cannot by themselves carry out all village level development programmes in the absence of local level initiative and participation. The local people must have a sense of belonging in the schemes. Involvement of GPs in a coordinating role in various projects of line departments would be a way forward for convergence.
- Constitutional representation of weaker section
- Close intimation with Executive and the people
- Strong network

Linkage of PRI in Extension System

- Involved in various committees
- Research prioritization
- Reviewing
- Social auditing
- Impact assessment in their respective areas.
- The PRIs should act as a coordinating, monitoring and evaluation body.

Sustainable Development Goals and Panchayats

- The twin objectives of the PRI as envisaged by the Constitution of India are to ensure local economic development and social justice.
- Many of the SDG targets are within the purview of these functions listed in the Eleventh Schedule.

- Various flagship programmes such as Swachh Bharat Abhiyan, Make in India, Digital India, Skill India, and Jan Dhan Yojana which are at the core of the SDGs and local governments play a pivotal role in many of these programmes.
- The Gram Panchayat Development Plans (GPDP) initiated after the recommendation of the Fourteenth Finance Commission paves the way for the Panchayats to link planning with the SDGs.
- For localization of SDGs, the Ministry of Panchayati Raj (MoPR) has prepared a 'Draft Vision Document for Achieving SDGs'. It has mapped roles of Panchayats in terms of SDGs and centrally sponsored schemes (CSS).

What can a Gram Panchayat Do?

- Micro, small and medium enterprises within the panchayat area
- Enterprise opportunities in the village
- Employment opportunities for different categories and degrees of disabilities
- Identify and track Potential candidates to set up enterprises, Skills of interested candidates
- Take steps to empower communities and community-based organizations to participate in activities
- Ensuring equal participation of women in local governance and decision making
- Value added products from agriculture, animal husbandry, pisciculture, non-timber forest produce
- (Handbook on Sustainable Development Goals and Gram Panchayats.)

Role of PRI in National Livestock Mission

Sub-Mission on Skill Development, Technology Transfer and Extension
The extension machinery at field level for livestock activities is not adequately strengthened and effective. The farmers are not getting the relevant technologies in time and not able to adopt the technologies. The development and adoption of new technologies and practices requires linkages amongst different stakeholders involved in the sector. The sub-mission will provide a platform to develop, adopt or adapt the technologies including frontline field demonstrations in collaboration with farmers, researchers and extension workers, etc. wherever it is not possible to achieve this through existing arrangements.

The Mission has a General Council (GC) at National level under the Chairmanship of Union Agriculture Minister.

Composition of GC

Minister of Agriculture	Chairperson
Ministers of:- Food Processing Industries; Environment & Forests; Finance; Panchayati Raj; Rural Development.	Member
Secretaries of Departments / Ministries of:- Animal Husbandry, Dairying & Fisheries; Agriculture and Cooperation; Agricultural Research and Education; Food Processing Industries; Expenditure; Financial Services; Health & Family Welfare; Environment & Forests; **Panchayati Raj;** Rural Development; Medium, Small and Microenterprise; Development of North Eastern Region; Biotechnology.	Member
Representatives of:- Animal Rearers Associations; Poultry Associations; Federations of Dairy Co-operatives; Food Processing Industry; Compounded Feed Industry (Maximum 5, to be nominated by the Chairperson).	Member
Joint Secretary (APF) & Mission Director (NLM).	Member-secretary

Social Audit

- The Mission envisages concurrent, continuous system of social auditing through the PRI/ similar recognized bodies, like Urban Local Bodies, etc, where PRI is not there.
- The Gram Sabha may be the body for primary level social auditing at village level.
- Panchayat level social audit committees may be constituted.
- The committees may conduct the audit at regular intervals, and may present the report in the Gram Sabha or appropriate authority like BDO etc. in cases where PRI is not present.
- (National Livestock Mission, Operational Guidelines (Revised as on 27.04.2016),

ATMA-Activity Mapping for Panchayati Raj Institutions

PRIs needs to be involved in the formulation, prioritization of activities & identification of beneficiaries at grass root level.

An illustrative Activity Mapping for involvement of PRI

Activity Category	**Union Govt. (MOA,DAC)**	**State Government**	**District Level**	**Panchayati Raj System**
				Distt,/ Intermediate/ Village Panchayat
Framing Sectoral Action Plan	Policy Formulation. Comments of Ministry of PRI suitably incorporated in the policy.	Implement policies formulated by GOI.	Aggregating Sectoral Action Plan in to District Action Plan	PRI institution from village level is involved in preparing the Sectoral Extension Work Plan along with other Stakeholders and farmers. Preparation of Block Action Plan in consultation with BTT and BFAC. Selection of Cafeteria activities.
Identification of Beneficiaries		Monitoring of beneficiary identification	Identify beneficiaries with active involvement of PRIs for training, demonstration and other farmer oriented activities.	Identify beneficiaries with active involvement of Farmer Friends for all beneficiary-oriented activities under the Scheme.
Conduct of Farm Information Dissemination Activities			Organization of exhibitions, Kisan Melas, use of Print & Electronic media, Field Days, KisanGosties, etc.	Actively involved in selection of area of specialization, venue, actual organization.
Monitoring & Evaluation	Review of performance, follow up & feedback	Review by IDWG in which PRI rep. is a member	ATMA GB in which CEO, Zila Parishad is a Vice Chairman	By Farmers Friend, BTM, ATM in association with PRI

(ATMA Guidelines, 2014 Under NMAET)

Conclusion

- PRI is the local level democratic Institution dedicated for rural Development
- Panchayati Raj Institutions can play a vital role in sustainable development of rural area.
- As Animal Husbandry, Agricultural Extension etc. comes under PRI, the extension activities for overal
- Changes in farming system, PRI should be involved in participatory planning and management process.
- Utilization of local resources is very important for Livestock and agricultural development and PRI should be made guardian of these resources.
- PRI should be more proactive in protecting the farmers' interest.
- The line dept officials of that particular level must attend the meeting of PRIs as well as Gram Sabha to discuss about different schemes and clarify the doubts of villagers.
- PRIs should mediate with financial institutions, Banks, cooperatives on behalf of the marginalized farmers for accessing formal credit.

29

Integrated Homestead Farming Towards Household Livelihood Nutritional Security and Conservation of Agro-Biodiversity

Dipak Kr. Ghosh

Horticulture (PSMA)
Bidhan Chandra Krishi Viswavidyalaya

Homestead is a small scale, supplementary food production system; it has the potential to produce high value crops including various spices condiments by and large for the household members. A typical home garden is an adjunct to the house, where selected trees, shrubs are grown, not only edible fruits / vegetables, but also for medicinal, ornamental, socioeconomic and ecological benefits. Homestead exhibit a multi tired canopy structure somewhat identical to the tropical evergreen forest formations. The vertical stratification provides a gradient in light and relative humidity, which creates different niches for enabling various spices/groups to exploit them .Mostly shade tolerant crops constitute the lower stratum, the shade intolerant trees the layer and spices with varying degree of shade tolerance in the intermediate strata .These multi strata system are structurally and functionally the closest mimics of natural forests yet attained The structural and floristic diversity of tropical home gardens are perhaps aided by the biophysical environment, socio-culture factors and economic consideration. Home gardens are suitable for resources poor situations and have economic advantage such as low capital and labour costs, increased self-sufficiency, risk avoidance and even distribution of labour. The published inventories suggest that food crops, medicinal plants, ornamental, fruits, multipurpose trees and folders crops abounds in the home gardens. Along with the crop, animals and birds are also reared for milk, meat and eggs making the homestead an integrated enterprises .The system has evolved because of the climatic conditions, the nature of precipitation and the soil conditions, as also the low per capita availability of land. The homestead farming is unique since there is livestock –crop integration with flow of inter-activity resources making it an integrated production system.

Food and nutrition security is a high priority on the global agenda or Sustainable Development Goals .The global agenda of integration of the Food Security Cluster and the Global Nutrition Cluster highlighted the need for developing strategies and sharing best practices in support of food security and nutrition needs for crisis affected households and populations3. There is strong evidence that linkages between food security and nutrition need to be considered in the design and delivery of emergency response4. As illustrated in the UNICEF Conceptual Framework. *M*aternal and child under nutrition have multiple immediate causes operating at individual level, underlying causes operating at household level, and basic causes operating at the societal level. This framework is applicable in Pakistan, where the causes of chronic malnutrition and food insecurity are complex, and compounded by frequent, unpredictable shocks including natural disasters & conflicts.

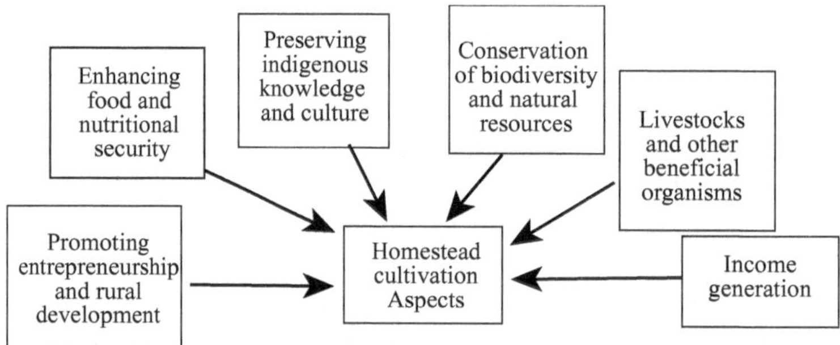

Perspective of the homestead farming

Homestead represents one of the functionally most diverse land use systems around the tropics. They are known for stable yields, varied products, and continuous or repeated harvests directly (producing edible fruits nuts, grain, rhizomes and tubers, leaves, flowers etc.) or indirectly (facilitating enhanced and /or sustained production) .All home gardens are also associated with varies service functions such as site enrichment, micro climatic modification and nutrient cycling. Considering the shrinking average land holding and also the requirement of in situ conservation of bio-resources and the commonly available homestead situation of West Coast region, development of suitable technologies for homestead farming with a concept of encouraging the number of tertiary producers of such valuable resources with far reaching utility through commercial means is the need of the hour. Some of the advantages of homestead farming are:

- The homestead farming increases whole farm productivities (land, labour and input).
- Ensures food and nutritional of the farm families throughout the year.

- Reduces stress periods in the farm
- Increases the profitability of the farming enterprises.
- Enhances the cash flows in the farm families.
- It provides the farmers a subsidiary source of income through potential crop/ integrated enterprises.
- It increases and sustains productivities of existing system cultivation.
- It encourages maximum utilization of available family labour.
- It creates an integrated business enterprise in micro level.

Different kind of benefits derived from homestead farming

Social benefits: Activities of homestead farming are labour intensive, which creates on-farm man days most of it in the production process is contributed by the farmer himself and also his family members. It gives year round availability of nutritious and seasonal food. Seasonal migration is reduced .Fodder fuel shortage is also minimized.

Economic benefits: The input cost is reduced, so net income increases. As income is diversified that is from different sub-systems, risk is reduced. The income has time wise and source wise diversified, i.e. the farmer is getting income throughout the year from different sources, which reduces the dependency on a single system.

Health Benefit : Fresh vegetables fruits, spices in one's own backward will make the citizens healthier. Chemical and fertilizer consumption will reduce as compare to commercially grown increasing The Nutritive value of the food stuff. Physical stress while moving in town will be reduce due to soothing land scape, shade during not sunshine, improved air quality and increase in thermal comfort Pesticide free foods and vegetables are obtained. Aesthetic value, satisfaction of growing plants and eating fruit of plants which are self-grown.

Ecological benefits: Soil health will be improved, percent organic carbon increased and the fossil fuel dependency as all the variable inputs are produce within the farm. The diversity is huge as various types of crops, creepers climbers, strategic crops etc. are cultivated within the farm. As large numbers of local crops are introduced, soil micro/macro fauna will be increase. Each and everything is recycled within the system, it is actually a zero west farming system. As it is diversified, it is disaster resilient.

Planning for Homestead farming

At present Homestead is practiced in a haphazard manner, without any scientific base, which leads to poor returns. There are no other components excepts and vegetables in many of the gardens at present .Therefore there is a need of scientific planning and establishment of Homestead gardens, So that there will be more output per unit area .Also there should be integration with other components like Animals, Mushrooms, Bee keeping etc. So that the family is more self-sufficient and independent.

Generally the size of a garden depends on the area available in the house compound. Before the actual layout the available area should be properly fenced .The irrigation channel from the water source and path should be so planned and preferred that it covers the whole area of the garden .Bunds can be used for growing root crops .The final selection of fruits and vegetables crops depends on likes and dislikes of the family However, in order to furnish a constants supply and avoid the glut, they can be staggered and planted on home scale .Important criteria will be choice of nutritious fruits and vegetables only those fruits and varieties should be selected which may have optimum performances and preference under local agro-climatic conditions.

Crops rotation for vegetables can be so worked out that at least 4-6 kinds of vegetables are also available .each plot should have a separate rotation so that period of harvest in different plots does not overlap .The same can be used in all the three seasons in a year. Suitable modification in the choice of plan of layout and selection of fruits and vegetables can be made in relation to the land available, adaptability of crop varieties, choice of family, etc. The main aim in lay out is the most economic utilization of space .Different root crops like Radish, carrot, beetroot and collocation can be grown on the ridges separating individual beds or on both sides of irrigation channels .Cucurbits like bitter gourds, sponge gourds, ridge gourd and snake gourd can be grown on the fences in summer and rainy seasons. Perennial crops like drumstick, curry leaf plant sand quick growing fruits like papaya and banana should located on one side .Tall grown vegetables should be grouped together it must be born in mind that the garden should be furnish a constant supply but avoid glut of any one crop .When space is the limiting factor for selecting vegetables, some basic principles can be followed .Vegetables which are costly not easily available in the market should be given priority over the vegetables which have shorter shelf life for upkeep of quality like spinach, mint etc. Further, vegetables which produce a larger amount of edible material in proportion to the space occupied should be given priority over the vegetable which have shorter shelf life for upkeep quality like spinach, mint etc. Further, vegetable which produce larger amount of edible material proportion to the space occupied should be given priority .before the actual implementation of the homestead farming, it very essential to assess the existing situation and the resource potential so as to plan a system on scientific lines.

Important points to be considered while planning homestead farming.

1. Area allocation for each crop/component should be based on the requirement of light, canopy Coverage, rooting pattern, nutrient demand, yield potential, family requirement market demand during different periods of the year.
2. Generally growing a mixture of different crops base on requirement of light in a multistoried pattern like tall growing species, medium statured ones, bushes and the surface creepers will utilized the solar radiation efficiency at different elevation.
3. Spacing of the fruits / perennial plants and vegetables should be as per the canopy .closer spacing will result in lanky growth, reduction in yield and quality.
4. Glyricidia plants should be planted all along the boundary so as to serve as a live fence .The plant being legume also fixes atmospheric nitrogen and serve as a regular source for supply of green leaves for mulching the valuable fruits trees.
5. Mulching with green or dry leaves for fruits and vegetables checks weed growth, checks evaporation losses the soil temperature, increases the microbial activity and adds organic matter.
6. As grafts grow dwarf, yield early and give high yield with good quality, all the perennial crops / fruits trees should be planted by use of graft only.
7. A cafeteria of medicinal plants should be part homestead farming. A variety of 10-15 medicinal plant species like Neem,Tulsi, Coleus, Kalmegh, Lemon grass, Stevia, Amritvel, Sarpagandha, Aloevera, etc., should be planted and maintained at regular intervals.
8. The organic matter content of the garden should be well maintained through recycling of wastes and bio-resources.
9. Vermi composting unit should invariable be a part of the garden so that the unit gets sufficient organics on a continued basis at reasonable cost.
10. Vegetables crops should be grown as per the season and preferably in rotation.

Subsidiary components in homestead farming

Depending on the resources available in the garden, family requirement and the market demand, the following additional components can be integrated:

Backyard poultry rearing : In most of the homestead farms, although backyard poultry can easily be practiced, many of the farms does not venture into it .Even if they practice, the bride are local type poor in weight, egg laying type and they are reared by free range system and are not properly cared. Up-gradation of local birds with introduction of breed of dual purpose nature i.e. for eggs as well as the meet is more beneficial to the farmers to generate additional income. The bred is also suitable for backyard rearing and can be easily maintained with kitchen and other farm west .In the study conducted, it was observed that 100 percent of the eggs produced were consumed by the households, thus enhancing the overall nutrition of the farm family .poultry manure with richest source of nutrients into the fields.

Goat rearing : Goat is a prolific breeder with a capacity to increase the herd size within a short span of time .improved breeds of goat like Osmanabadi with higher fecundity and growth rate can be maintained even in the backside shelter of the homestead with ease. Since goat eats all types of leaves, the lopping of the commonly available trees may be used for feeding the goats. However, care has to be ensure to not to be loose the Animals so as to avoid damage to the homestead garden.

Dairy: Rearing of milch crows is the easiest way of converting wastes into resourceful products. Improved breeds of dairy cows like Jersy X Sindhi cross, Holstein, Friesian, Gir, etc, .are widely adopted and can give better profits Cultivation of improved varieties / hybrids of forage grass and legume mixtures on farm bunds and using for dairy on a regular basis can bring down the production cost of dairy with enhanced profits. Balanced feeding with regular check-up of the animal for infertility problems can bring greater dividends.

Piggery: In areas where there is a demand for pork and sausages, the pig rearing will be highly successful . The pigs under goods managements can bring in higher profits with increase body weight gain in short periods. Improved cross breeds like Large White Yorkshire X Local with higher litter size and growth can be maintained even with house hold kitchen waste and can form a source of income for the house hold under emergency situation of cash requirement.

Mushroom cultivation: Production of Oyster (paddy straw) mushrooms can be practiced in all most all the homestead without problems. The major ingredient for mushroom production viz. paddy straw is normally available with most of the places and the production can be taken with provisions for protection from sunlight and upkeep of the humidity .As this is a short duration enterprise, the intermittent returns can be established through tying up with a regular market outlet.

Vermi-composting : The supply of fertilizer in the rural areas and their cost is increasing day-by-day .Continuous use of chemical fertilizer is also affecting the soil quality and the productivity of land. Recycling of available bio-resources and on-farm production of vermin-composting also helps to provide required essential plant nutrients to homestead farm. Besides, use of organic manures also improves the water holding capacity of soil and there by reduces the water requirement of the crops.

Bee Keeping: Due to a variety of flora under homesteads with varying flowering periods during different months of the year, beekeeping can easily be practiced .Initial colonization of the honey bees requires proper identification of site, installation of proper bee hives and attracting the queen honey bee. The nectar yielding plants can also be planned as a regular source of food for the honey bees .Care has be ensured to avoid dissertation of colonies by the honey bees. Due to the medicinal value of the honey, the family can be benefited with proper planning.

Plant Nursery : Assessing the local needs of planting material and planning for graft progenies in important crops of demand can fetch greater dividends . A small area in the homestead with facility for protection from the direct sun shine and rain fall with availability of irrigation can better be utilized especially for rare plants to earn more income. The seasoning in production can better be planned depending on the so as to have continuity in product ion during different months of the year.

Azolla Growing, Value addition/ processing, Handicrafts making etc. can also be taken up.

Establishment of Homestead system

Land shaping : The farmers need to level and smoothen the shape of the land so that raised portion of the plot is excavated and the soil so excavated can be used to raise a section of the low lying land to make it suitable for growing vegetables throughout the year . Since, the farmers are intensively oriented on economic, social and nutritional benefit of homestead farming in the long run, necessary measures of soil conservation, rain water harvesting and prevention of runoff water and soil erosion need to be taken up priority basis.

Space allocation : The need of land and water for different components like crops, livestock, fish and other enterprises varies .The most interesting aspect of this homestead farming is that every portion of the land need to be used for cultivation . For example, in one homestead farm, about 50 percent of the land is kept for growing vegetables, 20 percent for plantation and fruit crops, 15 percent for rearing of cattle and poultry and 15 percent for cultivation of fodder and other components .General farming practices and fruits cultivation being easy for integration, the low land is used for growing vegetables that give them a good income throughout the year .

Crop cafeteria for different types of space under homestead farming

Bou boundary through live fencing: All along the boundary, nitrogen fixing trees like Glyricidia can be planted for enriching the soil and also for supplying food fodder and fuel through lopping at regular intervals.

	Kharif Season	**Rabi Season**
Sunny Space	Bitter gourd, long bean, snake gourd, cucumber, bhendi, amaranthus, colocacia	Knolkhol, clusterbean, palak, raddish,amaranthus, methi, chilli, brinjal, onion, long bean, knolkhol
House roof	All cucurbits	Pendal bean
Trellis	Perennial-Little gourd, pumpkin, bittergourd,snakegourd,bottlegourd, ridgegourd	Perennial-little gourd
Land below trellis	Ginger, turmeric, colocacia,	Perennial leafy vegetables
Pond bank	Cucurbits	Long bean, water melon
Slightly Marshyland	Banana, mint	Banana
On trees	Perennial-black pepper Annual-cucurbitaceous vegetables	Perennial-black pepper

Integration between cattle shed-compost pit-vegetable garden: Cattle are raised essentially for milk. Cow urine and cow dung are used for making compost or vermin compost in permanent pits or on a plastic sheet laid on the ground. Compost, especially vermin compost serves as excellent manure for the vegetable garden. Cow urine and cow dung are also used in the ponds as manure.

Integration between cattle shed-biogas pit-kitchen-vegetable field: With only a small investment, a biogas can be a very useful intervention. Instead of using cow dung and urine directly in the compost pit, it may be transferred to the bio gas unit. THE gas generated may be transferred to the kitchen for use as a fuel or for lighting gas lamps. The slurry which is collected in a separate may be used in the vegetable garden field as excellent manure.

Awareness regarding agro-chemical and organic inputs: Farmers need to be trained and made aware to reduce, rather stop use of chemical pesticides and emphasis need to be laid on use of organic, manures, green manures, vermin-compost, extract of varies plants and weeds or ash as organic herbicide etc.

Seasonal cultivation of vegetables: Many of the vegetables are season bound and need to be selected for better productivity. The market also plays a crucial role in selection of crops for each season as there will be a wide variation in price structure. The vegetables that form a part of the homestead in western region are red amaranthus, brinjal, chillies, cluster beans, okra, Radish, Drumstick and different varieties of gourds including cucumber and pumpkins. Sweet potatoes, vegetables cowpea, onion are also grown to some extent.

Flower production for aesthetic value and profits: The cultivation of seasonal and perennial flowers offers a great scope especially aces like Goa where there is a great demand due to booming tourism. Even a small land allocation on a continuous basis especially in frontage of the household will not only beatify the outlook of the house but also makes the availability of fresh flowers for special occasions of the household.

Processing and value addition of homestead produce: It is very much important that the tiny produce developed at the homestead with lot of care finally is more useful for the end user with better returns for this, processing of the produce by following proper techniques, their value addition and proper marketing is very much crucial.

Utilization of homestead grown vegetables: The study on homestead farming revealed that among the annual production of vegetables, a major portion was consumed by the household. In terms of nutrition a huge amount of vitamin A and also surplus quantity of vitamin C were produced .Except niacin and riboflavin good amount of thiamin, calcium and iron were also produced. Thus only from a small homestead garden, the widespread deficient vitamins (vitamin A and C) could be successfully mitigated . The total income was 2.5 times higher than the production cost, there for, homestead vegetable production was economically viable, and in addition farmers obtained healthy food and created good relation through free distribution of vegetables among relatives and neighbors. Moreover, most of the sale proceeds from vegetables were owned by women, which they used for purchasing of small household items and for children education.

Family labour based production system: Availability of family labour is very crucial for the success of homestead farming. The study on homestead farming revealed that family labour utilization was enhanced with homestead gardening. Further, a job oriented variation was also observed among the male and female members of the family. In land preparation, sowing and marketing, male had a major role while for intercultural operations, harvesting and cooking women had the major role.

Development of Homestead models for different holding size : Based on the data collected and the interactions with the clients, model homestead units for different holding sizes of the household are attempted keeping in view the family requirement, marketing potential and the resource situation including part or full time availability of the family members to work in their gardens. As the majority of the households have a holding of 500, 1000 and 2000 m^2 in the region relevant models to suit to these holdings were attempted. These models although are apt for Goa situations could also be used in other parts of the country with suitable modification. The details of economics of different components crops for a models homestead of 500 m^2 and 1000 m^2 and 2000 m^2 are given below. The economics varies depending on the number in each of the components crops /enterprise. The models have been developed along with allocation of the land for varies components like vegetables, flowers, plantation crops, medicinal plants, fruits plants, vermi composting, mushroom shed, as well additional components like apiculture, fish aquarium, poultry rearing, etc. The crop / enterprise combination can be selected based on housed requirement, area of holding size, availability of water for irrigation, work force, marketing potential, etc.

Enhancing Income Model				
Increase in Agriculture Productivity	Diversification towards high value crops	Increase in crop intensity	Market Linkage for farmers	Adopting Integrated Farming System

Balancing nutrition through homestead farming: In India nearly 29 per cent of the population lives below the food consumption based poverty line, lacking sufficient resources to afford diet of 2, 122 kilocalories per person per day, along with other basic necessities. Apart from the prevailing deficit in total calories intake, the normal diet of the people is seriously imbalanced, with inadequate consumption of protein, fat, oil, fruits and vegetables, and with more than 80 per cent of calories derived from cereals. Women and children are especially vulnerable to their greater nutritional requirements. It is also reported that vitamin c, iron and other mineral nutritional deficiency are widespread resulting in different types of diseases, hampering physical growth and retarding brain development.

Food is the basic necessity of our life. Most people eat what they like or because it is warm or out of habit. Choice of food is not influenced by the awareness of nutritive value. Food is a prerequisite of nutrition. Nutrition includes everything that happens to food from the time it is eaten until it is used for varies function in the body. We now realize quality of our health depends upon the nourishment that we provide to our body.

Animal foods which are the richest source of many micronutrients, including Vitamin A, are beyond most people`s means in the country. Hence, promoting the production and consumption of comparatively cheap vegetables and fruits is an important strategy for combating nutritional deficiency. Per day at least 200 g of vegetable is needed for an adult man / woman, whereas the people are consuming only around 25 gm/head/days. However, research findings also suggest that lac of nutritional knowledge contributes to the problems to the problems of malnutrition. Fruits and vegetables play on important role in the balanced diet of human being by providing not only the energy rich food but also provide vital protective nutrients. They are not only adorning the table, but also enrich health from the most nutritive menu and toned up the energy and vigor of a person. They have a vital role to play on the foods and can admirably supplement the main cereals.

The consumption of these items in sufficient quantities provides taste, increases appetite and provides fair amount of fibers, which are required for maintenance of good health and are beneficial in protecting against diseases. They provide valuable roughage which promotes digestion and helps in preventing constipation. The intake of these categories of in our diets is from satisfactory more so in low income groups. Nutritionally fruits vegetables occupy an important place in human diet for the valuable minerals and fats content in them. Some of them are good source of carbohydrates (sapota, banana. Bread fruit, jack fruit etc), minerals calcium and iron (all vegetables, dates and raisin), vitamin A (mango, papaya, green leafy vegetables) vitamin B complex (apple, apricot, grapes and other vegetables) vitamin C (aonla, guava, citrus and vegetables).

In order to have fresh fruits and vegetables in kitchen, it is better to have homestead garden in the house compound .Fruits and vegetables obtained from market lack much freshness and deteriorate in the food value besides their exorbitant price. Therefore the best quality of the fresh produce can be had from one`s own nutrition garden as the time interval between the harvest and the consumption become the least. Further, working in the gardens is a pleasure and means of recreation and possibly family enterprise in which in all members have due share to spend the leisure hours .Further, the gardening will also help in giving an exercise to the body and soothens the mind which inturn will also help to keep the family members healthy and happy.

Nutritional demand met by the homestead vegetable production

	Per capita recommendation of vegetable as per ICMR (for normal male adult)	Per capita mean availability of nutrients (g/ person/day) through homestead farming	Excess /deficit (g/ person/day)
Energy(cal)	170	45	125
Protein(g)	17	6	11
Fat (g)	3.5	0.7	2.8
Calcium(mg)	750	300	450
Iron(mg)	25	16	9

Important horticulture source of nutrients

- Calories:-Tapioka, sweet potato, yam, potato, colocasia, onion plaintain breadfruit, jackfruit, pumpkin, banana, peas, etc.
- Proteins:-Peas, Cowpeas etc.
- Vitamins :- A – Carrots, spinach, amaranthus, methi leaves, drumstick leaves, pumpkin, mango, papaya, passion fruit, tomato, etc..''
- B-Complex: - Peas, broad beans, tomato, banana, grapes fruits, bhendi, capsicum and other vegetables.
- Vitamin C: - Aonla, leafy vegetables, tomato, orange, lemon, guava, mango, etc
- Calcium:-Curry leaves, drumstick, spinach and all the other leafy vegetables, custard apple, etc.
- Iron;-All leafy vegetables, dates, raisins, guava, etc.

Thus, homestead garden help in nutritional security of the farm family and also supplement the needs of the vulnerable group (pregnant and lactating mothers and children below five years), to overcome the malnutrition and micro nutrient deficiency and other health consequences. Further, it improves the nutritional value chain by means of production, availability and stability of food production.

Because food supply is the primary aim of the home gardens, vegetables and fruit yielding trees are most frequent there. In a study of the home gardens in Southern Kerala it was found that the gardeners grew 28 fruits, 21 vegetables and 12 spices and condiments. Some of these are seasonal crops, while others are perennials. Besides meeting the calorie requirements of the gardener and his family, they are also important sources of minerals and nutrients.

The results of the project study revealed that nutritionally, the homestead farming met a sizeable portion of the mineral and vitamin requirement of the household family members although the carbohydrate, protein and fat requirements were only met partially. The family nutrition was much improved through a mix of vegetables, including tuber crops, fruits, spices, plantation crops and medicinal plants. Further, a mixed vegetation around the household also brought a change in the local micro- climate with long term benefits on health of family members.

30

Extension Strategy to Develop Integrated Farming System (IFS) Model for Better Livelihood

Bimal Kinkar Chand

Directorate of Research, Extension & Farms
West Bengal University of Animal & Fishery Sciences

Introduction

Farmers work hard to earn a living. However, not all farmers make money, especially small family farmers. There is very little leftover after they pay for all their inputs (seeds, livestock breeds, fertilizers, pesticides, energy, feed, labour, etc.). However, the Integrated Farming Systems (IFS) has enabled farmers to develop a framework for an alternative development model to improve the feasibility of small sized farming operations. The ''modern'' technologies have been widely used to enhance the productivity per acre of land to ensure that there is enough food for the increased global population. Due to the indiscriminate and erratic use of chemical pesticides and fertilizers, our food and ecosystems have been poisoned. On the contrary, the integrated farming system uses the integrated approach to farming compared to monoculture approaches. It refers to agricultural systems that integrate agriculture with horticulture, livestock, fishery, agro-forestry, etc. and known as integrated bio-systems. In this system, an inter-related set of enterprises is used so that the "waste" from one component becomes an input for another part of the system. This reduces costs and improves production and/or income. Since it utilizes waste as a resource, farmers not only eliminate waste but they also ensure an overall increase in productivity for the whole farming system.

Integrated farming tries to imitate nature's principle, where not only crops but also varied types of plants, animals, birds, fish, and other aquatic flora and fauna are utilized for production. The basic principle is to enhance the ecological diversity:

- By choosing the appropriate cropping methodology with mixed cropping, crop rotation, crop combination and inter-cropping so that there is less competition for water, nutrition and space and by adopting eco-friendly practices
- By utilizing a multi-story arrangement so that the total available area is used effectively and there is a high level of interaction between biotic and a biotic components
- By integrating a judicious mix of agricultural enterprises like dairy, poultry, piggery, fishery, sericulture etc. suited to the given agro-climatic conditions and socio-economic status of the farmers can bring prosperity to the farming operations.

Concept of Farming System

The term "system" is derived from the Greek word "synistanai," which means "to bring together or combine." Likewise, the farming system denotes a complex inter-related matrix of soil, water, plants, animals (livestock/fish), implements, power, labour, capital and other inputs those are controlled in parts by farming families. These are influenced to varying degree by economic, institutional and socials forces that operate at many levels. Therefore, farming system is the result of a complex interaction among a number of interdependent components. Farm activities interact with market forces (socio-economic) and ecosystem (biophysical) for purchasing inputs and disposing outputs by utilizing and degrading natural resources (land, water, air, sunshine etc.). A farming system has Inputs, Processes and Outputs.

INPUTS - these are things that go into the farm and may be split into Physical Inputs (e.g., amount of rain, soil, seeds, fertilizer etc.) and Human Inputs (e.g., labour, money etc.).

PROCESSES - these are things which take place on the farm in order to convert the inputs to outputs (e.g., sowing/stocking, weeding, farm management, harvesting etc.).

OUTPUTS - these are the products from the farm (i.e., rice, wheat, milk, egg, meat, fish, etc.) Depending on the type of farming (e.g., arable/pastoral, commercial/subsistence), the type and quantity of inputs, processes and outputs will vary. You need to make sure you are able to define and give examples of Inputs, Processes and Outputs in farming systems.

Farming systems research (FSR) originates from the inter-dependence and inter relationships of natural environment within the farming system. In FSR the farmers by participating in the research process help in the identification of the research problems as well as take part in testing the possible solution. In the past decades, farming system research has emerged as a popular and major theme in international agricultural research. FSR approach involves following principles.

- Viewing the farm as a whole,
- Identifying the farming system, the interacting component and delineating boundaries,
- Systematic investigation of the nature and extent of interdependence among the enterprises and identifying constraint,
- Applying the modern technical know- how to the system so as to make it yield optimum results,
- Studying the equity gender income, employment and resources use efficiency, and
- Dealing with the issue at integration level through analysis and solution of problems towards sustainable farming system development.

Integrated Farming System: Key Features & Benefits

The overarching feature of IFS is to ensure total utilization of land and water resources of the farm resulting in maximum and diversified farm output with minimum financial and labour costs. In IFS, the different enterprises interact eco-biologically, in space and time, are mutually supportive and depend on each other. Thousands of small and marginal family farmers in resource-poor regions in Asia and Africa are embracing this system to diversify farm production, increase cash income, improve the quality and quantity of food produced and the exploitation of unutilized resources. The benefits provided by IFS are summarized below:

The schematic presentation of farming system is illustrated below.

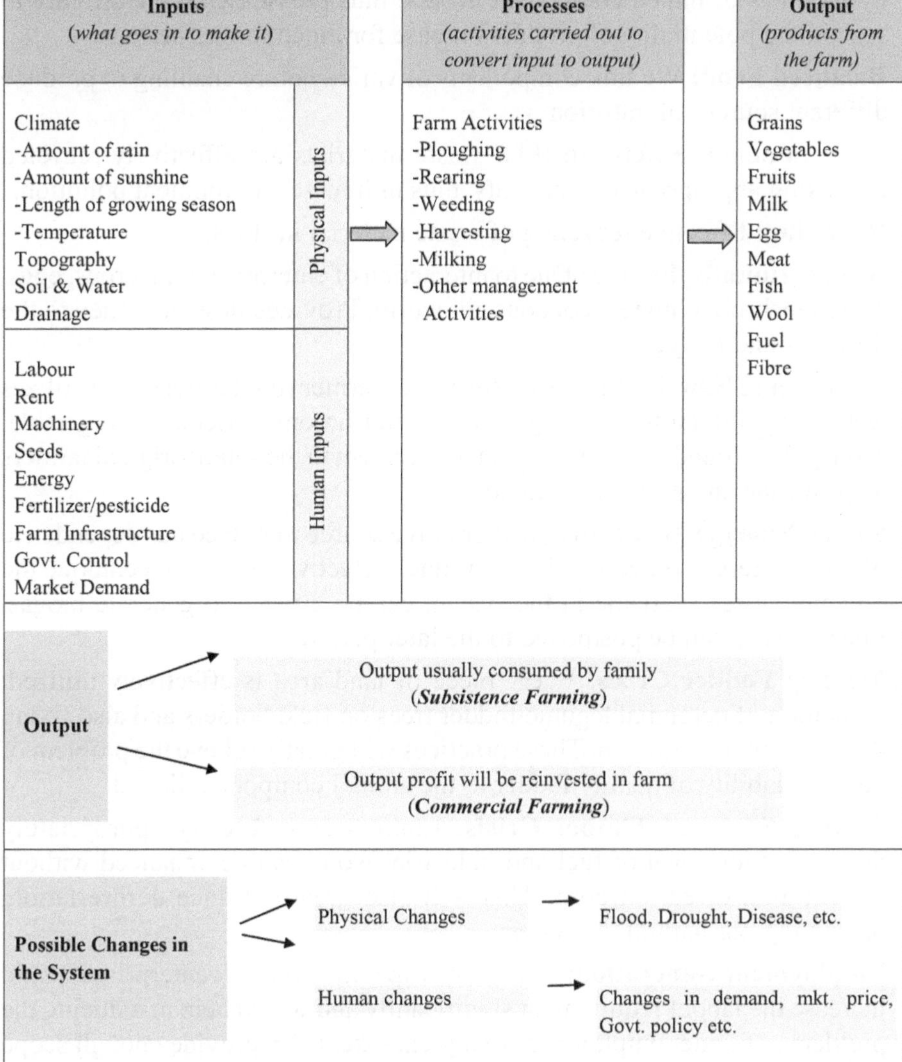

Fig. 1 Schematic Presentation of Farming System

- **Productivity:** IFS provides an opportunity to increase economic yield per unit area per unit time by virtue of intensification of crop and allied enterprises.
- **Profitability:** Use waste material of one component at the least cost, thus reduction of cost of production and form the linkage of utilization of waste material, elimination of middleman interference in most input used. Working out net profit B/ C ratio is increased.

- **Sustainability:** Organic supplementation through effective utilization of by-products of linked component is done thus providing an opportunity to sustain the potentiality of production base for much longer periods.
- **Balanced Food:** We link components of varied nature enabling to produce different sources of nutrition.
- **Environmental Safety:** In IFFS waste materials are effectively recycled by linking appropriate components, thus minimize environment pollution.
- **Recycling:** Effective recycling of waste material in IFFS.
- **Income Rounds the year:** Due to interaction of enterprises with crops, eggs, milk, mushroom, honey, cocoons silkworm. Provides flow of money to the farmer round the year.
- **Adoption of New Technology:** Resources farmer (big farmer) fully utilizes technology. IFS farmers, linkage of dairy / mushroom / sericulture / vegetable. Money flow round the year gives an inducement to the small/ original farmers to go for the adoption technologies.
- **Saving Energy:** To identify an alternative source to reduce our dependence on fossil energy source within short time. Effective recycling technique the organic wastes available in the system can be utilized to generate biogas. Energy crisis can be postponed to the later period.
- **Meeting Fodder Crisis:** Every piece of land area is effectively utilized. Plantation of perennial legume fodder trees on field borders and also fixing the atmospheric nitrogen. These practices will greatly relieve the problem of non-availability of quality fodder to the animal component linked.
- **Solving Fuel and Timber Crisis:** Linking agro-forestry appropriately the production level of fuel and industrial wood can be enhanced without determining effect on crop. This will also greatly reduce deforestation, preserving our natural ecosystem.
- **Employment Generation:** Combing crop with livestock enterprises would increase the labour requirement significantly and would help in reducing the problems of under employment to a great extent IFS provide enough scope to employ family labour round the year.
- **Agro-industries:** When one of produce linked in IFS are increased to commercial level there is surplus value adoption leading to development of allied agro-industries.
- **Increasing Input Efficiency:** IFS provide good scope to use inputs in different component greater efficiency and benefit cost ratio.

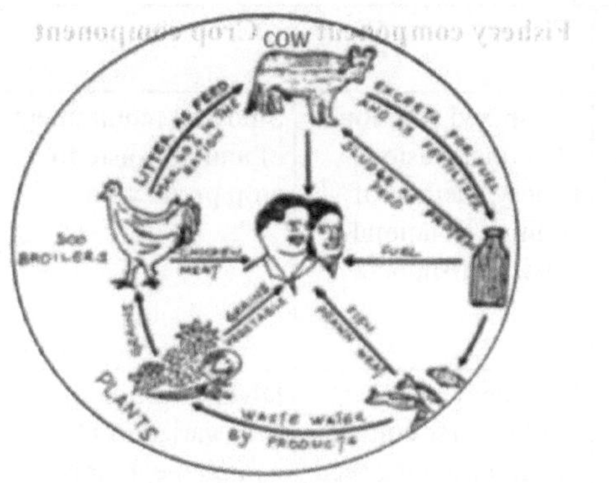

Fig. 2 Resource flow in IFS

Micro-level interlinking among the components in IFS

IFS is an integration of many sub-systems e.g., crop, livestock and fish which are linked to each other in such a way that the by-products/wastes from one sub-system become the valuable inputs to another sub-system and thus ensures total utilization of land and water resources of the farm resulting in maximum and diversified farm output with minimum financial and labour costs. The conceptual framework of micro-level interlinking in IFS is explained in the table given below.

Table 1: Conceptual Framework of micro-level interlinking in IFS

Micro-level attributes	Livestock component	Fishery component	Crop component
Space utilization	Use of pond dyke top for livestock shed	Use of pond water surface for duck, use of space over the pond water margin for growing creeper vegetable through hanging platform	Use of pond dyke (top, inner slope & outer slop) for crop production, use of top of the animal shed for growing creeper crop.
Recycling of nutrient	Recycling of crop byproducts / fodder for livestock production	Use of livestock waste as manure for fish production, use of crop byproduct / fodder for fish food	Use of livestock wastes in crop production, use of fishpond sediments and water for crop production

(Contd.)

Micro-level attributes	Livestock component	Fishery component	Crop component
Nutrient concentration	Standardization of livestock number in integrated system to generate required quantity of animal waste for fish & crop system	Optimized addition of animal waste in fishery, method of addition of animal waste in fishpond	Study on requirement of animal waste for crop production
Diversity	Increasing diversity of livestock may complement other farming system. For example, increased amounts of mono-gastric waste may be valuable for planktivorous fish	Efficiency of multispecies culture in exploiting the feed available in different aquatic niches	Diversification in crop variety may complement other farming system. For example, the fish like grass carp and ruminants may compete for limited amounts of grass
Environmental compatibility	Environment friendly disposal of animal waste	Efficient use of water for fishery, livestock and crop production	Promote organic farming through use of manure, control of pest due to free grazing of poultry & duck
Productivity	Increase in livestock production through crop byproduct and fodder	Increase in fish production through pond manuring	Increase in crop production due to sufficient water and manure.
Economic efficiency	Livestock as major source of cash in smallholder systems. Having a variety of livestock types improves versatility with respect to cash flow and risk aversion	Poly-culture and perennial water increase opportunities for strategic marketing	Returns to labour are often attractive. Integration reduces market risk and improves flexibility

Livestock-Fish Integration

The basic principles of livestock-fish integrated farming system are the full utilization of livestock farm wastes and conversion of waste in to valuable fish protein. The manure from livestock helps in production of planktons which forms the feed for fishes in the pond. Further, the spilled over feed or undigested/semi-digested food derived from the livestock manure may also be utilized as direct feed for fish.

The advantages of Livestock-Fish Integrated Farming are as below.

- Waste products of the animals are used for fish production.
- Feed residues can be eaten directly by the fish.
- Costs towards manure collection, storing and transportation are avoided.
- Saving of land otherwise needed for housing the livestock (if the housing is above the fishpond).
- Provide good solution to problems of environmental pollution caused by animal waste.
- Improve the environment for manure producing livestock.
- Saving of livestock feed cost due to the natural food, e.g., aquatic insect/ worms/plants for ducks.
- Improve the operational efficiency of the farm through better use of manure, joint use of feed storage, processing and transportation facilities.

The popular livestock-fish integrated farming systems are:

- Duck-fish integrated system
- Poultry-fish integrated system
- Pig-fish integrated system
- Sheep/Goat-Fish integrated system
- Cattle/buffalo-fish integrated system
- Rabbit-fish integrated system

The livestock manures contain major inorganic nutrients (N, P, K) as well other trace elements viz. Ca, Cu, Zn, Fe, and Mg. Waste output in the form of urine and faeces varies considerably in quantity and quality. Again, the distribution of nutrients (N, P, K) in faeces and urine also vary for different livestock. The nutritive values of different animal excreta are given below.

Table 2 Nutritive values of different animal excreta

Animal	Excreta	Moisture (%)	Organic matter (%)	Nitrogen (%)	Phosphorus (P_2O_5) (%)	Potash (K_2O) (%)
Cattle	Faeces	80-85	14.0	0.3	0.2	0.1
	Urine	92-95	2.3	1.0	0.1	1.4
Pig	Faeces	85	15	0.6	0.5	0.4
	Urine	97	2.5	0.4	0.1	0.7
Goat	Faeces	10	-	2.7	1.7	2.9

(Contd.)

Animal	Excreta	Moisture (%)	Organic matter (%)	Nitrogen (%)	Phosphorus (P_2O_5) (%)	Potash (K_2O) (%)
Rabbit	Faeces	10	37	2.0	1.3	1.2
Poultry	Faeces	78	25.5	1.4	0.8	0.6
Duck	Faeces	81	26.2	0.9	0.4	0.6

Table 3 Livestock units for integration with Fish Farming

Particulars	Cattle	Pig	Poultry	Duck	Rabbit	Goat
Qty. of dung/ha water area/yr. (tonne)	15-25	15-20	10-15	10-15	5-10	5-10
Qty. of dung/ animal/yr. (kg)	5000-10000	500-600	20-25	30-45	15-18	150-200
Nos. of animals to be reared for dung/ha/yr.	3-4	30-40	500-600	200-300	300-500	40-50
Stocking density of fish (no. of carps/ha)	5000-6000	5000-6000	5000-6000	5000-6000	5000-6000	5000-6000
Fish (tonne/ha/yr.)	4-5	4-5	4-5	4-5	4-5	4-5
Milk/Meat production (kg)	3000-5000	4000-5000	1240	500-750	900-1500	600-900
Egg production (nos.)	-	-	70,000	18,000	-	-

Checklist for Animal-Fish Integration

- Type of Animal and Fish?
- Consider religious and social taboos: demand for animals and/or their products marketing difficulties.
- Production cycle of animal and fish?
- Consider waste availability and requirements for fish, changing climate and ability of pond to use wastes.
- Feeding regime of animals?
- Quantity and quality of food to animals: amount of waste food available to fish, frequency of feeding, animal feeds grown on the farm or purchased.
- Is the animal waste fresh, diluted, well-rotted?
- Is some form of processing an advantage before use?
- Will the waste be sufficient to optimize fish production? If not are other fertilizer or feed supplements available?
- Effects of changing production of animal or fish on the management and profitability to the other?

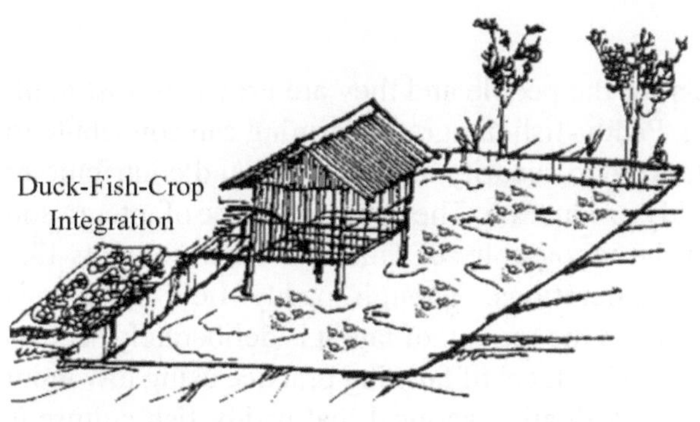
Duck-Fish-Crop Integration

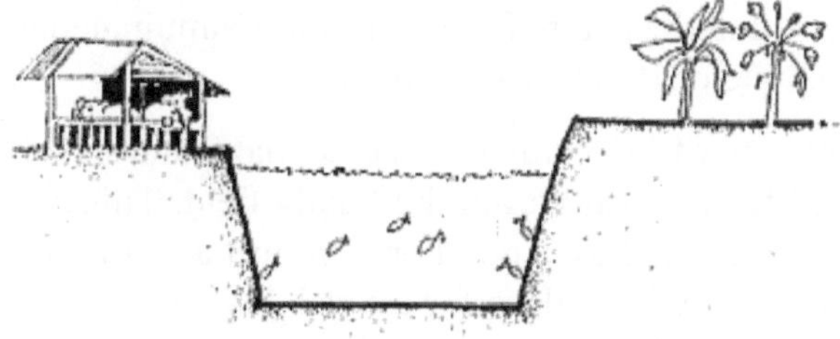
Pig-Fish-Crop Integration

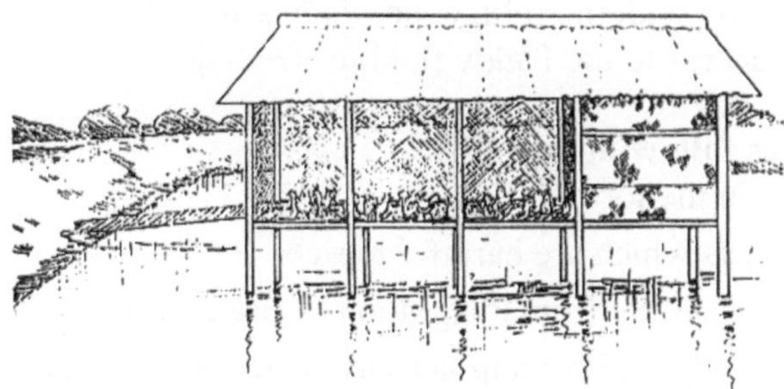
Poultry-Fish Integration

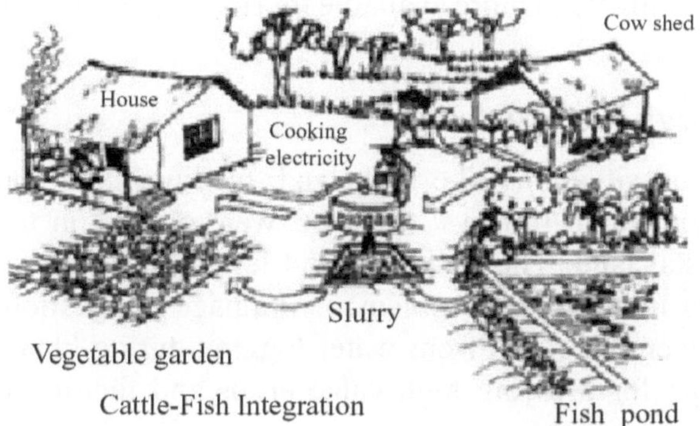

Cattle-Fish Integration

Paddy-Fish Integration

Paddy and fish are staple diets for the people and they are grown almost in all agro-climatic regions of India. Paddy-fish integrated farming can contribute to household income, contribute to food security and nutrition and contribute to improved sustainability of paddy production. The nature and type of integration vary largely depending upon the topography of land and other contexts like biophysical and technical considerations. Though paddy field fishery is recognized as traditional practice in the region, of late it is deliberately seen as a productive fishery. It is an extensive level of farming practice using low input technology. The cost and return evaluation showed that paddy-fish culture is more profitable than monoculture of rice. Generally, two production systems are recommended for culturing fish in the paddy fields. They are Simultaneous or Concurrent Method and Alternate or Rotational Method.

In Paddy-fish integration, creation of fish refuge is an essential feature. Fish refuge is a deeper area provided for the fish within the Paddy field. This can be in the form of a trench or several trenches, a pond or even just a sump or a pit. The purpose of the refuge is to provide a place for the fish in case water in the field dries up or is not deep enough. It also serves to facilitate fish harvest at the end of the Paddy season, or to contain fish for further culture whilst the Paddy is harvested. In conjunction with the refuge, provisions are often made to provide the fish with better access to the Paddy field for feeding.

Paddy-Fish Integration offers following benefits.

- Additional food and income in the form of fish.
- Control of mollusks and insects which are harmful to rice.
- Reduced risk of crop failure resulting from integration of rice and fish.
- Continued flooding of the paddy and rooting activity of fish help control weeds.
- Fish stir up soil nutrients making them more available for rice. This increases rice production.

Crop-Fish Integration through Land Shaping

In land shaping, different land situations like high land, medium land and low (original) apart from farm pond/ furrows/ trenches, were created in the low-lying and degraded coastal land. The rising of land levels and creation of water-harvesting facilities reduced the problem of drainage congestion. The high land/ridges/ dikes were also free from water logging during kharif season, which provided scope for growing high-value crops and facilitated early sowing of rabi crops.

Land Shaping for Deep Furrow & High Ridge Cultivation: The 50% of farm land may be shaped into alternate furrows (3m top width × 1.5 m bottom width × 1.0 m depth) and ridges (1.5 m top width ×1.0 m height × 3m bottom width). The ridges remain relatively free from drainage congestion and low in soil salinity build up. Thus, ridges can be used for multiple crop cultivation and the furrows are useful for rainwater harvesting and fish cultivation along with rice (on remaining 50% of original low-land) during wet season. During dry season the ridges continued to be used for vegetable/fruit cultivation. The remaining original fields are used for low water requiring field crops with the rain water harvested in the furrows.

Land Shaping for Shallow Furrow & Medium Ridge Cultivation: About 75% of the farm land may be shaped into furrows (2.0m top width × 1.0 m bottom width × 0.75 m depth) and medium ridges (1.0 m top width × 0.75 m height × 2.0m bottom width) with a gap of 3.5m between two consecutive ridges and furrows. Thus, there will be three land situations viz. low land (medium furrow), midland (original farm land) and high land (ridge). The furrows can be used for rainwater harvesting as well as fish cultivation along with paddy in wet season. In dry season furrows can be used for rice cultivation. The ridges are free from water logging in wet season and suitable for cultivation of crops other than rice throughout the year. The original land is used for growing low water requiring.

Land Shaping for Farm Pond: The water balance analysis shows considerable scope for conservation of excesses rain water in on-farm reservoir (OFR). Soil water balance model developed for rain-fed rice cultivation showed that about 20% of watershed/ farm area may be converted to OFR to harvest excess rain water for utilizing to grow crops in rabi /summer, supplemental irrigation in kharif and freshwater aquaculture. The dug-out soil was used to raise the land to form high and medium land situations for growing multiple crops.

Land Shaping for Paddy-cum-fish Cultivation: Trenches of about 3 m width × 1.5 m depth are dug around the field with a ditch of 6m × 6m × 3m (depth) at one corner. The excavated soil is used for making dikes of about 3 m width × 1.5 m high around the field to protect the fishes to be grown in paddy-cum-fish cultivation. During kharif paddy-cum fish is grown on the original low land and vegetables on the dikes. During rabi/summer low water requiring field crops & vegetables are continued to be grown on the dikes, and low water requires crops on the original land with live saving irrigation given with rain water harvested furrows. Otherwise, the original lands may also be used for brackish water fish cultivation. At the end of the summer season the brackish water is drained out with the help of pre-monsoon rains. The land is again used for Paddy-cum-fish cultivation.

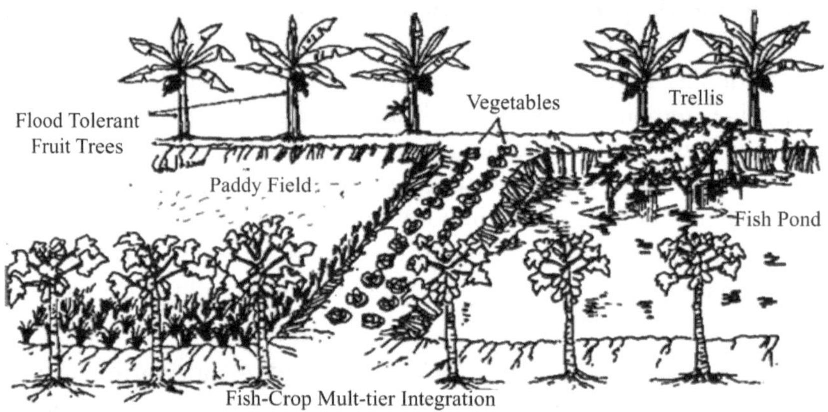

Effective Extension Strategies for IFS

Farmers are often excellent "researchers" and "extensionists". The "Farmer First and Last" (FFL) model is an alternative to the "Transfer-of- Technology" (TOT) model and more suited for IFS. It is based in the farmer's perceptions and priorities rather than on the scientist's professional preferences, criteria and priorities. When the research is done on-farm, the process is faster and there is a "natural selection" of technologies and priorities. The starting point is the scientific learning from and understanding of the resources, needs and problems of the resource-poor farmers and that the research stations and laboratories play a referral and consultancy role. This model is characterized by the use of informal survey methods, research and development within the farms, and with the farmers, and evaluation through the technology adoption. The farming system must be fully integrated in order to optimize the use of locally "available alternative" resources.

The approach for effective extension strategies for IFS needs to follow through a series of sequential steps.

- Identification of target areas with the relevant authorities,
- Establishment of a local task force consisting of SMSs, researchers, extensionists and trainers who will be responsible for implementing the programme,
- Preparation of appropriate technical and extension messages,
- Undertaking of a training needs assessment of extension staff and arrangement of the necessary extension support materials,
- Initial training of participating extension staff covering basic concepts to provide a framework on required skills and knowledge
- Extending hand-holding support to the participating farmers at field on IFS and continuous monitoring of activities.

Conclusion

Integrated farming systems offer unique opportunities for maintaining and extending biodiversity. The concepts associated with IFS are practiced by numerous farmers throughout the globe. A common characteristic of these systems is that they have a combination of crop and livestock enterprises and in some cases may include combinations of aquaculture and trees. It takes into account the concepts of minimizing risk, increasing total production and profits by lowering external inputs through recycling and improving the utilization of organic wastes and crop residues. There is a vast scope to improve the household profitability by judiciously utilizing family labour using innovative practices and ensuring multiple uses of various household resources. This is possible through women's empowerment through location specific trainings and critical need-based support. Developing women-centric IFS models is the need of the hour as men are migrating to rural non-farm sectors.

31

Value Added Livestock Products Marketing for Livelihood Empowerment

Subhasish Biswas and Sukanta Biswas*

Department of Livestock Products Technology & Marketing
**Department of Veterinary & A.H. Extension Education*
W.B. University of Animal & Fishery Science
Kolkata-700037, West Bengal, India

Value Addition in Livestock Product

Mankind has been utilizing different animal species from the dawn of civilization for a variety of purposes viz. production of milk, meat, wool, egg and leather etc. These products are either useful in raw form or in value added form. Value-addition describes economically adding value to the product by changing its place, time and form to characteristics that are more preferred in the market place. Another way of explaining is that what happens when you take a basic product and increase the value of that product, usually the price by adding extras in the manufacturing process, or by tacking on extra products and/or services.

Value can be added using one or two approaches i.e. first innovation (improving existing process, methods or services or creating new one). Second is Coordination i.e. arrangements among those who produce and market the products. Coordination links producers, wholesalers, retailers and consumers

Need of Value Addition

Adding value to farm commodities is becoming an important income-enhancing strategy for producers. Commodity prices will be similar in the future to what they have been in the past, but periods of excess supply and low prices will occur. New risk-management tools will need to be developed (Dobbins et al.). Many producers will look for ways to be economically viable through voluntary, incentive-based solutions. Producers' greatest opportunities may lie in activities that add value to their products and move their point of first sale downstream toward consumers. Adding value to bulk raw commodities is one way for producers to keep a larger share of the margins associated with further processing and market development. Progressive producers respond to market developments, determine what factors will drive the future of their industry, and use these results to their advantage by adapting to change.Value-added products can help dairy farming becoming a more viable enterprise, more visible to the public and open up new markets, but equally more risks involved when selling value-added versus marketing directly to your local milk cooperative.

Global Experience of Value Addition in Livestock Products

Global value chains, led by retailers and food processors, are increasingly dominating the agriculture and food sectors. Multinational retailers for example, work with importers and exporters and more and more, control how products are grown. Control of quality, food safety standards and traceability along the supply chain requires vertical co-ordination. A relatively small number of companies organize the global supply of food and link producers in developed or developing countries to consumers all over the world. Food safety is a global issue of increasing concern for governments, food producers, food processors and handlers, as well as consumers. There is a big gap in price fetched for the raw product by producer and finished products sold by retailer to consumers.

Four different methods can be used to add value to producers' raw commodities such as

1. Selling into open markets for normal distribution channels of marketing and processing,
2. Investing in a portfolio of food companies,
3. Using production or marketing contracts, and
4. Forming of producer-owned businesses.

Marketing

The key to the success of value-added products is to market a high quality product that is reasonably priced and available in a convenient location for the consumer to purchase. You must deliver your product with a consistent quality and have sufficient supplies to meet the demand. Remember that the consumer will react negatively to your product if you do not maintain your quality standards and/or timely deliver sufficient supplies.

Value-added products can be a good way to increase farm income, give farm more visibility and help to expand to new markets. Careful business planning and adhering to state regulations will also ensure the success of new venture.

Thus the key to the success of value-added products is to

- Market a high quality product that is reasonably priced and available in a convenient location for the consumer to purchase.
- Product must be delivered consistently and have sufficient supplies to meet the demand.
- A certification for food quality and safety.

Open Market Distribution and Processing Channel

Food marketing channels include all the institutions and processes by which food moves from the producer to the end user. Perishable products, such as fresh produce, move through shorter channels, whereas more storable products, like frozen pizza, utilize longer distribution channels. The purpose of middlemen has been to smooth the flow of goods from manufacturers or growers who produce large quantities of a few items to consumers who desire to purchase small quantities of many items. However, as retail chains have grown larger and more concentrated, food processors have found it advantageous to negotiate with and distribute directly to large retail customers (Connor, Schiek, and Uhl) et al. Over the last 20 years, food processors have provided innovative, easy-to-prepare foods with convenient packaging, because consumers desire product quality, variety, food safety, and nutrition. In addition, fulfilling consumers' desires will necessitate closer coordination and communication between producers and processors.

Preparation convenience is a key feature of foods purchased by busy, affluent households. In fact, the number of food service meals eaten away from home has increased by 50 percent in the last 20 years. Therefore six significant growth trends in consumer demand have been identified: more convenience, ethnic-identify foods, aging of the population, low-calorie foods, fresh foods instead of frozen or canned, and healthy natural foods (Connor et al.). Value-adding producers should focus on products that fill these consumer desires or market niches. By utilizing value-added precepts for business development, producers can identify the desires of consumers and target markets, rather than taking the commodity to the market and hoping that consumers will like it and use it. Target markets are tightening as retailers and consumers pay more for a narrower range of eating experience. Hitting these target markets means that value-adding businesses must know their consumers' desires.

Livestock Products Requiring Value Addition

Meat

Total meat production in India is 6.7MT and growth rate in meat production is 7.31%. Out of total animal slaughtered percentage of different livestock is as cattle 10.6%, buffalo 10.6%, sheep 24.1%, goat 58.8%, pig 95%, and poultry 90%. Per capita meat consumption is 5.5kg/person/year while world meat consumption is 42kg/person/year and 80.3kg/person/year in developed countries. Livestock contribution in GDP is 4.1%. India's trade in livestock & livestock products is in live form. India is not even contributing 1percent to global export of livestock market. India is thus very small player in global market. Total meat processing capacity of India is over 1million per anum, remaining meat sold in fresh and frozen form.

Value added meat products

Animal byproducts, traditional meat products, Enrobed meat products, Cured and smoked meat products, Dried meat products, Chunked meat products, Ground meat products, Designer meat, Emulsion meat products, Restructured meat products etc. There are few meat products with longer shelf life such as Cured & smoked chicken, chicken patties, chicken meat spread, chicken pickle, cooked chicken stock (one minute curried chicken, cost effective, instant use by working couple, old people and highly useful at the time of instant need. Meat is high in protein, low in fat, source of essential Amino Acid, good source of I, P, Cu, Zn & B12, Dark meat & skin is higher in fat then white

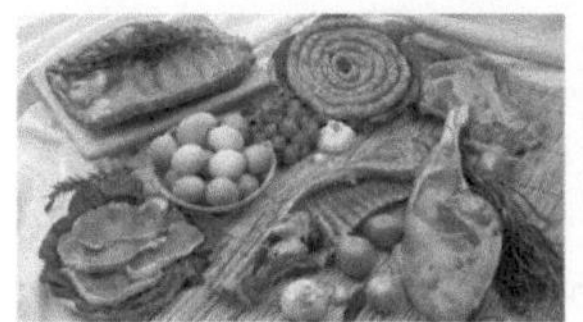

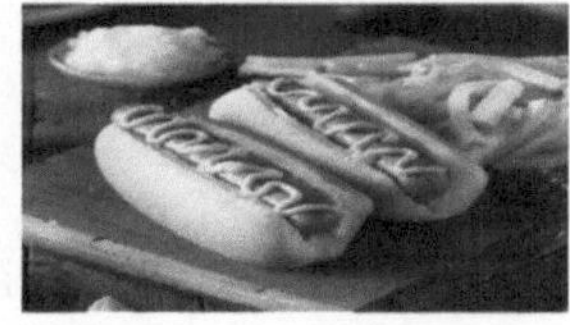

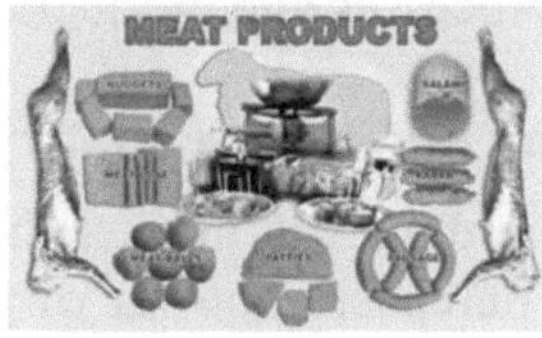

Value addition in Dairy

In case of dairy products, one can add extra value to milk by processing and marketing products, such as cheeses, packaged milk, yogurt, ice cream or butter.

Dairy Value Addition

For successful value addition the following points are necessary –quality of raw material, correct formulation, optimum processing, right packaging, storage stability, flavor and colour changes, nutritional value, product specification and regulation etc.

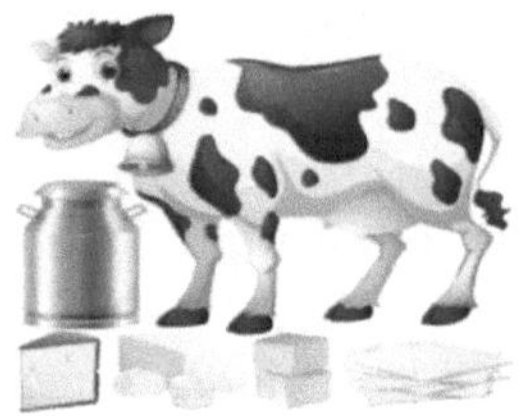
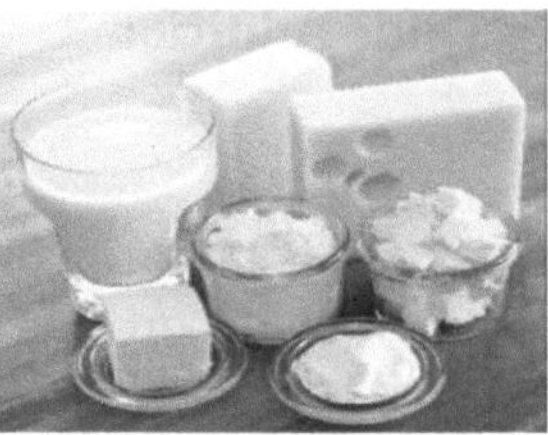

When considering the production and marketing of value-added dairy products, one should consider the capital outlay, time commitment, market share and the fact that your business may not make a profit in the first five years. Following point should be kept in mind while starting value addition to livestock products-

- Product you want to sell
- Target audience and how will I market the product
- Location(s) convenient to the consumer
- Profit potential of the product
- Consumer paying capacity
- Quality of the product?

Value-added products can help your farm become more viable, more visible to the public and open up new markets but there are more risks involved when selling value-added versus marketing directly to your local milk cooperative.

Farmers can take classes, or attend seminars on making the products that they are interested in marketing. Food technologists can also offer guidance on the processes and production of milk products.

Value Addition in Poultry

In the domestic market the consumption of poultry meat is low due to the low purchasing power of people. Just 25% population living in urban areas consumes about 75-80 % of eggs and poultry meat. The per capita consumption of egg is100 and poultry meat is 1.2 Kg per person per annum in urban areas. In rural area it is only 15 eggs and 0.15 Kg poultry meat. The output of eggs is increasing at the rate of 4-6 % and broiler at 8-10 % per annum. It accounts for about 3 % of the total GNP and 10 % of the total GNP attributed to livestock product with growth rate of 15-20%

Poultry sector is one of the fastest going segment of Agriculture sector in India. Driving this expansion are a combination of factors - growth in per capita income, a growing urban population and falling real poultry prices. Compared with meat, poultry industry has registered significant growth. India ranks fifth in the world with annual egg production of 1.61 million tones and18th largest broiler production. Indian poultry meat products have good markets in Japan, Malaysia, Indonesia and Singapore.

India has gifted the world the species like Red jungle and Silver jungle fowls, out of whose progenies, domesticated and crossbreed have emerged the "Pure lines" of today. Transformation has involved sizeable investments in breeding, hatching, rearing and processing. Farmers in India have moved from rearing non-descript birds to rearing hybrids which ensure faster growth, good livability, excellent feed conversion and high profits to the rearers. The industry has grown largely due to the initiative of private enterprise, minimal government intervention, considerable indigenous poultry genetics capabilities, and considerable support from the complementary veterinary health, poultry feed, poultry equipment, and poultry processing sectors. India is one of the few countries in the world that has put into place a sustained Specific Pathogen Free (SPF) egg production project. Some of the value added poultry products are : mention only the names salted chicken egg, Albumen rings, Egg roll, Egg crepe, Egg waffles, Pickled egg, Designer egg,

Some trends affecting poultry markets are -Consumer preference for convenience to save the time, attractive packaging, products for the children-funny shapes, convenient for microwave, preserving freshness etc.

Recommendations

As the poultry industry is among the fastest growing in the world, its potential to attract big-time foreign investment is negligible and that is why it needs greater integration, better cost-effectiveness and improvement in the distribution. Indian poultry industry needs good branding system in order to increase the consumption of chicken. More retail outlets, mass gathering and creating awareness home to home about the nutrient values of chicken and egg; Develop mechanism to counter anti-meat lobbies; Developing efficient, independent, authority for disease monitoring, biological quality control.

Livestock Niche Product Marketing

The farm share of profit in the food systems is falling. But there is an opportunity to turn that around. The "mass market" is breaking up in market segments – groups of consumers seeking unique products with specific attributes. Some are willing to pay premiums for those attributes. Many market surveys in US & Europe found that over half of consumers would pay a premium for food produced in a more healthful and environmentally sound manner. This offers an opportunity for farmers to go beyond producing cheap, undifferentiated commodities to adding value and earning premiums by delivering unique products that are highly valued by different groups of consumers. That may be food that tastes better. Perhaps it is locally produced and fresher or is produced in a way that improves its flavor. It may be food that is healthier or perceived as consistent with a healthier lifestyle – such as products raised without pesticide, hormones, and antibiotics. This is an area where products from indigenous livestock breeds have an offer to enhance farm incomes and make economic justification for raising indigenous breeds.

Future Prospects

Value addition of the livestock products is the best way to enhance the farmer's income. If farmers are directly involved or trained in value addition of different livestock products but the constraints such as Less preference for frozen meat by consumer, insufficient cold chain facilities, lack of well-organized marketing system, less demand for value added products, lack of infrastructure facilities for storage and processing, fluctuating export trade, high import duty etc. besides these constraints there are some challenges like poor process and marketing condition, microbial problem, bio-insecurity of products, quality deterioration and inadequate focus on quality & safety structure should be overcome

In summary, producers should stay attuned to the needs of the marketplace; they should see themselves producing consumer products instead of farm commodity products. To establish a value-added business, one must be very careful about:

- Start by choosing something you love to do.
- Establish good relations with customers to identify products that will appeal to them.
- Maintain consistent supply of high quality products.
- Make sure that products will be in high demand over the long term.
- Partner with people possessing good technical expertise.
- Carefully hire consultants with expertise, experienced project manager.
- Have a complete plan prior to start & make long-range plans.
- Plan on more time, effort, and expense than expected.

Way to Attract Indian Youth towards Family Dairy Business

In today's scenario youth are diverting from farm jobs to non-farm jobs. Therefore everyone should focus on how to attract youth to dairy farming or dairy business? There is only way to attract them towards dairy business by introducing new schemes as well as new technologies in dairy sector, giving some relaxation, different means of increasing income from dairy and paying more remunerative prices. The whole business of farming has to be commercially viable. Today's youth is modern, they go for commercial dairy farms, they build proper shed, milking through milking machines, good practices so that youth is interested in farming in a village.

Following are the strategies to be adapted to enrolled Indian youth for family dairy business-

- Government should allow free trade agreement with other countries.
- Dairy should be considered as the part of agriculture so whatever benefits agriculture sector gets that should arrive to the dairy sector too. The subsidized loans available for agriculture should also be available for dairy.
- Cooperatives are owned by the small milk producers, so they should be given relaxation from all kinds of taxation.
- Opportunities in the fields of animal husbandry should be introduced such as improved technologies of small-scale poultry and dairy farming can be introduced.
- Financing the dairy farming through bank under different financing schemes. Such as establishment of small dairy unit, purchase of dairy processing equipment's, transportation facilities of dairy products, cold storage facilities, vet. Clinics, dairy parlors or dairy outlets etc.
- Youth should realize that animal husbandry is a very attractive business with small land size or even for landless.
- Generate more employment opportunities in dairy sector.
- Such as Amul is launching innovative programmes like the "cow to consumer" to make the dairy sector "contemporarily cool" and commercially viable for today's youth who are moving to cities and reluctant to join the milk industry. In 1970, per capita of milk consumption in India was 111 gm and today it is 350 gm, it is growing at the rate of 2 per cent per annum. The demand for milk by 2050 would touch 540 million litres and to meet India's demand in the coming years there is a need to make the dairy industry commercially viable for India's youth, as said Sodhi.
- Codex alimentarius standards of food safety can be popularized in the case of perishable commodities. For this purpose, the young farmers should establish Gyan Chaupals or Village Knowledge Centers. Such centers will be based on the integrated use of the internet, FM Radio and mobile telephony.

Relaxation, in terms of regulation and policies, the industry seeks from the government?

The industry is going through a golden period as it is passing through a very excellent demand with good supply from procurement side. As far as the demand is concerned, urban India is buying more and more branded products whether it is wheat, egg or dairy product. The retail price of milk has increased around 60 percent in the last three to four years. Thus, the farmers are also getting handsome returns. It encourages them to increase their productivity. In India, milk production is increasing at the rate of 4.5 percent per annum while the demand is surging around 10-12 percent. So, it is good for the industry and the youth.

32

ITK: Relevancy & Need in Present Context of Animal Husbandry Development

Pranav Kumar

Division of Veterinary & Animal Husbandry Extension Education
Faculty of Veterinary Sciences & Animal Husbandry, R.S. Pura
Sher-e-Kashmir University of Agricultural Sciences & Technology of Jammu

Executive summary

The ITK system had been developed by the indigenous communities based on their experiences, continuous improvement through informal experimentation and transfer of such knowledge to next generations. The tried and tested rich ITK pertaining to agriculture, livestock and other allied sectors had been interwoven with the socio-cultural and traditional practices followed by them. Since time immemorial indigenous communities had been applying ITK in animal husbandry to increase milk production, fertility, retention of placenta, breeding, prolapsed, care for the young stock and preparation of indigenous livestock products. ITKs are often adapted according to the local culture and traditions, needs, and environment; they are very dynamic and continuously changing, and lay emphasis on minimizing the risks rather than maximizing profits. Indigenous knowledge of livestock rearing is often "*tacit*" and not necessarily expressed in the conventional form of scientific documentation. The origin and evolution of indigenous technical knowledge (ITK) in India has been reported since time immemorial. Since then, the knowledge, belief, skills and practices pertaining to diagnosis, treatment and management of animal and human diseases are imprinted and carried to future generations. In the light of evolution, the practice has come to limelight as an alternative low cost solution to conventional western medicine and readily practiced by ordinary farmers. Furthermore, it can be a major alternative to antibiotics use for the purpose of promoting growth and production performance of animals as well as for prophylaxis and treatment of common animal ailments. Therefore, it could be of great help in reduction of emergence of multidrug-resistant superbugs.

Introduction

Indigenous knowledge develops within a particular community and maintains a non-formal means of dissemination. Such knowledge is collectively owned, developed over several generations and subject to adaptation, and imbedded in a community's way of life as means of survival. Within the broad framework of indigenous knowledge, the contribution of Indigenous Technical Knowledge is remarkable. This knowledge plays imperative role in many grassroots innovations. Such knowledge is responsible for improvement in many important rural enterprises such as poultry. Despite the wide recognition of indigenous peoples' contribution to the world's cultural and biological diversity and sustainable development, many challenges still remain in the area of traditional knowledge and technologies. The term indigenous technical knowledge (ITKs) is also known as local knowledge and traditional knowledge. Traditional knowledge is based on the necessities, observation, instinct, trial, and error and is gathered over time, which is transferred from generation to generation. Indigenous technical knowledge refers to the unique, traditional, local knowledge existing within and developed around the specific conditions of women and men indigenous to a particular geographic area.

Indigenous technical knowledge is the local knowledge that the people have accumulated over generations that people have gained through inheritance from their ancestors. It is total knowledge based on old knowledge and experience of people in dealing with problems and typical situations in different periods of life and represents people's creativity, innovations, and skills. India is considered one of the richest due to its geographical diversities and many ethnic communities in terms of indigenous technical knowledge. All of these communities have some traditional knowledge. India has a wealthy heritage of traditional health control and different treatment systems that have been used for animals since time immemorial. ITK practices are environmentally sound and suited to specific local and environmental conditions. Innovation is the first attempt to carry out an invention in practice (Fegerberg, 2006). The knowledge inherently possess by the indigenous communities is used for purposes ranging from natural resource management, agriculture, medicine to other socioeconomic developments and thus it instigates the process of innovation. In the arena of grassroots innovation, it has been observed that most of the indigenous knowledge and technologies are at par with the modern knowledge and technology systems. ITK is momentous in many sustainable grassroots innovations which provide substantial substitutions for many modern systems and methods.

Concept and Definitions of Indigenous Knowledge

Indigenous Technical Knowledge can broadly identified as the knowledge, be it technological, know- how skills, practices and belief that a local community accumulated over generations of living in a particular environment. This knowledge system is vital for sustainability of natural resources and eco system since it comprises of components of local knowledge of species, environmental phenomenon, belief and practices in a way people carry out within an ecosystem (Cavalcanti 2002). World Bank (1997) also recognized that global knowledge have originated from indigenous people, therefore, the basic components of any country's knowledge system is its indigenous knowledge.

According to Atteh (1989) "it covers the whole range of human experience". Hence, as ITK is closely related to survival and subsistence, it provides a basis for local-level decision making in:

- food security
- human and animal health
- education
- natural resource management
- various other community-based activities

According to World Bank Report, 1998, the special features of indigenous knowledge are:

- **Local:** it is rooted in a particular community and situated within broader cultural traditions; it is a set of experiences generated by people living in those communities. Separating the technical from the non-technical, the rational from the non-rational could be problematic. Therefore, when transferred to other places, there is a potential risk of dislocating indigenous knowledge.
- **Tacit** knowledge and, therefore, not easily modifiable
- **Transmitted** orally, or through imitation and demonstration. Codifying it may lead to the loss of some of its properties.
- **Experiential rather than theoretical knowledge.** Experience and trial and error, tested in the rigorous laboratory of survival of local communities constantly reinforce indigenous knowledge.
- **Learned through repetition,** which is a defining characteristic of tradition even when new knowledge is added. Repetition aids in the retention and reinforcement of indigenous knowledge.
- **Constantly changing,** being produced as well as reproduced, discovered as well as lost; though it is often perceived by external observers as being somewhat static.

- Traditional knowledge (TK), indigenous knowledge (IK), traditional ecologic knowledge (TEK) and local knowledge generally refer to knowledge systems embedded in the cultural traditions of regional, indigenous, or local communities. These kinds of knowledge are crucial for the subsistence and survival and are generally based on accumulations of empirical observation and interaction with the environment. Indigenous technical knowledge (ITK) is a body of knowledge built up through generations of by a group of people living in close contact with nature (Adam, 2009). On the other hand Buresh and Cooper (1999), have defined indigenous technical knowledge as consisting of facts, experiences, practices, resource management strategies and production systems developed through trial-and-error during several millennia in a given community, nation or region.

The need to study ITK

It is observed that only limited number of technologies generated by State Agricultural Universities and ICAR is being adopted by the farmers, which indicate that the farmers are still in touch with their Indigenous Technical Knowledge (ITK). In this context, it is pertinent to identify and preserve these traditional knowledge / techniques in order to sustain the productivity and protect the ecosystem. Documentation of ITKs and their further refinement, validation and propagation among different stakeholders will also help to develop alternatives to ecologically damaging agricultural and animal husbandry practices, which will lead to sustainability in the long run. The resource constraints of livestock farmers and escalating cost of high- tech dairying make it imperative to seek an alternative in the form of blending of indigenous knowledge with modern animal rearing practices.

Attempts to impress researchers with the need to study traditional animal husbandry practices were already made in the late sixties (Verma and Singh, 1969). The study and appreciation of ITK is important because:

- ITK may have scientific basis and its technologies could be transferred to other similar farming situations; documentation and screening of ITK is necessary before the valuable information is lost forever;
- ITK may be an alternative, a substitute or a complement to modern technology;
- ITK may generate ideas for future research;
- It is often easier to secure adoption of ITK than modern technology.

India & ITK

India being a developing country with rich ethno-veterinary knowledge is sought to be a 'EVP hub' owing to practice with decades of experiences.

Since time immemorial, the practice is mainly based on the use of plant formulations and other locally available cheap ingredients. Livestock raisers and local people with a strong knowledge of veterinary medicine usually follow traditional ways of classifying, diagnosing, preventing and treating common animal ailments. The traditional medicines that are commonly used for animal healthcare can cut down costs considerably. Moreover, they are readily available to the ordinary farmer.

ITK regarding animal husbandry

Indian livestock farmers, over centuries, have learnt to rear animals and produce food crops and animal products to survive in difficult environments, where the rich tradition of Indigenous Technical Knowledge has been interwoven in the society in which they live. The enhancement of the quality of life of the Indians who in great majority live in and depend on livestock and agricultural production systems would be impossible by keeping this rich tradition of ITK aside.

ITK regarding animal husbandry is considered as old as domestication of livestock itself. Unfortunately, these age old practices, which were in practice widely throughout India, are seldom documented scientifically; consequently, they are now in danger of extinction. (*De Amitendu, et al*, 2004).Since independence all efforts in India had been exclusively focused on modern science based livestock breeding and management and promotion of allopathic-based veterinary services, entirely under control of the state. There had been a serious neglect and disapproval of ITK and practices to the extent that majority of the Indian society is not only unaware and unfamiliar with the ancient knowledge and literature but also extremely skeptical and cynical about it (Rangnekar, 1998). Livestock breeding and management programmes of the government and formal education curriculum of animal husbandry exclusively rely on and emphasize on knowledge and inputs of modern science from outside and remain extremely skeptical in acknowledgement and wider dissemination of indigenous knowledge research system (IKRS) (Ravikumar, et al, 2017).

Genesis of ITK/ Ethno veterinary practices in India

The history of ethno-medicine perhaps dates back to 4 millennia ago. It is believed that during the period of Hamburabi (2000 BC), the physicians had knowledge of more than 250 medicinal plants and 120 mineral salts. The veterinary and animal husbandry practices of the ancient India find mentions in Rig veda and Atarvaveda. Books written by Salihotra (1800 Bc) and Charak (2300 BC) and Palikapaya (1000 BC) described treatment of animal diseases using medicinal plants. The two great Pandavas-Nakula and Sahadeva, had expertise in treatment and management of horses and cattle, respectively. The ancient Indians also had distinction to establish the first state funded well-equipped veterinary doctor in the world, lived around 1800 BC in Northern India.

Sources of Indigenous Traditional Knowledge

The sources of the traditional knowledge mainly derived from the human experiences, beliefs and practices which are collected from several sources. There are also some semi-recorded information such as manuscripts, photographs and folk literature. Ancient literatures like the Vedas, Puranas, religious books, grey literature, ethno-botanical texts and archaeological deposits give detail account of the life of the ancient people and the method of living in a prosperous way. Again these sources also give information about bio-techniques, medicinal knowledge, breeding techniques, agricultural farming systems, human and animal healthcare techniques, religious and astrological guidelines and cultural artifacts. Some of the indigenous traditional knowledge is available in written form in primary, secondary and tertiary sources of information. But most of the indigenous traditional knowledge are undocumented and are available orally or in memory of the group of the community of a region or area.

In India, ITK and ethno-veterinary practices are common since time immemorial. The knowledge are imprinted and carried to future generations in the form of text manuscripts, by word of mouth and most of the folk health practices largely remain undocumented. A few oldest existing book of ancient era form the asset or repository of livestock health care practices in India. It includes Asvayurvedasiddhanta (Ayurvedic practices for horses), Asvachikitsita (therapeutics of horses), Asvavaidyaka (medicines of horses), Hastyayurveda (Ayurveda of elephants) (Tiwari and Pande, 2010). The contemporary India classifies ethno-veterinary systems on the basis of caste, religion and ecosystem. Therefore, sophistication, characteristics and intensities of these systems differ greatly among individuals, societies and regions.

Strategies to combat antimicrobial resistance in Indian scenario through ITKs

Antimicrobial resistance (AMR) refers to the decrease in sensitivity of the microorganism to the antibiotic, clinically evident either as an increase in MIC (minimum inhibitory concentration) or total insensitivity.

Major concerns of antimicrobial resistance

The increasing AMR incidences globally can be attributed to certain factors that are critically responsible for the spread of AMR. These include the lack of awareness regarding the use of antibiotics and their aftereffects in dairy farmers, poultry breeders and other stakeholders. It generates the major factor related to antibiotics-induced AMR improper drug and dose regimen that includes the dose, dosing interval, duration of treatment and the formulation. Use of too high or too low dose, over prescription of drugs, and incorrect duration of prescription usually intensifies the problem (Ayukekbong*et al.* 2017, Bello-López *et al.* 2019). Lack of awareness further leads to the indiscriminate use of antibiotics for treatment of diseases and as growth promoters. Indiscriminate use of antimicrobial is usually the primary driving force for antimicrobial resistance (AMR) in animal husbandry, removing the sensitive population and allowing proliferation of the mutant strains. It is the genesis of three critical conditions that determine the spread of AMR presence of a resistant mutant in the bacterial population; chances of vertical or horizontal transmission of resistance genes; selection pressure of antibiotics (Drlica 2007). In Indian scenario, lack of facilities to detect drugs of choice and perform antibiotic sensitivity to support the selection of effective drugs further contribute to AMR spread as it has been reported in food borne pathogens, wild birds, domestic animals and humans (Kumar *et al.* 2010, Kumar *et al.* 2011, Kumar *et al.* 2013, Malik *et al.* 2013, Suman *et al.* 2020).

ITK based treatment: an alternate therapy

The use of indigenous traditional knowledge (ITK) based treatment can be an alternate therapy. It requires the development and validation for cost effective, safe and easily available alternate medicines. The action plan should focus on innovation in the treatment through research and development of newer drugs including ITK based alternate medicine.

Organic Livestock Production: as a Model for reducing On-Farm Antibiotic Use

Organic methods can serve as a model for successfully eliminating the non-therapeutic use of antibiotics in livestock production. Certified organic production is also the best way to combat antibiotic resistance and protect the health of farm workers, communities and consumers because the organic standards strictly regulate antibiotic administration in livestock. As a result, organic livestock production contributes to reductions in overall antibiotic usage, particularly at non-therapeutic doses, and relieves the selective pressure that drives the proliferation of antibiotic-resistant bacteria. In addition to prohibiting antibiotic use, organic standards require organic producers to follow animal husbandry practices that support the health of the animals. For instance, they must develop a healthcare plan for their animals that focuses on disease prevention.

Keeping Animals Healthy without Antibiotics using ITKs

Organic's prohibition on use of antibiotics in livestock relies on the establishment of practices that prevent disease like supplying a nutritious and complete diet, choosing breeds naturally resistant to pests and diseases, maintaining strict levels of hygiene cleanliness in housing, and reducing stress. When these preventive practices failed, organic farmers turn to indigenous technical knowledge and natural disease control measures, like botanical extracts and minerals. However, when illness necessitates treatment with antibiotics, organic producers cannot withhold treatment to preserve the organic status of an animal, and, if treated, the animal and its products must be used after the withdrawal period of antibiotics used.

ITK and Ethno veterinary practice: An alternative treatment approach

India being a developing country, where nearly 80% of the population is below poverty line, mainly adopts agrarian economy. Animal agriculture is now a growing concern as it can satisfy unmet needs of the poor and can provide some income to the family. Being poor and weak, they can hardly afford for their own living, while to think for better animal living is still a long way to go. The practice is a cost effective and dynamic solution to the poor farmers for whom, fulfilling the basic amenities are always priority. Also it can be a major alternative to antibiotics use for the purpose of promoting growth and production performance or for prophylaxis and treatment of various pathogenic organisms. This way it could be of great help to reduce the emergence of multidrug-resistant pathogens or superbugs and to avoid antibiotic residues in food of animal origin, like meat, milk and egg. The constitutional ingredients of ethno-veterinary medicine are easily and locally available, easy to prepare and administer. Furthermore it has covered ever areas of veterinary specialization and all livestock species.

Importance/Relevance of indigenous knowledge

In the recent years, the role of IK in a range of sectors is being talked about. It includes intercropping techniques, pest control, crop diversity, and seed varieties in agriculture; plant varieties, and fish breeding techniques in biology; traditional medicine in human and veterinary healthcare; soil conservation, irrigation, and water conservation in natural resource management; and oral traditions and local languages in education. The realization of IK's contribution to these sectors has led to an increasing interest in it by academicians, and policymakers alike. Many government and non-governmental organizations, as well as international organizations such as the World Bank, International Labor Office, UNESCO and FAO are now appreciating the role; IK can play in achieving sustainable development in a country. This interest is also apparent in the policies and programmes of various countries.

Indigenous people can provide valuable input about the local environment and how to effectively manage its natural resources. Outside interest in indigenous knowledge systems has been fuelled by the recent worldwide ecological crisis and the realization that its causes lie partly in the overexploitation of natural resources based on inappropriate attitudes and technologies. Scientists now recognize that indigenous people have managed the environments in which they have lived for generations, often without significantly damaging local ecologies (Emery, 1996). Many feel that indigenous knowledge can thus provide a powerful basis from which alternative ways of managing resources can be developed. Indigenous knowledge technologies and know-how have an advantage over Science in that they rely on locally available skills and materials and are thus often more cost-effective than introducing exotic technologies from outside sources.

According to International Institute of Rural Reconstruction (1996), local people are familiar with indigenous knowledge system and so do not need any specialized training. The following are some of the features of indigenous knowledge, which have relevance to conservation and sustainable development:

- **Locally appropriate**: indigenous knowledge represents a way of life that has evolved with the local environment, so it is specifically adapted to the requirements of local conditions.
- **Restraint in resource exploitation**: production is for subsistence needs only; only what is needed for immediate survival is taken from the environment.
- **Diversified production systems**: there is no overexploitation of a single resource; risk is often spread out by utilizing a number of subsistence strategies.
- **Respect for nature**: a 'conservation ethic' often exists. The land is considered sacred, humans are dependent on nature for survival, and all species are interconnected.
- **Flexible**: indigenous knowledge is able to adapt to new conditions and incorporate outside knowledge.

- **Social responsibility**: there are strong family and community ties, and with them feelings of obligation and responsibility to preserve the land for future generations.

(*Source*: Dewalt, 1994)

The fact that indigenous technical knowledge is still in existence in many parts of the world, strengthens the argument that it has potential to help solve problems facing farmers. Farmers use this knowledge to modify new technologies to suit their diverse needs. If indigenous technical knowledge is recognized by technology developers then it can help in forming a basis for technology generation and development.

Based on these findings, indigenous technical knowledge has the potential to supplement present day farming system by means of better technology adoption and extension service reception since there are no hindrances from age, education or gender regarding dissemination.

Improve agriculture technology planners and developers should collaborate with farmers in a participatory manner, to develop, test and use appropriate channels to disseminate these technologies, which in turn will supplement their current work.

Indigenous Traditional knowledge and its role in-coping the climate change:

Indigenous Traditional Knowledge (ITK) is developed over a period of time through accumulation of experiences and intimate understanding of environment. This knowledge is gradually vanishing due to population pressure and industrial development. Traditional crops and cropping practices are becoming extinct, of which modern farming practices are major contributors. Further climate change is a significant change in the statistical distribution of weather patterns. The Intergovernmental Panel on Climate Change Third Assessment Report 2001 concluded that current knowledge on adaptation to climate change is limited and emphasized the need for research on viable adaptation measures. India is vulnerable to climate change as the majority of its population depends on agriculture, which is climate sensitive. Agriculture in India is involved in domestic food supply, employment and cash income. Recognizing the challenges to mitigate climate variability promotes more sustainable and resilient agriculture. The traditional knowledge for ecosystem management and use of natural resources is gaining credence as a key weapon to fight against climate change. Understanding the ITK will help sustain farming practices preventing plant genetic erosion and environmental deterioration. It contributes to sustainable food security and conservation of variety and variability of animals, plants and soil properties. There is a need to strengthen dissemination of indigenous knowledge and integrating with modern approaches in climate change resilience.

ITK/Ethno-veterinary Practices: A game changer in reducing antibiotic misuse in livestock

Antimicrobial resistance (AMR) is a worldwide problem created due to the excessive and indiscriminate use of antibiotics in human, animal and plant health. About 90 per cent of the antibiotics used end up in the environment, affecting the quality of water, soils, and biodiversity. AMR makes it harder to eliminate infections from the body as existing drugs become ineffective. In India, the annual rate of antibiotics use in the past five years has risen by 6-7 per cent. *Tackling a Crisis for the Health and Wealth of Nations* was published on the request of the UK Prime Minister to address the growing global problem of drug-resistant infections. It states that drug-resistant infections will kill an extra 10 million people a year worldwide and that the total world Gross Domestic Product cost of antimicrobial resistance will be $100 trillion.

One of the immediate challenges regarding AMR is to reduce the use of antibiotics both for human and animal health care. As antibiotics find their way through the food chain, there is an urgent need to focus on reducing the use of antibiotics in veterinary practice by working with veterinarians, farmers and dairy cooperatives. It is a established fact that ITK/ ethno-veterinary practices (EVPs) are efficacious and safe in preventing and curing certain clinical conditions in dairy animals and thereby reducing antibiotic residues in milk.

Use of Indigenous Technical Knowledge (ITK) or Ethno-veterinary practices (EVP) to reduce antibiotic drug residues in bovine milk:

The indiscriminate use of antibiotics in human medicine, agriculture and animal health, have resulted in the emergence of antimicrobial drug resistant (AMR) microorganisms (Nisha, 2008). Most of the antibiotics used in humans, crops and livestock end up in the environment. It is estimated that by 2050 AMR will cause 10 million deaths per year (O'Neill 2014). There is no effective and strategic implementation of government regulation in India to control antibiotic use in humans and domestic animals, in agriculture and other activities like horticulture and fisheries. Against a background of emerging endemic zoonotic diseases and higher occurrence of non communicable diseases (NCDs) the immediate attention of the all the stake holders to replace fragmented approaches by holistic strategies is warranted. Local healers and some farmers have experience in traditional veterinary health care, better known as indigenous technical knowledge or Ethno-veterinary practices

(EVP). They use the locally available medicinal plants for prevention and treatment of animal health conditions.

Study Report on ITK

The University of Trans-disciplinary health sciences and Technology, along with Tamil Nadu Veterinary and Animal Sciences University has documented EVPs from 24 locations in 10 states and rapidly assessed them using Ayurveda. It has established that 353 formulations out of 441 are safe and efficacious. *The study reports that In-vitro* antimicrobial activity of the extracts of the herbal formulation against mastitis had inhibitory activity against Escherichia *coli* and *Streptococus aureus.* Clinical study using traditional formulation for mastitis showed that somatic cell counts, electrical conductivity and pH of the milk became normal within six days, indicating cure of mastitis. It has been also reported that traditional medicine can be used during dry periods to reduce the incidence of mastitis and reduce the retention of placenta.

Adopting ITK/ EVPs to combat infectious and other clinical conditions in livestock has been identified and tested as a key game changer in reducing the use of antibiotic and other veterinary drugs in veterinary practices. It has also been shown that ITK/EVP was extremely helpful for the farmers during the novel corona virus lockdown period as these formulations could be prepared and used by farmers themselves for the well-being of their cattle.

Challenges faced by ethno veterinary practice in present arena

In current scenario, with increasing population the forest area is decreasing. The era is shifting towards western ends discouraging the aforestation and prefers more to readily available drugs. Also youths of India showing little interest towards this practice owing to disbelief and large communication gap with previous generation. Day by day, India is losing experienced persons as they are growing old and poor and there is no encouragement to pass this rural wisdom to next generations. Also, not a single Indian policy or regulation is framed till now to protect this traditional, indigenous rural wisdom. No one is aware of protecting this practice. So it is fading away in the mask of western medicine. The introduction of modern practices also made it difficult for the younger generations to appreciate and use the beliefs and practices of their forefathers. Despite recent efforts to promote the use of ethno veterinary knowledge worldwide, much information is only documented in field reports and scientific publications.

It is, obviously, most important for the local community in which the bearers of such knowledge live and produce. Development agents (CBOs,

NGOs, governments, donors, local leaders, and private sector initiatives) need to recognize it, value it and appreciate it in their interaction with the local communities. Before incorporating it in their approaches, they need to understand it – and critically validate it against the usefulness for their intended objectives.

Lastly, indigenous knowledge forms part of the global knowledge. In this context, it has a value and relevance in itself. Indigenous knowledge can be preserved, transferred, or adopted and adapted elsewhere. The development process interacts with indigenous knowledge. When designing or implementing development programs or projects for agriculture or any related field, three scenarios can be observed- The development strategy either-

- Relies entirely or substantially on indigenous knowledge,
- Overrides indigenous knowledge or,
- Incorporates indigenous knowledge.

Planners and implementers therefore need to decide which path to follow. Rational conclusions are based on determining whether indigenous knowledge would contribute to solve existing problems and achieving the intended objectives. In most cases, a careful amalgamation of indigenous and foreign knowledge would be most promising, leaving the choice, the rate and the degree of adoption and adaptation to the clients. Foreign knowledge does not necessarily mean modern technology, it includes also indigenous practices developed and applied under similar conditions elsewhere. These techniques are then likely to be adopted faster and applied more successfully. To foster such a transfer a sound understanding of indigenous knowledge is needed. This requires means for the capture and validation, as well as for the eventual exchange, transfer and dissemination of indigenous knowledge.

Limitations and Strengths

In the modern era of evidence based veterinary medicine, many professionals question the usefulness, applicability and adaptability of ITK/EVM. It is argued that the traditional practices lack scientific evidences and may not be as effective as claimed. Some practices are harmful or not readily available. No doubt, many of the concerns relating to ITK/EVM practices are true to an extent, but like other systems of medicine, EVM has both limitations and strengths.

The major limitations for EVM include

- ITK/EVM are often not as fast-working and potent as allopathic medicines. They may therefore be less suitable to control and treat epidemic and endemic infectious diseases. Further, effectiveness of EVM practices is questionable against emerging infectious diseases.

- Majority of the traditional animal healthcare practices are unregulated and prone to be affected by abuse and quackery due to concealment, distortions and misleading claims. A large proportion of conventional practitioners, whether in human or animal health care, are therefore skeptical about the value of alternative practices.
- Certain ITK/EVM practices can be harmful if used improperly or without appropriate knowledge and study. Even herbal preparations that are safe for use in some animal species may be toxic to others. For example, garlic which is recommended to reduce blood cholesterol in human can cause anaemia in dog. The white willow (Salix alba) preparations used for treatment of fever, rheumatic arthritis and headache in human can be fatal for cat, as felids cannot metabolize salicylic acid, a metabolite of salicin present in willow bark.
- Lack of documentation, inappropriate scientific validation and failure to disseminate and promote evaluated practices for field application adversely affect development and full utilization of EVM by the end users.
- The underlying science of ITK/ EVM is poorly researched and understood.
- No formal degree/ diploma/ courses on alternative system are available in the academic curricula in many countries including India.
- The diagnosis of disease and identification of underlying cause are inadequate
- Depleting medicinal plant resources and seasonal availability of certain plants is making ingredients unavailable for preparing medicine.
- Rapid decline in experienced traditional healers and pastoralist communities. Young generation is not keen to use EVM, probably due to lack of information and interest or rural exodus.

The evaluated veterinary traditional healthcare and management practices as well as herbal and holistic medicines are increasingly accepted as an important viable solution to address animal health problems not only in developing countries but in western countries as well. In general, though abuse and quackery exist, the application of traditional practices can be a pragmatic response in the areas without adequate veterinary services because of following advantages:

- ITK/Traditional knowledge has been generated and acquired by resource users in a diachronic (long term) time scale through observations and practical experience and are compatible with the local situation and less dependent on use of external inputs.
- In general, farmers are more comfortable to receive healthcare from known, trusted people (ethno-vets or extension specialists) who speak the same

language and have better understanding of local conditions than those who are alien to their socio-cultural background.

- Most traditional practices are easy to adopt; whereas the modern technologies may or may not be compatible with the existing situation of the farmers and they may need external input and special skill for field application. For example, indigenous knowledge based technology such as applying turmeric and coconut or mustard oil for treatment of wounds can be easily adopted and applied by local people; rather than using antibiotic and antiseptic treatment. Thus acknowledgment of value of traditional knowledge empowers local herders/farmers to try to solve disease problems of their livestock in a cost-effective way.
- ITK/EVM may be a potential tool to create better understanding between vets and extension personnel and communities. It can ensure proper health and productivity of animals in the areas where modern veterinary services are not readily available.
- Validated ITK/EVM practices, seems to be the most realistic choice for financially poor stock raisers who can neither afford nor have access to expensive high-tech modern healthcare practices.
- ITK/EVM research and developments have practical applications for cost-effective ways to control several economically important health problems such as internal or external parasitism, whether related to epidemiology, diagnostics and therapy, or to comprehensive disease control methods leading to integrated pest/disease management.
- Low-cost ITK/EVM remedies may ensure freedom from pain and diseases concerning welfare of animals with low market value (sheep, goat and poultry). Regardless of economic status of the stock raisers, these animals are likely to suffer for want of treatment involving high cost modern drugs.
- Proper application and adoption of ITK/EVM treatment approaches can provide a plausible answer to side effects of conventional drugs. These can limit any unnecessary use of antibiotics and other chemical drugs to overcome residue problems and the growing resistance of micro-organisms.
- The traditional animal healthcare and husbandry practices are well integrated with local environment and needs. Therefore, EVM practices and technologies are generally cost-effective, environment-friendly and sustainable to a specific area. For example, traditional herd- grazing and pasture management involve practices that do not over-exploit the natural carrying capacity of the land. There are several examples when substitution of some traditional practices has resulted in serious ecological impacts.

- ITK/ EVM provide a highly intricate indigenous knowledge systems pertaining to animal husbandry that have been developed by several pastoral societies to 'shape' their animals according to their own specific breeding goals and animal utilization. For example, the indigenous strategies for safeguarding and developing their valuable genetic resources include a variety of social mechanisms such as stock-sharing arrangements to prevent inbreeding and favoring birth of upgraded offspring; careful selection of breeding males with long list of favorable traits; castration to ensure that only best male reproduces and study the genealogy of their animals.
- Traditional practices constitute a potential knowledge resource for novel ideas and hypotheses. For example, understanding of zoo- pharmacognosy can provide ideas for developing grazing practices to prevent disease and discovery of medicinal use of plants as well as discovery of novel drug molecules. It is reported that 25% of conventional drugs and 120 pharmaceutical substances are plant derived and 41% of the Pharmaceutical development has herbal origin.
- EVM practices may effectively prevent occurrences of diseases thereby avoiding financial loss in the form of treatment cost and production losses.
- Strengthening of ITK/EVM and recognition of the age-old status of healers (ethnovets) give rise to a new approach referred to as 'participatory epidemiology', which promises to improve epidemiological surveillance in remote areas while simultaneously encouraging community participation in disease control to exchange professional information and also document their composite knowledge and experience.
- ITK/EVM may be an effective resource for community development and to protect the right of ethno-vets and owners of traditional knowledge at community level.
- ITK/EVM bridges the gap between natural resources and their human management for the future, as it characteristically promotes traditional practices and facilitates conservation, protection and propagation of floral biodiversity.
- ITK/EVM supports emerging agri-business opportunities such as organic animal husbandry and herbal farming. It is expected that the current global herbal market valued at US$120 billion would raise to nearly US$7 trillion by 2050. India ranks the world's second largest exporter of herbs (8.13% share) after China (28%).

Approaches in preservation and protection of ITKs

If ITKs to be used in farming system along with frontier technologies developed by agricultural and veterinary scientists, it would be more practical and not only the farmers would adopt it quickly but also increase the beneficiary, practicability and acceptability of these grassroots technologies.

I. Process and methods of ITK analysis

A. Identification and collection of ITK: methods and techniques

- Documentation of oral histories
- Agro-ecosystem analysis
- Conducting documentation workshops
- Continuous interactions during on-farm experiments
- Survey method
- In-depth interview of farmers.

B. Documentation

Types of documentation

- Documenting large variety of practices without scientific validation
- Documenting prevalent practices and comparing them with traditional ones
- Documenting the practices/details of experimentation on a specific aspect and understanding the various linkages
- Documenting the practices evolved to mitigate specific problems of farming or for sheer survival under conditions of ecological and economic stress
- Documenting practices that had evolved in response to specific external interventions

Methods and Techniques

- Notes
- Photos
- Audio-recordings
- Video-recordings

C. Testing and Validation: method and techniques

- Prepare a list of all the collected ITK practices
- Decide the continuum for rating the rationality of ITK with specific weight ages
- Send the list of ITK practices to experts for their opinion and judgment on each practice.
- Calculate the weighed mean score of individual practices.

- Select practices above mean score as rational.
- Clinical trial for ethno veterinary related indigenous knowledge

II. Preservation of ITKs

Efforts should be made to preserve various plants which have economic importance in terms of preventive and curative properties. In many situations, lack of knowledge for processing herbs, lack of time to document and validate ITKs and knowledge of suitable development of suitable dosage forms hinder the wider use of ITKs for field applications.

III. Indigenous Traditional Knowledge and Digital Library

Library plays a very significant role in acquisition, organization and dissemination of knowledge in any subject. Libraries available in rural areas are the sources of such indigenous traditional knowledge and can act as a key agency in local community for collection, organization and preservation of local culture. It is essential to identify such rural libraries existing in the state and the sources of information available in those libraries. After identifying and collecting such information, the appropriate technology can be used for capturing that knowledge in variety of media such as audio, video, digitized and electronic database. All such knowledge available in libraries may be digitized in systematic classification, cataloguing and indexing so that effective retrieval can be made. Whenever required retro-conversion of those documents can be done for developing the digitized format. The traditional knowledge digital library developed with the objective to protect the ancient and traditional knowledge of the country helps in preventing exploitation such as bio-piracy and un-ethical patents.

IV. Recent efforts for conservation of indigenous technical knowledge

(a) Launch of Traditional Knowledge Digital Library (TKDL)

Documentation of traditional knowledge is also acknowledged as a means of giving due recognition to the traditional knowledge holders. This particular aspect of documenting formulations in the Ayurvedic system of medicine in India in the shape of Traditional Knowledge Digital Library (TKDL) is already on. The scope of the TKDL work relates to the transcription of 35,000 formulations used in Ayurvedic system of medicines. These details are being converted into Patent Application Format and will include description, method of preparation, claim and the usage of the bibliography. The retrieval will be based on the Traditional Knowledge Resource Classification (TKRC) and International Patent Classification (IPC).

The original Sanskrit text is translated and presented in French, German, English, Japanese, Spanish and Hindi through unit code technology that is language independent. The total number of pages in each language will be 1, 40,000. The local names of plants are converted into botanical names and Ayurvedic descriptions of diseases into modern medical terminology. The TKDL will eventually cover other indigenous system like Unani, Siddha, Naturopathy, folklore etc. The documentation of such traditional knowledge in a digitized format would, it is hoped prevent patenting of knowledge, which is already in the public domain. Work on such libraries is also being pursued in WIPO where a specialized Task Force including representatives from China, India, the USPTO, and the EPO are examining how such libraries can be integrated into the existing search tools used by patent offices.

In India, preparation of village- wise Community Biodiversity Registers (CBRs) for documenting all knowledge, innovations and practices has been undertaken in a few States.

(b) The role of Information and Communication Technologies in the disseminating of indigenous knowledge

Indigenous knowledge is a profound, detailed and shared beliefs and rules with regards to the physical resource, social norms, health, ecosystem and cultural livelihood of the people who interact with environment both in rural and urban settings. Information and communication technologies play major roles in improving the availability of indigenous knowledge systems and enhancing its blending with the modern scientific and technical knowledge.

ICTs can be used to:

- Capture, store and disseminate indigenous knowledge so that traditional knowledge is preserved for the future generation
- Promote cost-effective dissemination of indigenous knowledge
- Create easily accessible indigenous knowledge information systems
- Promote integration of indigenous knowledge into formal and non-formal training and education
- Provide a platform for advocating for improved benefit from indigenous knowledge systems of the poor

Organizations promoting ITK/ Ethno veterinary practices

A number of non-profit and non-governmental organizations (NGOs) are functioning across the globe for identifying preserving and disseminating indigenous knowledge including ethno veterinary medicine practices. Here, a select list of organizations and its web sites are given for use.

ANTHRA: ANTHRA is a registered Indian NGO, founded by women scientists 1992. It focuses primarily on issues of livestock development, in the wider context of sustainable natural resource use including ethno veterinary practices. The URL of ANTHRA is http://www.anthra.org

Assisi Acupuncture: This websites is operated by Ann-Si Li, a veterinarian who combines allopath with alternative veterinary medicine in her small-animal practice. The site gives information about veterinary acupuncture and traditional Chinese medicine. Information can be downloaded from www. assisiacupunctureltd.com

Livestock and Range land Knowledge base (LRKB): The (LRKB) is an electronic platform for learning and sharing the experience gained from investing in rural (livestock) development for poverty reduction. It provides appropriate interactive knowledge tools to policy makers, projects design and project management staff. Currently there are 38 livestock projects analyzed in detail in LRKB, including projects where animal health was a major component http://www.ifad.org/Irkm/index.htm.

League for Pastoral Peoples (LPP): The LPP is an advocacy and support NGO for pastoralists who depend on common-property resources. Together with its Indian partner organization Lokhit Pashu-Palak Sansthan, LPPruns a camel project in Rajasthan that integrates both Western and local methods of animal healthcare. LPP initiated the LIFE network www.pasroralpeoples.org

Life: It is a network that seeks to conserve domestic animal diversity by building on farmers' and pastoralists' indigenous knowledge and institutions within the context of local and regional development. Their site provides information on the network's aims and activities, www.lifeinitiative.net

Network: It is a British NGO and promotes participatory livestock development. Their site presents information, an electronic magazine and contract addresses relating to community-based animal healthcare. It also contains the proceeding of the international conference on ethno veterinary medicine held in Pune, India, in November 1997, www.Network.org.uk. Ethno veterinary is an area which requires detailed information about ethno-botany and plants.

Centre for International Ethno-medical Education and Research (CIEER)

The CIEEF is a non-profit educational and research organization developed to establish a focal point for the exchange of ethno-medicinal knowledge and to establish an international network of ethno-botanical researchers. The site features bibliographies, databases, publication, online courses, research projects, a web directory, and more pertaining to medicinal plants and it can be browsed at www.cieer.org

Guide to Economic Botany Links: This Guide is designed to answer some of the queries received at the Centre for Economic Botany, Royal Botanic Gardens in Kew, UK, about useful & poisonous plants and to acts as a resource for the wider ethno-botanical community, particularly students. Coverage of medicinal plants. To use the site, turn your browser to http:// www. Rbgkew .org. uk/ scihort /eblinks

Herb Walk: This is an online community where people talk about herbs. The site contains also a discussion forum on herbs for pets. Very useful site for those who interested in ethno veterinary medicine which is available at www. herbwalk.com

Medicinal Plants for Livestock: This site is established by the animal Science Department of Cornell University in the USA. If focuses on medicinal plants for livestock and discusses topics such as their safety and efficacy. It is available at www.ansci.cornell.edu/plants/medicinal

Validation of ITK: QuIK (Quantification of Indigenous Knowledge) method

Validation of ITKs can be done through QuIK (Quantification of Indigenous Knowledge) method by some identified persons who were experienced in particular ITK(s), using the method (QuIK) developed by Anne K de Villiers in 1996. The basic premise of this method is that farmers know and understand the environment in which they farm and that answers to many questions can be found in the collective experience of the farming community and doing informal experiments over years. It can be used to unpack the practices of successful farmers, so that information can be disseminated to a wider group of farmers. QuIK methodology represents a rapid and relatively cheap way to elicit indigenous technical knowledge.

Farmers who are experienced in the particular ITK can be taken for validation. In QuIK, matrix ranking is combined with an interview schedule to elicit numerical data from experienced farmers. The matrix can be designed through preliminary discussions with farmers and then obtained as part of a systematic process to obtain quantitative data. The experienced respondents will be asked to weigh the ITK(s) in comparison with modern veterinary drugs for its performance on different criteria and effectiveness (How many animals are cured?, cost effectiveness, quickness in healing, ease in preparation, side effects and availability). The respondents can be asked to put required numbers of pieces of stone out of 10 in each block of matrix. Unlike others, in case of side effects, the greater value of stones indicates fewer side effects. The same matrix will be used to interview a number of farmers and the data from each farmer will be treated as an independent result. Then the data can be put in the statistical analysis (a standard analysis of Variance, ANOVA).

Data collected from the respondents on several criteria will be subjected to one-way analysis of variance (Snedecor and Cochran 1989). Analysis can be carried out separately for each group of data under each criterion under a particular disease studied. To test the difference of means among alternatives, Duncan's Multiple Range Test as modified by Kramer (1957) can be followed. The linear model ANOVA can be used,

$$Y_{ij} = \mu + t_i + e_{ij}$$

Where, Y_{ij} = Observation of jth respondent to i^{th} alternative

μ = Overall mean

t_i = Effect of ith alternative

e_{ij} = Residual, distributed with mean "0" and variance "1"

Way forward

ITK/EVM may be a potential tool to create better understanding between vets and extension personnel and communities. It can ensure proper health and productivity of animals in the areas where modern veterinary services are not readily available.

Proper documentation, validation and transfer of tested technologies for field use

Use of any healing practice without scientific assessment may be harmful to the patients and may erode their confidence as well as of the professionals as well. Hence, proper documentation and validation of traditional knowledge are essential steps for appropriate blending of ITKs with modern technologies and to provide effective solutions to meet the global demand of cost-effective eco-friendly safer technologies for management of livestock health. These steps are crucial to revive confidence in EVM by establishing the scientific rationale of the traditional wisdom and knowledge in the present era of 'evidence based veterinary medicine'. Documentation and validation of ITKs are also important to address Intellectual Property Right (IPR) issues. Even the validated EVM practices remained confined to research publications, reports, books and conference proceedings. Further, the clinical evidences provided in support of EVM practices often lack in conducting controlled trials. Even the claims about therapeutic efficacies of herbs are mainly based on in vitro testing and supported by information derived from published literature without high quality controlled clinical investigations.

Conclusion

Indigenous knowledge is not yet fully utilized in the development process. Conventional approaches imply that development processes always require technology transfers from locations that are perceived as more advanced. Inaccessibility, cost and emergence of superbugs associated with use of conventional western animal health care system have encouraged constant use of cheap, safe, time tested and local resources based traditional rural wisdom. Furthermore it has raised immense contemporary relevance for treatment of both human and animal diseases. Though not as potent as modern allopathic medicine, it can be used to treat common and chronic diseases as well as initial stage of critical diseases, as an antibiotic alternative. Thereby, reduce the cost of treatment and avoid emergence of superbugs. Therefore, it is important to focus on the conservation of this rich ethno-veterinary wisdom which could serve as a source of future treatment remedies. Documentation of these practices and ethno-medicine used by tribal and rural people could be of great help to avoid fading memory.

Rediscovery of ITK as adaptive management of natural resources offers prospects for scientists to address the problems. Documentation of such ITK provides tools for networking, sorting, visualizing and analyzing information as well as projecting long term trends as that efficient solutions to complex problems are obtained. There is urgent need to mainstream traditional healers in the animal healthcare services by incorporating knowledge of modern veterinary sciences. Young traditional healers may be trained by local NGOs and Agricultural University. Validation of several traditional treatments can be done in collaboration with Universities and Research Institutions. The plant species used for animal health care by the traditional healers, suggest that many of the diseases can be treated using local resources, therefore, establishing the fact of eco-m system management. These practices enhance the use of local available inputs and support economic growth of rural people. Sharing of indigenous knowledge could be very useful to protect the environment from degradation, sustained production, promote landscape heterogeneity and generate employment opportunities.

It is high time to consider ITK as complementary to scientific knowledge especially in its capacity to provide non-commercial solutions to location specific problems. It is necessary to understand that the information from so called scientific research alone is not enough to solve most problems in livestock farming.

33

Climate Resilient Farming Adaptation & Mitigation Strategy for Livestock Farming

Bikash Kanti Biswas

Directorate of Research, Extension & Farms
West Bengal University of Animal and Fishery Sciences
68 K B Sarani, Kolkata-700 037, India

Milk, meat, eggs and their products have been the important part of the human diet in almost all countries of the world. These are highly nutritious and provide vital nutrients absent in typical starchy staples which dominate poor people's diets. On global scale, animal meat, egg and milk provide 80% of animal protein intake.

The livestock sector requires a significant amount of natural resources and is responsible for about 14.5% of total anthropogenic greenhouse gas emissions (7.1 Gigatonnes of carbon dioxide equivalents for the year 2005). Methane, mainly produced by enteric fermentation and manure storage, is a gas which has an effect on global warming 28 times higher than carbon dioxide. Nitrous oxide, arising from manure storage and the use of organic/inorganic fertilizers, is a molecule with a global warming potential 265 times higher than carbon dioxide. The carbon dioxide equivalent is a standard unit used to account for the global warming potential. Mitigation strategies aimed at reducing emissions of this sector are needed to limit the environmental burden from food production while ensuring a sufficient supply of food for a growing world population.

Man's relentless pursuit of material comfort and happiness has engendered an irreversible harm to the environment in the form of climate change. In India, agriculture and allied activities constitute the single largest component of Gross Domestic Product (GDP) contributing nearly 25% of the total. The tremendous importance of this sector to the Indian economy can be gauged by the fact that it provides employment to two-third of the total workforce. The possible effects of climate change on food production are not limited to crops and agricultural production. Climate change will have far-reaching consequences for animal husbandry also. Climate change, as some of the studies suggest, may alter the distribution and quality of India's natural resources, enhance water insecurity, reduce agriculture productivity, enhance exposure to extreme weather events, and pose even unforeseen health risks. This in turn is most likely to adversely affect development of the economy that is closely linked to the natural resource.

Livestock is a key asset for poor people, fulfilling multiple economic, social and risk management functions. The impact of climate change is expected to heighten the vulnerability of livestock systems and reinforce existing factors that are affecting livestock production systems, such as rapid population and economic growth, rising demand for food (including livestock) and products, conflict over scarce resources (land tenure, water, bio-fuels, etc). For rural communities, losing livestock assets could trigger a collapse into chronic poverty and have a lasting effect on livelihoods. The direct effects of climate change will include, for example, higher temperatures and changing rainfall patterns, which could translate into the increased spread of existing vector-borne diseases and parasites, accompanied by the emergence and circulation of new diseases. In some areas, climate change could also generate new transmission models. The consequences of gradual warming on a global scale and the associated physical changes will become increasingly evident, as will the impact of more frequent extreme weather events.

Livestock GHG emissions

The livestock production system contributes to global climate change directly through the production of GHG emissions, and indirectly through the destruction of biodiversity, the degradation of land, and water and air pollution. Livestock contributes 9 % of all GHG emissions measured in CO_2 equivalents. There are three main sources of GHG emissions in the livestock production system: the enteric fermentation of animals, manure (waste products) and production of feed and forage (field use). Indirect sources of GHGs from livestock systems are mainly attributable to changes in land use and deforestation to create pasture land. Mitigation of GHG emissions in the livestock sector can be achieved through various activities, including:

- Different animal feeding management.
- Manure management (collection, storage, spreading).
- Management of feed crop production.

Potential Impacts of Climate Change on Livestock

Factor	Impacts
Water	Water scarcity is increasing at an accelerated pace. Not only will this affect livestock drinking water sources, but it will also have a bearing on livestock feed production systems and pasture yield.
Feeds	**Land use and systems changes** As climate changes and becomes more variable, niches for different species alter. This may modify animal diets and compromise the ability of smallholders to manage feed deficits. **Changes in the primary productivity of crops, forage and pastureland** Effects will depend significantly on location, system and species. In C4 species, a rise in temperature to 30-35° C may increase the productivity of crops, fodder and pastures. In C3 plants, rising temperature has a similar effect, but increases in CO2 levels will have a positive impact on the productivity of these crops. For food-feed crops, harvest indexes will change, as will the availability of energy that can be metabolized for dry season feeding. In semi-arid rangelands where the growing season is likely to contract, productivity is expected to decrease. **Changes in species composition** As temperature and CO_2 levels change, optimal growth ranges for different species also change; species alter their competition dynamics, and the composition of mixed grasslands changes. For example, higher CO_2 levels will affect the proportion of browse species. They are expected to expand as a result of increased growth and competition between each other. Legume species will also benefit from CO_2 increases and in tropical grasslands the mix between legumes and grasses could be altered. **Quality of plant material** Rising temperatures increase lignification of plant tissues and thus reduce the digestibility and the rates of degradation of plant species. The resultant reduction in livestock production may have an effect on the food security and incomes of smallholders. Interactions between primary productivity and quality of grasslands will require modifications in the management of grazing systems to attain production objectives.
Livestock Health	Vector-borne diseases could be affected by: (i) the expansion of vector populations into cooler areas (in higher altitude areas: livestock tick-borne diseases) or into more temperate zones (such as bluetongue disease); and (ii) changes in rainfall pattern during wetter years, which could also lead to expanding vector populations and large-scale outbreaks of disease. Temperature and humidity variations could have a significant effect on helminth infections. Heat-related mortality and morbidity could increase.

Impact of Climate Change on Animal Resources of West Bengal

Livestock Productivity: The Temperature Humidity Index (THI) relates animal stress with temperature and humidity. Livestock are comfortable at

THI between 65 and 72, under mild stress when THI is between 72 and 78 and under severe stress when it is above 80. The livestock in West Bengal is already experiencing medium to high stress levels. Increase in temperature levels in the future may make the entire West Bengal region with THI > 80. The daily milk yield decreased around 2.2 kg/day when the THI values increased from 65 to 73. However, in the warning to critical range of THI of **70-72**, performance of dairy cattle is inhibited and cooling becomes desirable. At THI of 72-78, milk production is seriously affected.

Impact on production systems: There is normally a decrease in milk production for animals under heat stress. This decrease can be either transitory or longer term depending on the length and severity of heat stress. These decreases in milk production can range from 10 to >25%. It has been estimated that with a temperature rise of 1.0 or 1.2°C with minor change in precipitation during March – August, (Region 23- HADCM3 A2/B2 scenario) milk productivity is likely to be marginally affected and during other months productivity will remain relatively unaffected. The negative impact of temperature rise on total milk production for India has been estimated about 1.6 million tons in 2020 and more than 15 million tones in 2050. An average adult cow or buffalo producing 10-15 lit milk per day requires about 40- 45 lit/day as drinking water on hot days and about 40- 60 lit for other related work thus requiring a minimum of 100 lit/ day/ animal. An organized animal farm following standard management practices and disposal of animal wastes requires additional water about 50- 100 lit/day/animal. Any loss in water availability will certainly lead to decline in milk productivity.

Impact on animal growth and reproduction: Heat stress due to temperature or temperature-humidity impairs reproductive functions and efficiency of almost all livestock species. Various studies have shown that heat stress challenges the reproductive performance of cattle and buffaloes such as altered follicular development. Further, possible climatically associated shifts in animal breeding time and offspring born could occur in cattle and buffaloes under different agro-climatic conditions. Rising temperatures negatively impact growth and time to attain puberty of livestock species; it is likely to slow down from a growth rate of 500g/day or more to 300-400 g/day of growing cattle. Crossbreds are more sensitive to rise in THI than indigenous varieties. Analysis of the potential direct effects of climate change and global warming on Murrah buffaloes indicated that a temperature rise of more than 2°C over existing temperatures in 2050s will cause higher incidence of silent estrus, short estrus and decline in reproduction efficiency of buffaloes. Such impacts are also expected on indigenous cattle varieties in West Bengal.

Impact on physiological responses and functions: The sensitivity of livestock to increasing ambient temperatures under open ambient conditions and in climatic chamber have been evaluated by exposing Zebu, crossbred cattle and Murrah buffaloes to warm/hot ambient temperature (26-40 °C) and low/cool temperatures (6-16°C) at NDRI Karnal. Body heat storage increased beyond their capacity to tolerate heat particularly on days, when THI exceeded 80 during summer and hot-humid conditions. The study also revealed that Zebu animals under hot dry/hot humid conditions have better heat tolerance than crossbreds or buffaloes. The sensitivity of buffaloes to temperature rise above 35°C was observed to be higher than either Zebu or crossbreds. The physiological responses, such as respiratory frequency, heart rate and energy expenditure doubled or trebled for an increase of 1.0°C in temperature.

***Effect on feed and fodder availability*:** Water scarcity not only affects livestock drinking water resources, but also it has a direct bearing on livestock feed production systems and pasture yield. Rising temperatures also have an additional impact on the digestibility of plant matter. Raised temperatures increase the lignifications of plant tissues and thus reduce the digestibility and the rates of degradation of plant species. This not only affects the health of an animal but also results in the reduction in livestock production which in turn has an effect on food security and incomes of small livestock keepers. Studies have shown that dry matter intake decreases in animals subjected to high temperatures. This depression in dry matter intake can be either short term or long term depending on the length and duration of heat stress. In West Bengal there is already a severe shortage of feed and fodder. The fodder requirement is around 615 MT/year, as against this, availability is only 248 MT (40%). The area under permanent pastures and other grazing land is less than 0.1 per cent of the. Total reporting area under fodder land is only 1.08% in West Bengal. There is acute shortage of good quality fodder seeds in the State. The two main feed ingredients viz., maize and soybean are required to be imported from other states.

Animal diseases and livestock health: Climatic conditions favorable for the growth of causative organisms during most part of the year due to temperature rise will facilitate spread of diseases in other seasons and also increase area of spread. Higher temperatures and changing rainfall patterns can enhance the spread of existing vector borne diseases and macro parasites, accompanied by the emergence and circulation of new livestock diseases. Climate change will modify the dispersal, reproduction, maturation and survival rate of vector species and consequently alter viral and bacterial disease transmission. In some areas, climate change is likely to generate new transmission models. Temperature and humidity variations could also have a significant increase in helminth infections, protozoan diseases such as Trypanosomiasis and Babesiasis. Some of the viral diseases (PPR or RP like diseases) may also reappear affecting both small ruminant populations as well. Frequency and incidence of mastitis and foot diseases affecting crossbred cows and other high producing animals may increase due to increase in number of stressful days.

Adaptation Strategies for West Bengal in Livestock Sector

Strategy	Actions
1. Encourage breeding of small ruminants for livelihood security.	i. Assistance to small and marginal farmers to buy Bengal Goat, Garole Sheep, Ghungroo Pig/ Improved breed and Broiler chicken ii. Assist in establishing small farms iii. Undertake Male exchange programme of Black Bengal goat to arrest inbreeding depression iv. Undertake research to genetically upgrade Bengal goat, Garole sheep and Ghungroo pigs.
2.Strengthen disease investigation system	i. Develop disease forecasting systems ii. Establish disease surveillance system iii. Undertake research studies on a. the causes of diseases related to climate and b. the nature of emerging diseases due to emergence of new pests and vectors c. developing control measures by involving livestock research institutions.
3. Preventive health measures	i. Prepare long term strategies where by 100% population of the livestock get regularly vaccinated (large and small ruminants) ii. Set up Animal health camps to make people aware of adopting different control measures.
4. Improved cattle sheds for alleviating heat stress in livestock	i. Support farmers to augment their cattle sheds vis-a-vis Water sprinklers to enable them to have evaporative cooling and increase the air circulation in sheds so that cool air is retained, undertake evaporative cooling; ii. Create special community ponds to allow them to wallow in the ponds
5. Feed and fodder development	To combat fodder shortage fodder development needs to i. have an additional impetus from the government by promoting mixed crop system, growing fodder on waste land, agro forestry etc. ii. Supporting farmer cantered fodder banks. iii. Undertake mineral mapping in different regions to assess mineral status and accordingly supply specific mineral mixture to farmers for growing fodder.

6. Enteric fermentation	Decreasing methane emissions from ruminants is one pressing challenge facing the ruminant production sector. Strategies for reducing this source of emissions focus on improving the efficiency of rumen fermentation and increasing animal productivity. A large number of mitigation options have been proposed (e.g., diet manipulation, vaccines, chemical additives, animal genetic selection, etc.) with different efficiencies in reducing enteric methane.
7. Dairy development	For enhancing the milk productivity even with increase in temperatures, extensive Artificial Insemination of the indigenous stock of the State has to be undertaken. Popularization of local adopted and up-graded breeds can be done.
8. Capacity building of farmers for effective adaptation to climate change	Strengthen Extension to provide advisory on Adaptation practices vis a vis i. right shelter for animals to protect them for heat stress, ii. right grazing practices that would enable the animals to be protected from heat, iii. the practices for identifying disease and mitigating them iv. creating feed mixes with proper nutrients for enhancing mild productivity, etc.
9. Risk management	Coverage of agriculture insurance may be extended to animal husbandry as well, especially for small and marginal farmers. i. Feasibility of the same needs to be studied before it can be launched. Other forms of risk management for farmers can be explored. ii. Extend coverage to at least 5% of the small and marginal farmers.

Summary and Conclusions

Climate change will have significant impacts on livestock sector. There is still a great deal that is not well understood concerning the interactions of climate and increasing climate variability with other drivers of change in livestock. Livestock sector is substantial users of natural resources and globally they contribute to global warming, while at the same time they make contributions to the livelihoods of millions of poor people in rural households, almost all of whom are in developing countries. Hence, it is critical to differentiate between survival emissions vis-à-vis luxury emissions. Responses to these changes must center on boosting adaptive capacity and resilience both of communities and the ecosystems on which they depend.

For most livestock keepers in the developing world, the variability of the weather patterns they experience is projected to increase. Changing climate variability may have critical effects on food security; in addition to impacts on food availability, variability may strongly affect the stability of food supplies and vulnerable people's ability to access food at affordable prices. Key to both of these broad issues will be the further development and refinement of impact assessment frameworks that can evaluate potential and implemented adaptation and mitigation options at regional and local scales, their effects on livelihoods, and the trade-offs that arise between income, food security and environmental objectives.

34

Entrepreneurship Development Training for Sustainable Livelihood Generation in Rural Areas

Amitava Biswas

Department of Agricultural Extension
Bidhan Chandra Krishi Vishwavidayalaya, Mohanpur, Nadia, West Bengal

Miles to go for uplifting the entire population above the poverty line. But the picture was different in ancient times. As life style was simple, all amenities required in daily life were available within the villages. In need social system used to spread its helping hand towards the distressed. But the stability of the system becomes disturbed by invasion of foreigners and exploitation of foreign rulers.

In the British period series of famines from 1875 to 1901, numbering 18 out of a total 33during the whole 19th Century , the Government was compelled to appoint some Commissions and imposed some acts and established Development Departments like Agriculture, Animal Husbandry and Veterinary irrigation etc. The journey for rural development stated from here by Government.

After 75 years of independence till now there is need for helping rural people for earning their daily bread. Though numbers of developmental programmes were launched in this period till there is gap between what is now and what ought to be.

In this circumstances entrepreneurship development training programmes may play crucial role in sustainable livelihood generation by building capacity of being rural entrepreneurs and at the same time by using newly trained trainees as change agent. It can strengthen the already existing extension system .

A myth that 'entrepreneurs are born and not made' But through experiences researchers comes to the conclusion that development of entrepreneurship is possible through planned endeavor. It is possible through required training for trainees as well as for the development of the entrepreneurial environment.

Entrepreneurship drives innovation and technical change, and therefore generates economic growth (Schumpeter, 1934). So, energetic, enthusiastic rural youth can be selected for Entrepreneurship Development Training Programme. Trainees can be selects among rural youth It is possible to develop his/her required skill by Entrepreneurship Development Training.

All farmers will not be the entrepreneur. If some representatives of them or other rural youth become motivated to be an entrepreneur, It will create an immense impact in the economy of the village because entrepreneurs will act as change agent at that area and can guide the farmers in crop planning and production practices and can arrange assured market facilities.

Generally farmers produce for home consumption and sell the surplus product to the market. If entrepreneur can be developed within the village the entrepreneur can collect the produce as raw material for his own product and sell it to the market. In this way he can l replace the middleman. Hence the farmers will be benefitted in two ways - by getting assured market and expected to be less exploited.

But most of the people try to avoid this venture of becoming an Entrepreneur due to fear of failure and risk. Because our formal education system do not teach to develop knowledge and skills required in running an enterprise. In formal education system qualities like creativity, risk taking perseverance and innovativeness which are some of the accepted entrepreneurial qualities are not encouraged. So in real field the 1st generation entrepreneur feels like 'fish out of water' in this unfamiliar situation. These dormant qualities are required to be aroused to an extent that people may start opting for entrepreneurial career.

In addition to that beginner entrepreneurs have to develop capability of suitable project formulation, writing project reports, providing plant machinery etc. and access to available facilities and resources required in launching his enterprise. These qualities are to be developed through appropriate training intervention. Proper Training will play important roles in initiating and accelerating the process of entrepreneurship development. The training will help to change the attitude, desire and motivation of the individual in the desirable direction, his capability to perceive the environment changes and opportunities as well as his ability to solve problems will be enhanced.

So, stimulatory support and sustaining efforts has emerged as precondition for the success of Entrepreneurship Development Programme.

Ability for enterprise management is another quality of a successful entrepreneur.

The knowledge about various aspects of management such as production, marketing, financial management etc. are very much important for entrepreneurs. Knowledge and skills regarding business management can be developed through proper training.

So, the objectives of "The sound training programme for entrepreneurship development should be able to help selected entrepreneurs to strengthen their entrepreneurial quality / motivation, analyze environment related to small industry and small business, selected project/product; formulate projects, understand the process and procedure of setting up of small enterprise, Know and can influence the sources of help/ support needed for launching enterprise, acquire the basic management skills, knew the pros and cons of being an entrepreneur; and acquainting and appreciating social responsibility/ entrepreneurial disciplines."

On the other hand, continuous quality raw materials from farmer's field are essential to run the enterprise smoothly. So, to get quality production, farmers are also to be trained in modern agricultural production system continuously. An Entrepreneur can play a pivotal role in connecting different development departments with the farmers for training and demonstration on crop production technology, assured supply of quality seeds and other inputs available in time. Financial support, continuous supervision and Technical advice for nutrition and protection from pest and dieses for both plant and animal are inevitable for sustainable livelihood generation. Derelict water bodies may be used for air breathed fish culture for extra Income. Community based integrated farming system advisory along with entrepreneurship development efforts may lead to success for sustainable livelihood development.

35

Frontline Extension System Present Status and Future Prospects in Development of Rural India

Nilendu Jyoti Maitra

Deputy Director of Research, DREF, WBUAFS, Kolkata – 700 037
West Bengal, India

Introduction

In agriculture, Knowledge and decision-making capacity determine how production factors like soil water and capital are utilized in judicious manner. Agricultural Extension System remains in central position for formulating and disseminating knowledge including hands on training to the farmers. Realizing the scope and importance of integrated working of inter relationship between research, education and extension functions, the ICAR established a section of extension education at its head quarter in 1971 which was later on strengthen and renamed as Division of Agricultural Extension. Extension Education plays an important role in most of the Agricultural Development project. Moreover, Agricultural Extension is part of system of factors which influence farmer's decision. It includes agricultural researchers, political authorities, farmer's organization, non-govt. organizations, farmers training centre and media. These actors assume the functions of research, information dissemination, training and so on. The primary goal of agricultural extension is to assist farming families in adopting their production and marketing strategies to rapidly changing social, political and economic condition so that they can, in the long term, shape their lives according to their personal preferences and those of community.

Major Extension System in India

India has experienced with different models of extensions for reaching the farm operators of the country. The broad typology of the extension systems are mainly Field Extension System and Frontline Extension System. The Field Extension System largely concerned with large scale agricultural technology dissemination to huge number of farmers whereas Frontline Extension System focuses on adaptation and frontline demonstration of new technologies and capacity building of the relegated stake holders. Thus, broadly there are five different categories of Institutional Extension System operating in the country by different agencies. These are field extension system through the Department of Agriculture and co-operation (DAC) and the related ministry of the Rural Development through its networks of Agriculture and related departments at State, District and Village level whereas frontline extension system by KVKs, ICAR Institutes, SAU, Services by different commodities board, agri business house and input agencies and also by voluntary organization of the country.

Frontline Extension System

Some of the major initiatives taken up by the ICAR is presented below:

1. **National Demonstration on major food crops:** It was launched in 1964 and was a nationwide project with a uniform design and pattern. The basic purposes are to show the genetic production potentiality of new technology of major crops and also to encourage farmers to adopt and popularize the technologies.

2. **Operational Research Project (ORP):** It was initiated in 1974-75 and aimed at disseminating the proven technology in a subject matter or area among farmers on water shed basis. It covered the whole village or a cluster of Village with a view to rapid spread of improved technical knowhow. Here, the performances of new technologies are tested on farmer's field at operational level.

3. **Lab to land:** It was launched in the country on 01.06.1979 for transfer of viable technologies from laboratories to farmer's field. Under this programme 50,000 farming families comprising of small and marginal farmers and land less labours were adopted by the ICAR through its Research Institutes and SAU for their economic upliftment. The basic idea is to bring the scientists farmers into a common forum and to introduce appropriate technologies, facilitating the diversification of labour used and creating supplementary sources of income in the field of agriculture and allied sectors.

4. **Institutes village linkage programme (IVLP):** It was started by ICAR in 1995 with special emphasizes on generating appropriate technologies by refining and accessing innovations for farm production system like commercial, green revolution and complex, diverse and risk prone. It was implemented through ICAR Institutes, SAU, ZRSs and KVKs following basket approach in cluster of villages.

5. **Technology Assessment and Refinement (TAR):** In the year 1995, the ICAR launched this innovative programme with emphasis on technological interventions towards stability and sustainability along with productivity of small production system. Through this programme, the productivity and profitability taking environmental issues and marketable surplus in commercial on and off farm production system were considered.
6. **National Agricultural Technology Project (NATP):** It was launched by ICAR in 1998 with the support of World Bank to strengthen and complement the existing resources to augment the output of the National Agricultural Research System (NARS). The major role of this component was to accelerate the flow of technology from research and extension to farmers, to improve the dissemination of location specific and sustainability enhancing technologies and also to decentralization of decision making authority at district level. Set up of privatization and sustainable public extension systems were also emphasized through this system.
7. **Agricultural Technology Management Agency (ATMA):** It was launched to strengthen research-extension-farmer linkages and to provide an effective mechanism for co-ordination and management of activities of different agencies involved in technology adoption or validation and dissemination at the district level and below developing new partnership with the private institutions including NGOs.
8. **National Agricultural Innovation Project (NAIP):** It was started in 2006 and overall objective is to facilitate the accelerated and sustainable transformation of Indian Agriculture in support of poverty, alleviation and income generation through collaborative development and application of agricultural innovation by the public organization in partnership with farmers groups, private sectors and others stake holders.
9. **Horticultural Mission:** It was launched under the 10th five year plan where Govt. of India contributes 85% and 15% share is contributed by the State Govt. This is a centrally sponsored scheme to promote holistic growth of horticultural sector through area based approaches. Through this programme, creation of employment opportunities among the skilled, unskilled and specially unemployed youths was emphasized.
10. **KVK Model (Research Extension Linkage at Grass Root Level):** With a view to integrate the Research, Output in the existing farming situation, the ICAR came up with a noble idea of establishing KVKs in rural districts of the country in the phased manner for reducing the gap

between technology generation and application in the field level. The first KVK in the country established in 1974 at Erstwhile Pondicherry and mandate of the KVK in the initial year of establishment was confined only in training. The effectiveness of these extension initiatives lays with varieties of Host Organization, SAU, Educational Institution, NGOs and in some instances the state department of agriculture in their contiguous operational areas with the active participation of multidisciplinary research scientists. The immense policy reforms in the KVK mandates and its activities were brought about only after a thorough realization of the importance of micro-ecological/farming situation perspectives of technological suitability and their tailoring and adoption. With a decision of establishing KVKs in all the rural districts of the country in X five year plan, the revised mandate of KVK became technology assessment, refinement and demonstration of technology/products. At present there is a network of 725 KVKs in the country with major mandates (XII plan) of Technology Assessment and Demonstration for its Application (TADA) and Capacity Development (CD).

The activities of KVK include

- On farm testing to identify the location specificity of agricultural technologies under various farming systems.
- Frontline demonstration to establish production potential of technology at the farmers' fields.
- Training of farmers to update their knowledge and skills in modern agricultural technologies, and training of extension personnel to orient them in the frontier areas of technology development.
- To work as resource and knowledge centre of agricultural technology for supporting initiatives of public, private and voluntary sector for improving the agricultural economy of the district.
- Provide farm advisories using ICT and other media means on varied subjects of interest of farmers.

The KVKs thus serve as the district level institution working with problem solving approach by involving team of multi-disciplinary scientist in their contiguous villages. They slowly roll out their activities in to reach out all the blocks and large number of villages through its various programmes. The experiences gained and information generated by their activities is shared with the district line departments through appropriate convergence mechanism. By utilizing the tools of farmer participatory researches, KVKs identify and prioritize the most significant problems in crop production, horticulture, animal husbandry, soil sciences, extension education and home science. Based on it, the interventions in the form of OFTs, FLDs and capacity building programmes are decided and executed in closed partnership with the farmers, farm women, and rural youth. The information thus generated are passed on to the main extension system of the district and the research system working in that area.

Specialized Programmes-Recent Initiatives:

National Innovation on Climate Resilient Agriculture (NICRA): This flagship programme is initiated by the ICAR and executed through different KVKs at village level. The main objective is to develop and demonstrate different climate resilient technologies in the field level so as to sustain the production potentiality of different crops even in extreme climatic aberrations. More emphasizes were given on natural resource management activities, demonstration of stress tolerant varieties/strains, fodder production, housing of small animal and birds, rain water conservation and institutional arrangements etc. Through this programme, Village Climatic Risk Management Committee (VCRMC) is constituted at village level to look after the programme in long run. A small weather station including custom hiring centre at village level is established for obtaining weather based agro advisories and forecast to make the farmers aware well ahead also to adopt coping mechanism against any adverse weather.

New India Manthan-Sankalp Se Siddhi: The country level awareness program named as Sankalp Se Siddhi was organized during the current year and total of 565 KVKs across the country organized these events with the participation of 4.5 lakh farmers. The programme was attended by 74 Union Ministers, 286 Hon'ble MPs of Lakh Sabha and Rajya Sabha, 111 Ministers of various States, 350MLAs and 391 Chairmen of Zila Panchayat. Besides, 178 district magistrate and 2176 bank officials also participated in this programme. Out of 565 programmes, 315 programmes were directly covered by Doordarshan and the event was telecast by 825 other channels including private channels. The major thrust of Sankalp Se Siddhi was to create mass awareness about government of India's commitment for doubling farmer's income by the year 2022.

Pre-Kharif and Pre-Rabi Campaigns: As per guidelines of ICAR and Ministry of Agriculture and Farmers Welfare, Government of India, pre-kharif and pre-rabi campaigns were organized during 2015-16 and 2016-17 by 438 KVKs with the participation of about 2.68 lakh farmers across the country for better planning and farmers' participation ensuring timely dissemination of knowledge and information, flow of technological inputs and effective crop management strategy.

Pradhan Mantri FasalBima Yojana (PMFBY): The KVKs created awareness about Pradhan Mantri FasalBeema Yojana (PMFBY) across the country for protecting farmers from production risks that happens through crop loss/ damage due to unforeseen natural vagaries and to stabilize the income of farmers by the adopting innovative and modern agricultural practices. It was informed that under this scheme farmer need to pay a very low premium for insuring their crops which is 2% for Khari/crops, 1.5% rabi crops and 5% for commercial and horticultural crops. Since last five years, a total of 725 KVKs across the country are organizing this event with the participation of Union Ministers of respective State Governments; Members of Parliament; Members ofLegislative Assembly and many Government and Non-Government officials benefitting more than 10 lakh farmers and farm women.

Attracting Rural Youth in Agriculture (ARYA):The ARYA project aims at attracting and empowering youth in rural areas to take up agriculture and allied sector enterprises for sustainable income and employment. It also envisages enabling farm youth to establish network groups to take up resource and capital intensive activities like processing, value addition and marketing. The trained youth groups are functioning as role model for other youths and demonstrate the potentiality of the agri-based enterprise and also give training to other farmers. Under ARYA, more than 1000 different enterprise units related to mushroom production, processing and value addition of Non Timber Forest Produce (NTFP), processing and value addition of lac, backyard poultry management, vermi-compost production, bee keeping, piggery, large cardamom production, fisheries, off season vegetable production, Integrated farming system (IFS), production of vegetable and fruit nursery, herbal jaggery making unit, commercial goat farming etc. were established during the year benefitting more than 3000 rural youth in the selected districts. Skill training was given to rural youth through various training programmes pertaining to the enterprise units allotted to each ARYA centre. Exposure visits were arranged to rural youth to different enterprise units being managed successfully as training and confidence building measure.

Farmer's FIRST project: The Farmer FIRST (Farm, Innovations, Resources, Sciences and Technology) initiative has been launched by ICAR to move beyond production and productivity to privilege the smallholder agriculture; and complex, diverse and risk prone realities of majority of the farmers through enhancing farmers-scientists interface. In this approach, farmer will be in a centric role for research problem identification, prioritization, conduct of experiments and its management in farmer's field conditions. It emphasizes on resource management, climate resilient agriculture, production management including storage, marketing, supply chains, value chains, innovation systems, information systems, etc. During the year 2016-17, the 51 centers have made several interventions at the field level in crop, horticulture, livestock, NRM, enterprise and IFS modules. Under crop module, about 151 numbers of technologies were demonstrated in which 16597 of number of farm households were benefited. Likewise, under horticulture, livestock, NRM, enterprise and IFS modules, 113, 105, 45, 28, and 11 numbers of technologies were demonstrated and 13017, 11398, 4370, 1852 and 1057 number of farm households respectively were benefited.

Mera Gaon Mera Gaurav (MGMG): This is an innovative flagship programme of ICAR and is operational and being monitored by eight zones in the country. Total 126 institutions including ICAR institutes and SAU's are working under MGMG programme which is monitored by ATARI, of each zones. During 2016-17, total 1226 groups were formed by involving 4774 scientists under ICAR institutes and SAUs. Through training, demonstration, literature, general awareness and linkages developed with other departments/ organizations lakhs of farmers from different villages were benefitted under this programme.

Skill development training in agriculture: Agriculture Skill Council of India (ASCI) has affiliated Krishi Vigyan Kendras (KVKs) for conducting skill development training in different qualifications packs (QPs)/job roles of 200 hrs or more duration. Maximum number of trainings organized in the job role of Mushroom Grower Small Entrepreneur, Quality Seed Grower, Gardener, Dairy Farmer - Entrepreneur, small Poultry farmer and Beekeeper etc.

Conclusion

Technology tailoring, technology potential demonstration and skill building are the key supplementation by the frontline extension system for robust performance of the field level main extension system of the country. The technology specific and situation specific feedback to the research system as offered by the KVKs, facilitate the researchers in planning and designing their more need based and appropriate research agenda. Some of the future programmes like VATICA (Value Adding and Technology Incubator Centre in Agriculture), KSHAMTA (Knowledge System and Household Agricultural Management in Tribal Areas) and NARI (Nutritional Sensitization and Agricultural Resource and Innovation) will also improve the agricultural production system in a sustainable manner. The national level information dissemination cum monitoring system through mobile app for covering the entire villages of the country through KVKs and other extension organizations are very much helpful for reaching to the grass root level with basket of innovative, climate resilient, demand driven, market led and sustainable technologies. Besides, the frontline innovative national level programmes being implemented through KVKs, SAU and ICAR institutes etc. are yielding the impressive dividends in the interest of farmers and country's food basket. However, the strongest sense of ownership development, convergence among the Line Departments, co-ordination with educational institutions, farmers centric approach and strong policy framework are required for overall development of the farming communities and other stakeholders, in particular and the Nation, in general.

36

Health, Health Education and Health Extension Practitioners

Chanchal Debnath

Department of Veterinary Public Health
W.B. University of Animal and Fishery Sciences, West Bengal

Being a Health Extension Practitioner, one should have a clear idea regarding some fundamental aspects like the nature of health, health education, health promotion and some related concepts. This will help them to understand the social, psychological and physical components of health and enable them to be a better health educator by considering these basic ideas while planning and carrying out a health education session.

Definition & concepts of health

As a Health Extension Practitioner, one's main target will be to prevent health problems in a community rather than to treat them. Malaria, diarrheal diseases, tuberculosis, pneumonia, HIV/AIDS, substance abuse and many harmful traditional practices are among the different health problems we generally see within our community setting.

In the Oxford English Dictionary health is defined as: **'the state of being free from sickness, injury, disease, bodily conditions; something indicating good bodily condition'**. Now if we consider a person from within our community who is healthy, and someone else who is not, in view of the above definition, we will definitely see that this definition fails to address few individuals who might have some infirmities or some individuals who look apparently good but with some mental sufferings or individuals who never do any exercises. Therefore, it can be said that health is not as simple as it has been defined here.

The perception of health is extensive and the ways we define health also rest on individual idea, religious beliefs, social values, customs, and societal class. Generally, there are two different outlooks concerning people's own definitions of health and as a Health Extension Practitioner we should understand them well: ***a narrow outlook*** and ***a broader outlook***.

Narrow outlook of health

Here health is considered as the absence of disease or disability or biological dysfunction. In this perspective someone is called unhealthy or sick when there is evidence of a particular illness. Social, emotional and psychological factors are not considered here to define unhealthy conditions. This view is narrow and confines the definition of health only to the physical and physiological competences that are essential to perform routine works. According to this definition, someone is healthy if all of his cells, tissues, organs and systems are running well and as such there is no apparent dysfunction of the body. According to this model the human body is comparable to a computer or any mechanical device — when something is not perfect with them, we take them to experts who maintain them. Physicians, unlike behavioral counselors, often concentrate on treatment and clinical interventions with medicine rather than educational interventions to bring about behavior change.

Now if we take up an example of a hypothetical situation where about one month before a farmer Anil lost both of his milk producing cows due to flood. So, he is now mentally traumatized. He was always lean but now he looks very thin. He cannot sleep, eat and even doesn't show interest to talk to anyone. Whether the narrow outlook of health applies to Anil here? The answer will be no, because it does not consider many of the social and psychological causes of ill health. Anil's grief is not an illness but it is definitely affecting his health.

In our work as a Health Extension Practitioner, we should diagnose the overall social, psychological and physical factors which affect the health of a community and should think about effective interventions accordingly.

Broader outlook of health

The broader outlook of health is wider as well as all-inclusive. The most widely used broader definition of health is given by the World Health Organization (1948), which defines health as: 'A state of complete physical, mental, and social well-being, and not merely the absence of disease or infirmity.'

This classic definition is important, as it includes all the vital components of health. This concept of health can help us as a Health Extension Practitioner when we are planning and implementing any health education activities at community level. It also well explains the state of health of Anil in our hypothetical example and now we can say that Anil is mentally upset. He does not have 'mental and social well-being'.

Physical health

Physical health, which is one of the many components of the definition of health, can be defined as the absence of any disease or deformity of the body parts. Physical health could be defined as the ability to perform day to day works without any physical restriction. The following examples can help us to recognize individual who is physically unhealthy:

- An individual who has been injured due to a road accident.
- A farmer infected by brucellosis and unable to do his farming activities.
- An individual infected by bovine tuberculosis and unable to perform his or her tasks.

Psychological or mental health

Again, health is not restricted to the biological intactness and the physiological working of the human body. Psychological health is also an equally important aspect of health definition. If someone in a community showing such a behaviour which may indicate that he is going through a phase of mental agony in his life; or if we think about Anil again, we can easily understand that sometimes it can be really difficult to tell from the outside if a person is suffering from some mental health issues. They may show some warning signs that suggest a lack of self-awareness or personal identity, or an inability of rational and logical decision-making.

So how do we recognize a mentally healthy person? The mentally healthy adult shows behaviour that proves awareness of self, who has purpose to their life, a sense of self understanding, self-value and a willingness to perceive reality and cope with its problems. The mentally healthy adult is dynamic, hardworking and prolific, continues with tasks until they are finished, rationally thinks about factors affecting their own health, reacts flexibly in the face of pressure, obtains pleasure from a variety of sources, and accepts their own limitations truthfully. The healthy adult has a capacity to live with other people and understand other people's needs.

In general, mental health of an individual is measured by observing the growth and maturity in three areas:

I. Cognitive,

II. Emotional and

III. Social.

The **cognitive component of a person** determines the ability of thinking and work things out. It also measures the learning ability of an individual as well as the level of awareness and to perceive reality. At a higher cognitive level, an individual shows good memory and can reason anything rationally and solve problems. He is also able to exhibit creativity through his work and have a sense of imagination.

The **emotional component** of health is measured by an individual's capability and skill of stating emotions like gladness, anger or grief in an 'appropriate' way. To explain these aspects if we consider another hypothetical situation where a high school student, before writing his examination, was found to cry hysterically. This might be due to his failure to resist himself in the worried condition; or he might have a profound emotional health issue. But, to explore the reality we should not instantly say 'oh this boy is having exam phobia'. Collecting details about someone's life is very important before drawing any conclusion in this situation. If we knew this boy regularly passed through examinations and were a calm person, then it would provoke us to think differently and indicating something requiring investigation; or possibly family conditions are related here-maybe a beloved one has just passed away.

The **social component** of health is determined by a person's ability to make and preserve 'acceptable' and 'proper' relations and communicate with other persons within the community. This component also measures satisfying interpersonal dealings and fulfillment of a social role determined by the ability to maintain their own identity while sharing, cooperating, communicating and relishing the company of his fellows. This is really vital when a person is engaging himself in friendships or taking a full part in family and community life. Following are some events that could have a social component and help towards building people's social view of health.

- Mourning when a close relative passes away
- Going to watch a movie or participation in a community assembly
- Observing customary festivals within one's society
- Going to a shopping mall
- Establishing and maintaining friendship.

Health education

As a Health Extension Practitioner, health education is among the most important tasks. The purpose of health education is to educate each and every member in a community to develop appropriate and effective ideas about their own health and the health of their family and their community. If Health Extension Practitioners are able to percolate the right health education messages, the people in asociety will conceive properly about their health problems and of measures of preventing those problems for themselves and their community. Health education is indispensible in developing a positive mind in order to support behaviour change voluntarily.

A good number of different educational methods and strategies are used in health education to enable people to make the right choice for themselves in relation to their health. Health education messages needs to be eye-catching and suitable for the target audience and will shift the people individually or as a group to take their responsibility in preventing exposure to disease. Therefore promotion of healthy practices in a community is very important. For example, we may consider those people who as a result of receiving health education messages are now deworming their animals regularly, or vaccinating their animals against different infectious diseases so that they are able to protect their animals from diseases.

An individual's behaviour determines his health problems; again it can also be the main way out. By using health education as a tool, Health Extension Practitioner may take advantage to help people to understand their behaviour and how this behaviour affects their health. Proper health education will support them to make their own choices for leading a healthy life. But Health Extension Practitioners should not force them to change. Behaviour change should come by regular persuasion about the fates of unhealthy behaviour and its subsequent effects on the health of the individuals, families and communities.

Foundation for health education

To understand the basics of health education we can use the famous quotation from Dr Hiroshi Nakajiima who was the Director-General of the World Health Organization. He once said, 'We must recognise that most of the world's major health problems and premature death are preventable through changes in human behaviours and at low cost. We have the know-how and technology, but they have to be transformed into effective action at the community level.' If we critically go through this quotation definitely we will be able to think of some examples from our own experience like the treatment cost and possible disability due to malaria, and think of the reduction to exposure to malaria by insecticide treated mosquito nets.

The rationale for health education is as follows:

1. To concentrate on the spread of transmissible and non-transmissible diseases within the community by using health education principles
2. Promotion of health and prevention of disease are two important strategies to cut down the health problems in a cost-effective way as compared to the cost spent for therapy

3. Maximum health issues in developing countries are simply preventable through generation of awareness and community involvement
4. The cause of most of the health problems is human behaviour and thereby the way for their prevention should be targeted upon through influencing it.
5. Health education is a tool to help people with symptoms of disease to ask for treatment
6. Health education methods and principles are also useful for adolescent and young age group to keep away from detrimental practices and behaviours like substance abuse, teenage pregnancy etc.

In this way we need to prepare a list of important health issues that will outline the rationale for health education activities. After that as a health extension practitioner we need to decide the item that will be the most important for us in our role as a health worker in our community.

Health promotion

The definition given by World Health Organization in its Ottawa Charter said that "process of enabling people to increase control over and to improve their health." is called health promotion. The objective of health promotion is to reduce the fundamental causes of ill-health so that there is a continuing decrease in many diseases. As a Health Extension Practitioner we are regularly involved in many such health promotion activities like routine vaccination, execution of nutritional interventions, distribution of different health related aids at community level and destroying places favorable for the breeding of vectors like mosquitoes etc.

Some Important Aspects of Health Education

Judging the pulse of a community

As a Health Extension Practitioner, we should know what are the priority health problems as well as possible resources within a community so that we can carry out our health education planning in the most effective way. For that at the very outset our main target will be to diagnose the issues and work out ways to solve those health problems. Just like clinicians go for a proper diagnosis of an individual's illness before it can be properly treated, the Health Extension Practitioner should diagnose or understand the behavioural, cultural and social background of a community before it can be properly changed. If the grounds of the unhealthy behaviours are well revealed this will be crucial to be able to intervene with the most suitable and effective combination of education, reinforcement and motivation.

People's participation

Every effort of health education is directed with an attempt to turn people's behaviour towards healthy practices. Any effort to implement health education in a community by changing people's behaviours will be most effective if the Health Extension Practitioner is closely involved with the individuals, families, community groups as well as *public* administrators and other **stakeholders** at community level.

Participation assists people to recognize their own needs for change and endorses the ability to select for themselves methods and strategies that will enable them to take action. The involvement of all community members is crucial to increase support and to be able to use nearby accessible resources. Participation will help us to utilize nearby resources as well as build local partnerships and use community members as educators and experts within their particular cultures.

To explain the importance of participation we may take the help of a hypothetical example. Suppose that in one of the municipal wards a Health Extension Practitioner observed more dengue cases than it had occurred earlier. While visiting the area he had observed that there is one place favourable for mosquitoes to breed. He now wants to start a health education programme to convince the community to destroy the mosquito breeding site. To become successful, participation of community leaders and other members of the community will be crucial for his health education session to destroy the breeding site. So, in his planning he will have to consider how to involve these key people before deciding how to conduct the session.

Use of various methods and materials

In general, people's behavior is very complex. In order to bring about any positive changes to achieve good health practices the Health Extension Practitioner is required to have knowledge of different educational methods and a diversified media that he could use to conduct health education sessions. A combination of educational methods is essential to grasp the attention of any audiences and convey the messages to their best effect.

To explain the importance of using multiple methods and materials in health education we may take the help of another hypothetical example where Sandeep is a Health Extension Practitioner, who often goes to the local panchayet to conduct health education assemblies. Whenever he goes for any session, he uses to carry different materials like posters, leaflets, charts *etc.*

After each session, he asks the participants in a feedback form about how the session has gone and always he is satisfied with the response received. One day Sandeep went to panchayet to generate awareness on cleanliness, but on that day he missed to carry her educational aids with him. After finishing the session when he received the feedback from the participants it was not as good as earlier. This kind of feedback that he received may not have been as good as he expected because he didn't use diverse educational aids and the session may have been uninteresting for the participants as only one method of communication – talking was used. If he had his posters and other materials, he would have been able to attract the mind of the participants in a better way.

Planning and organization

Any unorganized and unplanned health education sessions may well be a wastage of effort and time as well. Proper planning and organization is a prerequisite to conduct effective health education and distinguish it from other incidental learning experiences. The Health Extension Practitioner should determine in advance by asking himself different questions in the form of *what, why, how, who* and *when* of each health education session. It is quite significant to make the health education planning participant centric by including other people and groups as far as possible. Health education, starting from planning, through the operation, quality control and evaluation stages should always consider the dynamic and complete involvement of the concerned audience.

It always produce better results when members from a target audience are also included during planning of a health education programme because it helps to get supports which is very essential for a successful health education session. If participants feel they are also connected then they are more likely to think about the programme, apply different strategies and stay committed to it.

It is desirable to have proper scientific knowledge related to the topic or issues to be addressed before providing health education. For example, the health educator must know the current scientific knowledge on how COVID-19 is transmitted and details of various preventive means. Scientific knowhow is ever changing and any health education session should be well prepared with the up-to-date information about the subject. To explain its importance, we may take help again of a hypothetical example where Sandeep is a Health Extension Practitioner. While conducting a health education session on human brucellosis he said to his audience 'I think brucellosis might be transmitted from accidental needle pricking during vaccinating animals'. This was an improper planning from the part of Sandeep. The Health Extension Practitioner should *know* that brucellosis is transmitted from accidental needle pricking during vaccinating animals and there are ways that can reduce the risk. Health education activities should not be planned randomly but prepared based on scientific facts and figures. During teaching, if Health Extension Practitioner use any terms like 'I *think'*, *'most probably'etc.*, it proves lack of confidence in the part of the educator. A better way of putting this should be more confident and assertive. It is *correct* to say 'brucellosis can be transmitted from accidental needle pricking during vaccinating animals.' When we know something to be the cause always we should express it as a fact.

Audience segmentation

Any health education programme should be designed in a way so that it becomes audience-specific and targeting a particular group of people whom the Health Extension Practitioner wishes to reach. Proper selection of audience for each specific session of health education activities is necessary. For example, if someone is targeting to create awareness on prevention of accidental transmission of brucellosis due to needle pricking during vaccination of animals then the specific audience should be as many as possible of the auxiliary veterinary staff. If the objective is to create awareness on the importance of colostrum feeding then target audience could be farm managers and farm keepers. This kind of **segmentation** of audience yields better result from any health education programme.

Need-base assessment

Before starting of any health education programme an assessment about the real needs of the community is important to identify their problems. There is little or no use making an effort conducting health education on problems that are not pertinent for a community. Say for example if someone wants to create awareness on rabies in a local high school; his health education session might be useless unless he identifies what it is that the participants wish to learn. Another fact is that there is no use to explain a lay man about all the latest study on a particular health issue when they may only be interested in knowing simple facts about what the problem is and its solutions. In fact, overloading the participants with facts and figures might lose their interest on the topic.

Health Education activities should also consider current cultural beliefs and norms and slowly build up talking points to avoid any direct clash of ideas. This will allow people to become understanding and lead to the appreciation and the ability to take on fresh ideas. In general, the Health Extension Practitioner should ideally try to understand the culture of the community and introduce novel ideas with a natural ease and caution. Using opposing statements that may be contrary to existing local beliefs, culture and practices of a community should be avoided.

Motivation

Motivation is usually expressed as a psychological course or a wish for doing or rejecting something. These are the happenings within the person and not something done to a person by others. It involves the internal dynamics of behaviours, not external stimuli such as incentives. To apply this in health education, someone can use any motive-arousing conversation, but not through any other external factors. Rather than 'telling' people the best action they should take, Health Extension Practitioner should help them to learn about their health and give confidence and encourage them to take steps to get better. For example, if we are going to conduct a health education session among the farm keepers from a block thinking about importance of colostrum feeding in new born calves. *Our response to motivate them should include the following:*

1. Asking them what they know about the goodness of colostrums (this will help them to draw on their own knowledge and will align with their lives and concerns)
2. Repeating main issues time and again (this will allow people time to get into the messages and also help them compare this to their own knowledge)
3. Encouraging the participants who are responding (this will give values to people's views which will ultimately twist their mind in positive direction and help in further motivation)
4. Showing examples of some farmers who are getting benefit by adopting this practice (if participants see some real examples before them they will easily understand what they also can do to help themselves).
5. Giving demonstrations of how colostrums feeding should be done (will help them to understand how to start and that can be motivating and make behavior change hassle free).

37

Intellectual Property Right (IPR) & Technology Management for Commercialization of Animal Husbandry

***Samit Nandi*[1] *and Sukanta Biswas*[2]**

[1]*Department of Veterinary Surgery & Radiology*
[2]*Department of VAHEE*
W.B. University of Animal & Fishery Science, Kolkata-700037
West Bengal, India

Introduction

In India, the concept of commercialization of technology from R&D is relatively new in most sectors; especially in agriculture & animal Husbandry. The Government of India has recently announced the "National Intellectual Property Rights (IPR) policy (GOI, 2016a). The policy advocates promotion of a holistic and conducive ecosystem for catalyzing the intellectual property for economic, socio-cultural development and protecting public interest. The policy document put forth seven objectives namely i) IPR awareness: outreach and promotion, ii) generation of IPRs, iii) legal and legislative framework, iv) administrative management, v) commercialization of IPR, vi) enforcement and adjudication and vii) human capital development. The policy aims at strengthening the national initiatives such as- Make in India, Skill India, Startup India, Smart Cities, Digital India (GOI, 2016). The flagship program of the Government like Startup India aims at building a strong ecosystem for nurturing innovations and Start-ups in the country (GOI, 2016). Under this, Atal Innovation Mission (AIM) is the action plan envisaged with the focus on promotion of entrepreneurship and innovation in sectors such as manufacturing, agriculture, health and education (GOI, 2016).

Current Statutory IP Laws in India vis-vis Agri-based Technologies in India

The WTO-TRIPS agreement of 1995 (WTO,2016), which is binding on all member countries including India, provided for minimum norms and standards in respect of protection of IPR in several categories: patents, copyrights, trademarks, plant varieties, geographical indications, industrial designs, layout designs of integrated circuits, and trade secrets. This agreement led India to put in place a set of appropriate and compliant mechanisms and instruments. Some of the legal instruments passed by the Indian Parliament as part of compliance process to the TRIPS include The Patents Act, 1970 (39 of 1970), The Patents (Amendment) Act, 1999 (17 of 1999), The Patents (Amendment) Act 2002 (38 of 2002), The Patents (Amendment) Act 2005 (15 of 2005), The Geographical Indications of Goods (Registration & Protection) Act, 1999 (Office of Controller General of Patents Designs and Trade Marks,2016) and The Protection of Plant Varieties and Farmers Rights Act, 2001 (PPV FR Act) (53 of 2001) (PPV&FR Authority. 2016.) Apart from these, the Government of India also enacted an umbrella legislation called the Biological Diversity Act, 2002 (No.18 of 2003). (NBA,2008) as part of the country's commitment to Convention of Biological Diversity (CBD). There is no specific IPR Act to provide protection for undisclosed information (trade secret). The Indian Contract Act of 1872 and common law have provisions covering this with the Ministry of Law and Justice as the nodal agency. The broad institutional mechanisms, legislative provisions and potential returns to the stakeholders of agri-value chain are also depicted. Considering special nature of use of bio resources and traditional knowledge (TK) in agriculture, the various provisions and legal mechanisms for protection of these are also enumerated.

IP and Technology Management in ICAR System

The IP&TM scheme launched by the ICAR during 2008 is a driver towards implementation of the policy (ICAR, 2014). Capacity building of the manpower engaged in the scheme formed the primary focus of the initial implementation process leading to series of awareness building and sensitization programmes. These initiatives resulted in emergence of a pool of about 100 trained IP professionals across the system. Notwithstanding initial apprehensions on IP protection towards stimulate investment in research in agriculture (Kumar and Sinha, 2015), these initial steps of ITMU scheme grants led to the building of vibrant IP ecosystem in the NARES. In terms of visible gains, the numbers of filings under various IP categories have increased significantly in last ten years (ICAR, 2014c). The recent recognition of ICAR as an organization through grant of the „Thomson Reuters India Innovation award 2015 is yet another testimony to this fact (Thomson Reuters 2016). Thus a viable governance mechanism (ICAR, 2014a) gives a conducive environment for and necessitates an understanding of regulatory and statutory laws in the country for better positioning of technologies and related products and services in markets. Only then can it lead to trigger better opportunities for business in this sector.

Recent reports of agri-start-ups successfully bringing new technologies in markets signify this fact. For example, the success of Barix, a start-up advocating eco-friendly, low cost crop protection methods to increase crop produce and quality at low cost. (Amit Tiwari, 2016) There are other successful start-ups like BIOSAT which uses Biochar based organic Soil Amendment Technology as an soil additive, Nashik-based start-up, MITRA (Machines, Information, Technology, Resources for Agriculture) which works on improving mechanization at horticulture farms with the use of R&D and high quality farm equipment like sprayers. These instances are early-stage successes of technologies in agriculture leading to commercialization and setting of agri-start-ups. In the current ecosystem, start-up trend in India is picking up in academic and R&D institutions, where researchers are looking beyond just publishing or licensing technologies to the industry. This is also relevant for technologies applicable in agri and food sector.

IPR management incorporation into work systems is now regarded as highly productive and a necessity

Characteristics of patent: *An invention must have the following characteristics in order to be patent protected:*

- New invention-The invention must never have been made before, carried out or used before or made public before the date it is filed. It should be novel.
- Non-obvious and inventive- Sufficient advance in relation to the state of art before it can be considered worth patenting. It should involve an inventive step and when compared with what is
- Already known, it should not be obvious to someone with a good knowledge and exposure on the subject.
- Industrially applicable-It needs to be of use in some way. An invention should be applicable or used in some of kind of industry. This means that the invention must take a practical form of an apparatus or device or product such as new substance or method of operation.

Who can apply?

Application for patents can be made by any person claiming to be the true and first inventor of the invention or by his assignee or legal representative. An application for patent can be made by any of these persons either alone or jointly with any other person. Two or more companies as assignees may also make an application jointly.

Patent Law in India

Introduction of Patent Law in India took place in 1856 whereby certain exclusive privileges to the inventors of new inventions were granted for a period of 14 years. However, the formal Patent protection in India was introduced by way of Patent Act, 1911. Thereafter, various acts appeared on the patent law pattern. Presently, the provisions with respect to patents in India are governed by The Patents Act, 1970 and the subsequent amendments to it in a phased manner in 1999, 2002 and 2005.

What is patentable?

Patents are granted in respect of any invention in goods. An invention means any new and useful art, process, method or manner of manufacture, machine, apparatus or other article, or substance produced by manufacture, and also includes any new and useful improvement in any of them.

What is not patentable?

The patent Act, 1970 and amendment 2002 and 2005 specifies some areas that are not patentable, as under Section 3:

An invention which is frivolous or which claims anything obviously contrary to well established natural laws.

- An invention the primary or intended use or commercial exploitation of which could be contrary to public order or morality or which causes serious prejudice to human, animal or plant life or health or to the environment.
- The mere discovery of a scientific principle or the formulation of an abstract theory or discovery of any living thing or non-living substance occurring in nature.
- The mere discovery of new form of a known substance which does not result in the enhancement of known efficacy of that substance or mere discovery of any new property or new use e for a known substance or of the mere use of a known process, machine or apparatus unless such known process results in a new product or employs at least one new reactant.
- A substance obtained by a mere admixture resulting only in the aggregation of the properties of the components thereof or a process of producing such substance.
- The mere arrangement or re-arrangement or duplication of known device each functioning independently of one another in a known way.
- A method of agriculture and horticulture.

- Any process for the medicinal, surgical, curative, prophylactic, diagnostic, therapeutic or other treatment of human beings or process for a similar treatment of animals to render them free of disease or to increase their economic value or that of their products.
- Plants and animals in whole or any part thereof other than microorganisms but including seeds, varieties and species and essentially biological process for production of propagation of plants and animals; (The exclusions states “other than microorganisms” suggesting that microorganisms in principle have not been excluded from patentability).
- A mathematical or business method or a computer programme per se or algorithms; (This clarification relating to software is important as it suggests that if software satisfies conditions of patentable inventions and are linked to applications, etc., their grant should not be rejected).
- A literary, dramatic, musical or artistic work or any other aesthetic creation whatsoever including cinematographic works and televisions productions.
- A mere scheme or rule or method of performing mental act or method of playing game.
- A presentation of information and Topography of integrated circuits.
- An invention which, in effect, is traditional knowledge or which is an aggregation or duplication of known properties of traditionally known component or components.

Other provisions after amendments:

- To make the understanding of the term clearer, invention has been redefined as “a new product or process involving an inventive step and capable of industrial application.
- Recognition to an international patent application has been provided for. The international application is defined as an application for patent made in accordance with the Patent Cooperation Treaty (PCT).
- Any process for the treatment of plants to render them free of disease or to increase their economic value or that of their products is now patentable.
- The time for restoration of patent has been increased from 12 months to 18 months and as such an application for restoration of a patent ceased on or after 20th May 2003 can be filed within 18 months from the date of cessation.
- No person, without the permission of the Controller, can make an application outside India for grant of a patent for an invention relevant for defense purposes or related atomic energy. The current provision has been added for the safety purposes of the country.

- Patent application and other documents (except PCT international application) are now required to be filed only in duplicate. Documents can now be filed, one copy in electronic form with one hard copy (paper form).

Requirement for biological materials (in Section 10 of the IPA, 1970)

- The specification shall be accompanied by an abstract to provide technical information on the invention.
- If the applicant mentions a biological material in the specification which may not be described in such a way as to satisfy clauses requiring the disclosure with the best method of performing the invention such that any one trained in the art can reproduce the invention, and if such material is not available to the public.
- The deposit of the material shall be made not later than the date of the patent application in India.
- All the available characteristics of the material required for it to be correctly identified or indicated are included in the specification including the name, address of the depository institution and the date and number of the deposit of the material at the institution (as per the Budapest Treaty of which India is a signatory).
- Access to the material is available in the depository institution only after the date of the application for patent in India or if a priority is claimed after the date of the priority, and,
- Disclose source and geographical origin of the biological material in the specification, when used in an invention.

Definition of "chemical process"

- Section 5 subsection (a) and (b) of the non-amended Patents Act 1970 does not allow grant of product patents for foods, drugs, medicines or even to substances prepared or produced by chemical process including alloys, optical glass, semiconductors and inter-metallic compounds. Only process patents were allowed in these areas
- The text of the second amendment clarifies that for the purposes of Section 5 of the Act, "chemical process" includes biochemical, biotechnological and microbiological process

Other patentable subject matter, as per new amendment in 2005

- Since the Act does explicitly specify that any method relating to the treatment of plants is patentable it can be interpreted that the Act allows an invention to be patented that is merely a method of making plants free of disease. Also, a process for improving the plant's value or increasing the value of the plant's products is patentable.

- The living entity of artificial origin such as microorganism, vaccines are considered patentable.
- The biological material such as recombinant DNA, plasmids and processes of manufacturing thereof are patentable provided they are produced by substantive human intervention.
- The processes relating to microorganisms or producing chemical substances using such microorganisms are patentable.
- Patents are available for "processes or methods of production of tangible and nonliving substances" like enzymes, hormones, and vaccines
- Processes using bioconversion, microorganisms, biologically active substances, biotechnology, microbiology, and/or chemical substances produced by using genetically engineered organisms are patentable.
- Clones and new variety of plants are not patentable. But process / method of preparing genetically modified organisms are patentable subject matter.

The Trade Marks Act, 1999

In India the Trade Marks Act, 1999 (47 of 1999) was passed on 30thDecember 1999 and came into enforcement since 15 September 2003; before commencement of this Act, Trade & Merchandise Marks Act governed the protection of trademark in India, 1958, which is now repealed. The Act is in complete coherence with the provisions of Agreement on Trade Related Aspects in Intellectual Property Rights (TRIPs) of the WTO. In comparison to the earlier Act, the new Act covers the additional features as given below:

- It has enlarged the definition of trademark. It now includes shape of goods, packaging and combination of colours that can be adopted as a trademark.
- The Act provides for registration of trademark for services in addition to goods
- It provides for a single Register of Trademarks with simplified procedures for registration.
- The Act has simplified the procedure for registration of registered user (licensing of registered trademark).
- Provides for registration of collective marks owned by association of persons.
- Provides for establishment of an Intellectual Property Appellate Board for speedy disposal of appeal from Registrar orders and decision.
- Transferred the final authority for registration of certification of trademarks to the Registrar.

- Provides for enhanced punishment for the offences relating to trade marks on par with the Copyright Act, 1957 to prevent the sale of spurious goods.
- Prohibits use of someone else's trademarks as part of corporate names or name of business concern.
- Provides for filing of a single application for goods or services falling in more than one class (multi-class filing).
- Increased the period of registration and renewal from 7yrs to10yrs.
- Has made some trademark offences cognizable.
- Act has amplified the powers of the court to grant ex parte injunction in certain cases.
- There are other related amendments to simplify and streamline the administration of the trade marks law and procedures in the country.

What is the meaning of service and which aspects in Agri-Animal Husbandry are covered?

"Service" means service of any description which is made available to potential users and includes the provision of services in connection with business of any industrial or commercial matters such as banking, communication, education, financing, insurance, chit funds, real estate, transport, storage, material treatment, processing, supply of electrical or other energy, boarding, lodging, entertainment, amusement, construction, repair, conveying of news or information and advertising.

What is a Mark?

"Mark" includes a device, brand, heading, label, ticket, name, signature, word, letter, numeral, shape of goods, packaging or combination of colours or any combination thereof.

What is a trademark?

"Trademark" means a mark capable of being represented graphically and which is capable of distinguishing the goods or services of one person from those of others and may include shape of goods, their packaging and combination of colours; and a registered trademark or a mark used in relation to goods or services for the purpose of indicating or so as to indicate a connection in the course of trade between the goods or services, as the case may be, and some person having the right as proprietor to use the mark.

What is an associated trademark?

"Associated trademarks," means trademarks deemed to be or required to be, registered as associated trademarks under this Act. Where a trademark which is registered, or is the subject of an application for registration, in respect of any goods or services is identical with another trademark which is registered, or is the subject of an application of an application for registration, in the name of the same proprietor in respect of the same goods or description of goods or same services or description of services or so nearly resembles it as to be likely to deceive or cause confusion if used by a person other than the proprietor, the Registrar may, at any time, require that the trade marks shall be entered on the register as Associated trademarks.

What is a certification trademark?

"Certificate trademark" means a mark capable of distinguishing the goods or services in connection with which it is used in the course of trade which are certified by the proprietor of the mark in respect of origin, material, mode of manufacture of goods or performance of services quality, accuracy or other characteristics from goods or services not so certified and registrable as such under Chapter IX in respect of those goods or services in the name, as proprietor of the certification trademark, of that person. A mark shall not be registrable as a certification trademark in the name of a person who carries on a trade in goods of the kind certified or a trade of the provision of services of the kind certified.

What is a collective mark?

"Collective mark" means a trade mark distinguishing the goods or services of members of an association of persons (not being a partnership within the meaning of the Indian Partnership Act, 1932), which is the proprietor of the mark from those of others. In relation to a collective mark the reference in clause (zb) of sub-section (1) of section 2 to distinguishing the goods or services of one person from those of others shall be construed as a reference to distinguishing the goods or services of members of an association of persons, which is the proprietor of the mark from those of others.

What is a well-known trademark?

"Well known trademark", in relation to any goods or services, means an mark which has become so to the substantial segment of the public which uses such goods or receives such services that the use of such mark in relation to other goods or services would be likely to be taken as indicating a connection in the course of trade or rendering of services between those goods or services and a person using the mark in relation to the first mentioned goods or services.

Domain names and trademarks

The domain name system is essentially a global addressing system. It is the way that domain names are located and translated into Internet Protocol (IP) addresses, and vice versa. Domain names are the human friendly forms of Internet addresses, and are commonly used to find web sites, form the basis of other methods or applications on the Internet, such as file transfer (ftp) or email addresses. The domain names ending with .int are exclusively reserved for international organizations, and ending with .gov are exclusive to the government of USA. There are various levels of domain names such as- 1. gTLD is a generic top-level domain. It is the top-level domain of an Internet address, for example: .com, .net and. org. In addition were also selected by ICANN (the Internet Corporation for Assigned Names and Numbers) on November 16, 2000. These are: .aero (for the entire aviation community); .biz (for business purposes); .coop (for cooperatives); .info (unrestricted); .museum (for museums); .name (for personal names); .pro (for professionals); 2. ccTLD is a country code top-level domain, for example: .in for India. These ccTLDs are administered independently by nationally designated registration authorities. There are currently 243 ccTLDs reflected in the database of the Internet Assigned Numbers Authority (IANA). Domain names are while designed to serve the function of enabling users to locate computers (and people) in an easy manner, domain names have acquired a further significance as business identifiers and, as such, have come into conflict with the system of business identifiers that existed before the arrival of the Internet and that are protected by intellectual property rights. Domain name disputes arise largely from the practice of cyber-squatting, which involves the pre-emptive registration of trademarks by third parties as domain names. Cyber squatters exploit the first-come, first-served nature of the domain name registration system to register names of trademarks, famous people or businesses with which they have no connection. Since registration of domain names is relatively simple, cyber squatters can register numerous examples of such names as domain names. As the holders of these registrations, cyber squatters often then put the domain names up for auction, or offer them for sale directly to the company or person involved, at prices far beyond the cost of registration. Alternatively, they can keep the registration and use the name of the person or business associated with that domain name to attract business for their own sites. The conflict between domain names and trademarks has been the matter of great concern to transnational companies such as 'walmart' as well as Indian companies such as TATA and Satyam, etc.

Administrative steps in registration process

Applications for registration of trademarks are received at the Head office and its branches according to territorial jurisdiction. Applications are then examined mainly with regard to the distinctiveness, possibility of deceptiveness and conflicting trademarks. The registrar on consideration of the application and any evidence of use or distinctiveness decides whether the application should be accepted for registration or not, and if accepted, publishes the same in the official gazette i.e. Trade Marks Journal (published in CD- Rom). Within a prescribed period any person can file an opposition, a copy of which is served to the applicants who is required to file a counterstatement within two months failing which the application shall be treated as abandoned. Thereafter, the opponent leads evidence in support of his case by way of affidavit followed by the applicant's evidence also by way of affidavit in support of the application. After that the opponent files evidence by way of rebuttal. On completion of evidence, the matter is set down for a hearing and the case is decided by a Hearing officer. The registrar's decision is appealable to the Intellectual Property Appellate Board. The flow chart as given by the registry is given below:

Classification of goods and services

34 goods classes and 8 service classes has been identified in the Act for the purpose of application and registration.

Tips for selecting a good trademark

The trademark registry provides following tips for selecting a good trademark;

- If it is a word it should be easy to speak, spell and remember.
- The best trademarks are invented words or coined words.
- Please avoid selection of a geographical name. No one can have monopoly right on it.
- Avoid adopting laudatory word or words that describe the quality of goods (such as best, perfect, super etc.)
- It is advisable to conduct a market survey to ascertain if same/similar mark is used in market.

Concluding Remarks

Summarized below are few points for R&D professionals and technology developers engaged Agri-Animal Husbandry research in NARES to consider:

i. Current legal framework India affords several opportunities for R&D outputs with applications in agricultural PCS to be protected. Multiple IPs and portfolio building is possible and may be harnessed for building business models for technology developers.

ii. Compliances with regulatory bodies on use of agro-biodiversity and related knowledge is mandatory. These should form part of SOP for due diligence during the entire process of technology development and its transfer.

iii. Capacity building for R&D professionals in IP & technology commercialization should be intensified

iv. Technology developers or seekers for plant protection technologies should be encouraged through enabling ecosystem and enter as start-ups. These should form part of curriculum at University level in line with National IP Policy.

v. Encouraging the use of IP informatics for research projects proposals and execution as part of due diligence processes for understanding technology push and market –pull forces before R&D investments are made. This would more useful for technology development in SME sector. Thus, the early successes in transferring technologies as businesses signal positive returns on R&D investments. This is further accelerated through the fillip given by current GOI policies on innovation, incubation including building vibrant ecosystem for triggering start up culture in agriculture sector. Researchers and technology generators in agricultural sector need to recognize these opportunities and re-orient their R&D efforts. Such efforts will not only bring innovation to combat crop losses but also bring a more vibrancy and better returns in agribusinesses engaged in this sector.

38

Non-Governmental Organizations and Rural Extension Activities Correlative Factors

Biswajit Pal

Department of Rural Studies
West Bengal State University, West Bengal

Any kind of developmental programme needs a proper integration of different parts of the society i.e. stakeholders of that programme. Apart from the nodal body, many implementing agencies take part in the implementation, monitoring of those programmes. Non-Government Organizations are one of those who actively participated in developmental activities not only as an implementing agency but also in mobilizing the resources, proper utilizing that and also effectively utilizing the resource towards development. Non-Government Organization is an organization that is independent in nature, politically, socially unbiased and has a proper legal stand with developmental orientation.

Whenever we are talking about the NGO, always we are assuming an organization that is dependent on other financial or nodal intuitions but the fact is the resource mobilizing parts of an NGO are partially neglected. If we are taken into account the pre-independence era, different community-based organizations were self-funded and widely participated in development on large scale. In India development of rural India is a huge task and related to multi-factorial development like socio-economic development, improvement of quality of life, empowerment and awareness of citizens. People participation in governance is also an important developmental work that has not always been considered as a major one. This task of development is enormous and complicated and the government program alone is not sufficient to fix the problem. The governmental limitations, resources, working structure, time-bound and complicated paperwork rather delay and compromise the exact task-oriented operations. After independence, different sector or holistic development programmes and policies were developed and implemented on Community development, poverty alleviation, food security, employment generation, skill development, infrastructural development and overall development of quality of life and gross national income. Apart from This Panchayati Raj institutions have also been initiated to strengthen the local government, democracy and people participation. In these developmental efforts of the government, NGOs plays a catalytic role to implement the programmes, reducing the regional imbalances, minimizing the geopolitical barriers and enhancing people's participation. In this massive developmental task of the government, many NGOs play a vital role as collaborative agencies.

Evaluation of Non-Government Organization

We have to admit the fact of voluntarism in India is an age-old practice. Before the formal voluntary actions, village communities were the main institutions to meets the needs of the poor. With the effective engagement of the Christian Missionaries and some educated Indians different social movement was initiated by the renowned Indian persons. Social reformers like Raja Ram Mohan Roy, lswara Chandra Vidyasagar, Rabindranath Tagore, Dayananda Saraswathy, Kesava Chandra Sen, Ram Krishna Paramhansa, Sayyed Ahmed Khan, and Swami Vivekananda had focused on the social action against social evils and malpractices like Sati, prohibition of widow remarriage, etc. The First Voluntary Association in India (Atmiya Sabha) was started in Calcutta (Kolkata) in 1815. The other prominent associations that originated during this period were: the Unitarian Committee (1822), Brahmo Samaj (1828), Dharma Samaj (1830), Widows Remarriage Association (1850) and so on. In the later part of the nineteenth century, several voluntary organizations were originated by active middle-class persons focused on socio-economic and political perspectives of the country. The establishment of the Friend-in-Need Society (1858), Prathana Samaj (1864), Satya Shodhan Samaj (1873), Arya Samaj (1875), National Council for Women in India (1875), Indian National Social Conference (1887), The Rama Krishna Mission (1898), further strengthened the voluntary movement in India. The enactment of the Society registration act was one of the milestones and boosted voluntarism in society. In a later stage, we experienced the active involvement of CBOs in the Freedom movement.

The term "non-governmental organization" was first coined in 1945, when the United Nations (UN) was created. After the independence of India, the role of NGOs was not only limited to social development issues but also, they have participated actively in different policy development. Numbers of NGOs emerged in independent India and a large section of them followed the Gandhian philosophy of development. The second phase of NGO development was started during the 1960 s when it was felt that only governmental programmes were not sufficient to fulfill the needs of rural areas. Many community level voluntary associations were formed to work with the grassroots people and empower them in different developmental activities. Different state policies on NGOs have also impacted the formation of NGOs in a different state as a result a large number of NGOs were formed during this era. their role significantly changes with the change in the policies of the government through different plans.

Characteristics of NGO

NGOs are quite different from other types of organizations in terms of their structure, mode of operation and formation procedure. An NGO is voluntary in nature means all the members of the NGOs are involved in the NGO without any presumed remuneration or not on a profit basis. The NGO itself is not for profit organization that has a standing point to work for their objectives without any profit-making intention. The members of the NGO need a dedicated mental setup and developmental orientation. Every Ngo should have a social value that should work towards the public good. The activities undertaken by the NGO should improve the quality of living as well as the environmental condition. All the NGOs are independent in nature and not controlled by any public or private authority. But all the NGOs should have legal status as registered and trustworthy organizations.

The legal status of NGO

(a) Registration of NGO

(i) **Public Trust Registration:** A trust is a non-governmental organization wherein a property owner transferred his/her property to the trustee. In the case of public trust, the main objective of transferring property is to provide benefits to societies. Here the registration can be done through The Indian Trust Act of 1882. Usually, the purpose of a trust is aimed at providing relief from poverty, promoting education, medical aid, etc.

Advantages of Trust Registration

- Trusts can apply to get land from the government
- It gets long term taxation benefit
- Lesser audit formalities
- Trusts are eligible to apply for 80G certificate benefits
- Administrative autonomy

(ii) Society Registration

The most common form of Ngo we found is the NGO registered as a society. A society is a group of individuals who get together to deliberate, govern, and act jointly for a common good. The societies are formed based on the presumed idea of development and social involvement like the betterment of sports, music, culture, religion, art, education, and so on.

The societies are registered under the provision of the Societies Registration Act, 1860.

Advantages of Trust Registration

- It has a separate legal entity.
- A wide range of activities can be performed.
- Income tax benefits and exemptions
- Freedom to accept funds and donations
- Ease in property acquisition
- Distribution of leadership can be possible and maintained by all the members. It cal also dissolve easily without much paperwork.

(iii) Section 8 Company Registration

The third way to register an NGO is through the sanctioning of Section 8 of the Companies Act of 2013. These types of companies are established to promote community development through economic ventures. However, the earnings of this company are not used by the shareholders; rather it is used by the company for the promotion of social work. All profits generated during the course of its functioning have to be applied for promoting the objectives of the organization i.e. no dividend can be paid to the members of the company. The Section 8 Company is registered under the Ministry of Corporate Affairs, Govt. of India.

Advantages of Section 8 Company Registration

- No minimum capital requirement for the establishment
- It has a separate legal entity
- It can also categorize for tax exemption benefit
- No stamp duty during registration
- Easy transfer of ownership
- When compared with any other NGO structure, a Section 8 company is more credible. Nation wise operation area as registered centrally.

Difference between Society, Trust and Section-8 Company

Registration Process	Non-profit Company	Society	Trust
Law and Act applied for registration	Company Act	Society Registration Act	Indian Trust Act
Registering authority	Registrar of Company	Registrar or Deputy Registrar of Societies of the concerned state	Sub-Registrar of Registrar of Registration
Issue Name approval	Name approval is required before registration	Name approval required in the particular jurisdiction	No required
Time takes to form	3-6 months	1-2 months	2 days to 1 week
Eligibility of family members to be a member of the organization	Anyone can be a director	No	No such restriction
Minimum members/ Directors /Trustees	Two directors	Seven members	At least two trustee
Minimum members at the National level required	Minimum two Directors	Minimum 8 members from 8 different states	Minimum two trustee
Governing structure	General body of Directors/ Board of Directors	General Body/ Executive Committee	General Body/ Board of Trustees/ Executive Committee
Area of Operation	Throughout the Nation	State for State-level registration and National level when registered as a national level society	Can operate throughout India
General Body meeting	At least one AGM and 4 Board meetings in a year	As prescribed in the bye-laws	Not mandatory, regular meeting of the trustees
Status for Rights of vote	Basis of shareholding capacity of Directors	Equal among the members	Equal among the Trustees
Transfer of Directorship/ Membership/ Trusteeship	Can transfer	Non-transferable	Non-transferable
Foreign funding	FCRA required	FCRA required	FCRA required
Can members get payment	Can approve to get payment	GB/EC can permit to get payment	Cannot receive funds but can receive professional fees

(b) Foreign contribution regulation Act (FCRA)

Foreign contribution regulation Act 1976 or FCRA is a law enforced by the Ministry of Home Affairs, Government of India which regulates receipt of foreign contributions or aid from outside India to Indian territories. This act has been enacted to ensure that any activities related to political and national disturbances are not performed with the use of this foreign fund. The genuinely of the funding source and the funding for is very important in this provision. Regular compliance is limited to the filing of annual returns every year.

(c) Section 80G of Income Tax:

Any NGO can register them under this section to provide their donor with an income tax exemption. By this exemption one can donate to NGO can avail income tax benefits of the donated amount. Any NGO can apply to the Income-tax department for this and by fulfilling the required condition NGO can avail of 3 years provisional 80 G certification. Within these 3 years, the NGO needs to apply for revalidation for another 5 years.

(d) 12A of Income Tax

Any NGO, a Section 8 corporation or charitable trust can apply for registration under Section 12 A if it wants to get an exemption from income tax. NGO will categorize under the normal tax range without 12A certification.

Benefits:

Income tax is exempted for NGOs

It can avail benefits by taking grants from any Government agencies further, it can avail benefits of the FCRA Registration.

World Bank's operational directives (1989) classification

- Relief and Welfare agencies: They are more active during any disaster or natural calamities like flood, earthquake, drought etc to provide food, shelter, clothing, medicines, water and other essential services. Example: Red Cross.
- Technical Innovation Organization: Operate their projects to pioneer new or improved approaches to problems. They are also acted as field testers. Example: Aga Khan Foundation etc.
- Public Service Contractors: They are working with the government to help proper implementation of governmental initiatives. Example: Care, PHFI etc.
- Popular Development Agencies: Non-profit organizations in developed countries fund their counterparts in developing countries and work on self-help, social development, grassroots democracy. Example: OXFAM etc.

- Grassroots Development Organization: Working with the grassroots level and people-centric development and following the participatory approach of development. Example: SEWA etc.
- Advocacy Groups and Networks: They exist for education and lobbying. Checking malfunction, corruption at the height levels of the government or assisting the government on policy development. Example: Greenpeace, The Union etc.

Participation of NGO in rural Extension services:

As social motivator: NGO acts as a social motivator and act as a catalytic agent for any developmental program. The thought penetration techniques used by them has a huge impact on the proper implementation of successive developmental programs.

As field tester: A new technology, practices, knowledge needs to be tested in their real field of operations. Ngo plays a vital role in respect of test this 'New' as they have wide access to the rural society.

Rural empowerment: Empowerment of the society means empowerment of women, political empowerment, and cultural empowerment is an important factor for rural development and proper implementation of extension services. The 'needs' of people are identified in an empowered society. Here the activities of NGOs in different fields of operations ultimately work for empowerment.

As communicator: The NGO personnel can act as a communicator- a bridge between the implementing agency and the grassroots people to the utilization of all factors of communication and effectively widen the way further extension activities.

As a public service agent: Ngo as a public service agent works for the public organization. The Go-NGO collaboration is effectively utilized to promote and implemented different developmental programs.

As fund mobilize: It is one of the unique features of the NGO that they are mobilizing funds for the developmental services from all sources like government, private organization Big corporate houses as CSR fund, international development funds and the fund from donor NGOs. These funds are largely allotted for rural development issues and can effectively minimize the financial constraint for developmental programmes.

It is a fact that 132634 registered NGOs are enrolled themselves under the NITI Aayog monitored NGO Darpan portal for the effective and transparent operational management of the NGO nationwide. But it is also a fact that all the NGOs are operated and registered are not equally trustworthy, not financially sound. There are so many managerial lacunas. Local-level organizations have so many financial gaps compare to others, less involved in networks, less proper planning and strategies and lack of effective professionals. These imbalances within the NGOs lead to the non-operation status of some organizations. NGOs are the social organization that originated, formulated and maintained by the common people and in a bigger sense, all of us directly or indirectly are part of these social institutions. The people-centric organization can work properly and sustainably by effective participation of the basic unit of the society i.e. our family.

39

Paradigm Shift in Livestock Extension Attracting and Retaining Livestock Farmers by Creating Successful Marketing Models

P. Mathialagan

Tamilnadu University of Veterinary and Animal Sciences, Chennia Tamil Nadu

N. Vimal Rajkumar and P.Thilakar

Department of Veterinary and Animal Husbandry Extension Education Madras Veterinary College, Chennai

Introduction

Agricultural and Animal husbandry extension continues to be in transition worldwide. Governments and international agencies are advancing structural, financial and managerial reforms to improve extension. Decentralization, pluralism, cost sharing, cost recovery, participation of stakeholders in development initiatives and the decisions and resources that affect them – these are some of the elements in extension's current transition.

Public sector extension was severely attacked in the 1980s for not being relevant, for insufficient impact, for not being adequately effective, for not being efficient and, sometimes, for not pursuing programmes that foster equity. In the context of meeting the holistic needs of increasing agricultural production in a sustainable manner in India, agricultural extension has a crucial role to play. Reforms in the system envisaged an extension service which is more broad-based and holistic in content and scope and beyond agricultural technology transfer.

Agricultural extension programmes are very diverse from an international perspective as most are managed as public sector agencies and some non-governmental organizations (NGOs while many private firms and private organizations conduct extension programmes. In a competitive production environment, occasioned by the globalization policy, extension services must be oriented to markets and overcome the exclusive focus on production that ignored market demand and profitability as was the constraint of many past extension programs. Varied extension services are needed to help farmers remain competitive and profitable, diversify production, produce for niche markets, and move to higher-value products and more value-added production. A broader rural livelihoods approach requires extension services to deliver information on local organization development, micro- enterprise and non-farm employment, environmental issues, rural infrastructure, social programs, rural health and education, and other non-agricultural issues.

Integrated approaches connecting the design and delivery of programs across disciplines and sectors are instrumental to address such challenges, *Agricultural extension and advisory services (AEAS) refers to any organization in the public or private sectors (e.g. NGOs, farmer organizations, private firms etc.) that facilitates farmers' and other rural actors' access to knowledge, information and technologies, and their interactions with other actors; and assists them to develop their own technical, organizational and management skills and practices, so as to improve their livelihoods and well-being.*

Over the past few decades the role of AEAS has changed substantially, shifting away from a production oriented, technology transfer model to a greater emphasis on broader development objectives such as improving rural livelihoods through a demand-led, participatory and market-oriented approach. It is in the context of this paradigm shift that a potential role for AEAS in promoting market oriented information to the farmers.

Paradigms of Agricultural Extension

Agricultural extension has four paradigms namely: Technology transfer; advisory work; human resource and development; and facilitation for empowerment. Based on My Agricultural Information Bank (2011), these paradigms differ on the way communication takes place and why it takes place.

Technology transfer

Technology transfer is characterized by persuasive and paternalistic approach in communicating with farmers. It requires persuasive or convincing power because, here, extension is designed to recommend practice and technology for the specific needs of farmers and move the farmers to adopt such practice and technology while, it is paternalistic in a sense that it uses top-down approach

Advisory work

Advisory work, on the other hand, uses persuasive but participatory approach. It needs persuasive capacity to encourage the farmers to adopt the predetermined packages of technology based on the stated needs of the farmers. Moreover, advisory will not take place unless farmers raise questions or consulted extension worker about particular problem, thus, it is participatory.

Human resource paradigm

It is an educational and paternalistic approach. This paradigm originated from the universities doing extension works for those who cannot afford to study in the universities, hence providing knowledge and skills through education. It also allows the students to make their own decisions based on the knowledge they acquired. However, this paradigm still uses top-down approach, thus is it still paternalistic in nature.

Facilitation for empowerment

It is also an educational and participatory in nature. It is educational because it provides new information, practice and skills on how to increase the production and environmental protection while it is participatory because it involves farmers-to-farmers communication and interactive process to educate farmers.

As animal husbandry extension progress and shifts from one paradigm to another, the role of farmers or stakeholders also increases. In technology transfer, development is achieved by transferring modern research results to the traditional farmer. Farmers are treated as just mere recipients of programmed technology. In advisory works, on the other hand, farmers' capacity to identify their problems and to inquire for solutions to such problems is acknowledged. However, solutions provided by the extension worker are based on pre-determined packages. Hence, farmers still have no other choice but to adopt the prescribed solutions by the extension worker. While in human resource development, extension worker decides on the knowledge, skills and technology to be taught on the farmers but farmers are being equipped to be able to "know what to ask for… evaluate the appropriateness of technical information" and to be "responsible decision makers

Then, in facilitation for empowerment, extension worker is "no longer seen as the expert who has all the useful information and technical solutions." Here, farmers' knowledge, skills and creativity are acknowledged as major resources. Searching for solutions to problems is a collaborative work between extension worker and farmers.

Market-led Extension approach in Livestock sector

Market-led extension is an extension system operated on the Philosophy and principles of marketing to cater to the needs of clients. Strong network of marketing extension is very much necessary at all levels to effectively advise farmers on various aspects of marketing, advise on product, planning, marketing information, securing market for farmers, advise on informed market practices and advise on post harvest management practices.

Market-led extension as defined by Thomson means to extend the knowledge of marketing, and solution to the problems to those who are in a position to apply this knowledge in impressing marketing. Extension education involves the transfer of production technologies from lab to land, the market-led extension involves the transfer of marketing technologies to the shareholders or shareholder namely primary producers (farmers), the intermediaries and the ultimate consumers.

The objective of market-led extension is to appraise the producers, traders and consumers of various voluntary and regulating measures brought into force for the improvement of marketing system, so that they can all derive the benefits of marketing. The market-led extension is to educate the primary agricultural producers viz., the farmers, on what to produce? How much to produce? When to produce? And where to market? so as to make them realize remunerative prices with the involvement of least marketing costs. The marketing extension education must also do help the traders/intermediaries in what to buy? When to buy? From where to buy? How much to buy? And where to sell? So as to help them in buying, selling and handling the produce with least marketing cost and reasonable profit margin and to keep them going in their business.

Another target group of market-led extension is the ultimate consumers.The market-led extension again must help the ultimate consumers in buying right type of goods in right quantity and quality, in right place and time and in right price, with least costs involved, so as to derive the maximum satisfaction. The market-led extension education helps in improving the marketing efficiency, which is a single ration of output to input, by minimizing the marketing costs and maximizing the satisfaction at various stages of the vertically value adding agricultural marketing system.

A Proven Market Led Extension Model

Government of Tamil Nadu had announced the continuation of Scheme for Poultry Development (SPD)" in the non poultry backward regions of the State during the year 2013-14. Native chicken rearing was encouraged on a smaller scale wherein a flock size of about 250/500 birds can be profitably reared and marketed by the farmer himself. This scheme was focused on the production of commodity.

A study was conducted in this scheme in Tiruchirapllai district and from 17 blocks of Thiruchirapllai, Uppiliyapuram block was purposively based the fact the highest number of beneficiaries and success of the state sponsored Scheme for Poultry Development. All the scheme beneficiaries was chosen for capacity building programmes for recommended technologies in Desi bird rearing through various extension methods. From these scheme beneficiaries, one interested farmer was identified for establishment of hatchery unit, second farmer for slaughter unit. Further, five farmers was identified and trained for value added meat product preparations. Capacity building programmes and all the inputs needed to establish the respective units were distributed to the beneficiaries of the scheme. Follow –up activities and recording of the outcome of the scheme were carried out periodically by the research team.

Findings of the study

The economical, social and environmental benefits obtained by the beneficiaries in different components of the scheme in given below

I. Mini Slaughter Unit

i. Economical

Mr. C. Ramasamy, 47 years old tribal farmer with primary level of education from Kaanapaady Village of Uppiliyapuram Block in Thiruchirapalli district is one of the beneficiaries of this scheme. Basically he is an agriculturist and also rears four dairy cattle and two goats at his backyard. Previously he was one of the successful beneficiaries of State Poultry Development Scheme of Tamil Nadu. He owns poultry shed of 1000 birds capacity and through the scheme he reared and sold nearly 1000 birds in a span of two years. To market the adult birds, he owns a small meat retail outlet in his farm premises and sold 700 – 800 kg of meat / week for Rs. 200/ kg of dressed meat. Further, he also earned profit through selling of live birds. Under this scheme, Mr. C. Ramasamy attended a three days capacity building programme on "Poultry meat production and value addition" at Veterinary University Training and Research Centre (TANUVAS), Coimbatore. The training focused on hygienic slaughter of the bird, preparation of cut up parts, packaging etc. The training also imparted skills on preparation of value meat products.

Tamil Nadu Country Chicken Entrepreneurs Action Model (TNCC EAM)

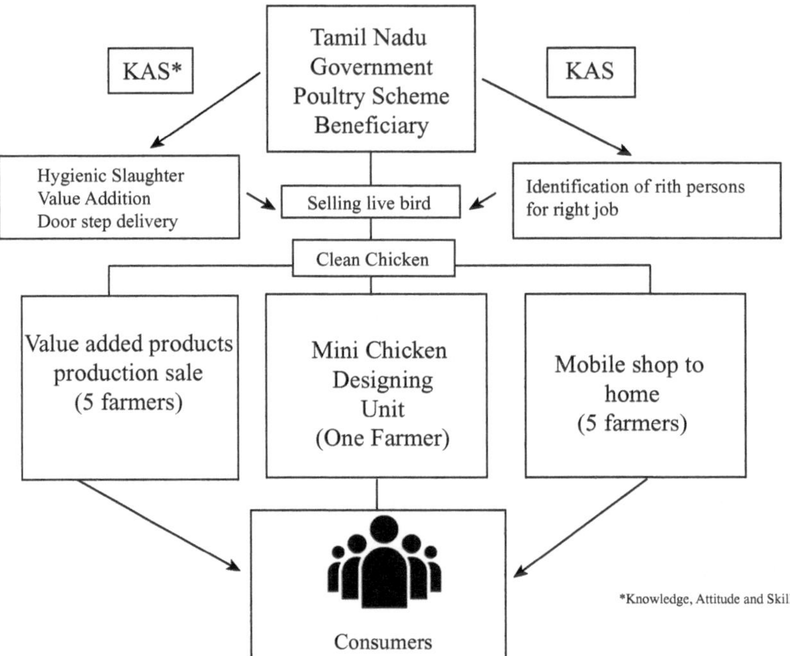

Then after he had established the Surya Chicken Processing Unit and is presently using all the poultry slaughter and dressing equipment and instruments viz., stainless steel knives, choppers, use of fly control unit, stainless steel dressing table, Teflon plates, provision of geyser for hot water and use of defeathering machine *etc.,* distributed through this project. The farmer is now producing hygienic chicken meat following scientific principles and selling 1000 to 1500 kg of meat / week as dressed meat and live bird for Rs.230 / kg and Rs. 200/ kg, respectively. He is now able to produce more quality meat in a shorter time with labour saving techniques and equipments and the quantity of meat sold has increased after the establishment of this Unit. The reasons for such increase in sales is that the consumer preferred wholesome meat with solid cut up parts, no fly in the retail outlet and no wood pieces in the meat after using the Teflon plate for cutting birds which he adopts in his new retail outlet

ii. Social

Many desi bird farmers and rural youth visit his slaughter unit and motivated to establish such unit in their farm premises. Presently, Mr. Ramasamy with the entrepreneurial skill is an opinion leader for Uppiliyapuram Block to disseminate the knowledge and skill acquired in successful establishment of chicken meat retail outlet.

iii. Environmental

The Food Safety Officer of Uppliyapuram Union, Trichy, Mr.Palanisamy, inspected the Unit and appreciated the role of TANUVAS, NABARD and the Department of Animal Husbandry in the establishment of this successful model unit in a village through this Project. He expressed that the Unit has been established as per the FSSAI norms and appreciated the use of stainless steel knives, choppers, use of fly control unit, stainless steel dressing table, provision of geyser for hot water and use of defeathering machine etc., The FSSAI license was issued to the unit. This ensures safety disposal of slaughter unit wastes and also provides wholesome meat to the consumer making the environment clean and green.

II. Hatchery Unit

i. Economical

Two beneficiaries for establishment of hatchery unit namely Mrs. V.Suba w/o Velusamy and Mrs. K.Thilakavathi w/o Kumar from Uppliapuram village participated in the training programme and imparted skills on operation of a Hatchery unit. Hands-on training on "Establishment of hatchery unit" for skill development was given to the beneficiaries.

The above said two beneficiaries were given each one fully automated incubator with capacity of 500 eggs containing setter and Hatcher in single compartment with power backup facility (1 KVA inverter with 24 volts battery).

Beneficiary-1: Mrs. V. Subha

The following table shows the hatchability performance of the incubator

	No. of Hatch	Total eggs set	Total chicks hatched out	Hatchability in percentage
Mrs. V. Subha	1st Hatch	150	130	86.66
	2nd Hatch	100	65	65.00
	3rd Hatch	36	13	81.25
	4th Hatch	15	13	86.67
	5th Hatch	50	40	80.00
	6th Hatch	40	15	37.50
	7th Hatch	25	17	68.00
	8th Hatch	64	48	75.00
	9th Hatch	30	23	76.67
	Overall hatchability			**72.97**

Beneficiary – 1 : Mrs. K. Thilagavathi

	No. of Hatch	Total eggs set	Total chicks hatched out	Hatchability in percentage
Mrs. K. Thilagavathi	1st Hatch	120	102	85.00
	2nd Hatch	35	27	77.14
	3rd Hatch	187	132	70.59
	4th Hatch	100	73	73.00
	5th Hatch	39	33	84.62
	6th Hatch	70	59	84.29
	7th Hatch	70	61	87.14
	Overall hatchability			**80.25**

The above said beneficiaries so far procured eggs from neighboring farmers and collected hatching charges of Rs.10/egg.

ii. Social

The two beneficiaries had collected eggs from nearly 25 farmers for a period of six months and hatched chicks for them in their hatchery unit. The beneficiaries also supported the State Poultry Development scheme farmers with supply of chicks as and when needed. Further, the beneficiaries show cased their hatchery unit in an Exhibition organized by State Department of Animal Husbandry and this made an eye opener for many desi bird farmers to establish hatchery unit for supply of day old chicks to needy farmers. This hatchery unit helped other needy farmers to produce quality chicks with high hatchability when compared using brooding hens.

iii. Environmental

The incubator operated in AC current is environmental friendly without causing any pollution to the environment. The unhatched eggs and broken shells were buried safely in barren lands without causing any hazards to the public and environment.

III. Meat And Meat Products Unit

i. Economical

Mrs. R. Dhanalakshmi, W/o Mr.V.Ravi, aged 45 years, who has studied only up to 6th standard from 359, Ambalakkaarar Street, O. Krishnapuram, Okkarai Post, Trichy who has a desi chicken unit, started a chicken meat outlet and is selling desi chicken meat up to 80 kg per week.

Under the scheme, she attended a three days capacity building programme on "Poultry meat production and value addition" at Veterinary University Training and Research Centre (TANUVAS), Coimbatore. Further, poultry slaughter and dressing equipment and instruments viz., stainless steel knives, choppers, use of fly control unit, stainless steel dressing table, Teflon plates, provision of geyser for hot water and defeathering machine were given. She is also supplied with gas stove, utensils, hot box and other necessary vessels and equipments to prepare and sell various poultry based value added meat products. By acquiring necessary skills on value added meat product and with the help of the equipments supplied in this scheme, the individual has established a retail meat product sales outlet on the main road and has now started to produce and sell chilly chicken and chicken soup. Presently she now sells 50 cups of chicken soup and 1.5 kgs of chilly chicken every day. To prepare 50 cups of chicken soup, she spends Rs.400 (cost of chicken meat, vegetables and other masala items) and by selling she get Rs. 1000 (Rs.20 per cup). The net profit is Rs. 600 for 50 cups of chicken soup. Similarly, she spends Rs.350 to prepare 1.5 kgs of chilly chick which includes cost of chicken meat, egg, masala items, oil etc. She gets Rs.680 (Rs. 40 / 100 gms of prepared 1.7 kgs of chilly chicken) by selling chilly chicken and net profit is Rs. 330.

ii. Social

Being women entrepreneur she spends her leisure time fruitfully and adds additional income to the total family income. This helps her family to invest more on agriculture and allied farming activities thereby increasing the livelihood status of the family as a whole. So, this motivated other women in the nearby villages and hence they can start their own enterprise.

iii. Environmental

In the meat and product preparation unit, the slaughter wastes and other cooking waste are properly disposed without affecting the agriculture lands and hence this unit is an environmentally friendly.

Conclusion

The study revealed that the beneficiaries in the study area gained economical, social and environmental benefits thereby making native chicken rearing as an ideal livelihood option for the landless and marginal farmers. Thus a market-led approach of conceptualizing a model of linking various beneficiaries' viz., parent bird rearers, hatchery unit, slaughter unit and value added product unit would help in continuous supply of inputs among them and making native chicken rearing a commercial sustainable venture. Through the years, extension shifts its focus from one function to another as a response to the changing goals of the government leading to the emerging issues in agricultural sector. For decades, extension used top-down approach wherein the extension system decides on what should be provided to the farmers based on their perceived needs but now, it shifted to bottom-up or participatory approach giving importance to the farmers in planning, implementing and making decisions about extension works. This new paradigm broadens the role of farmers by being not just recipients of extension services but as co-implementers of these services. It recognizes the significant contribution of farmers' knowledge, experiences, and potentials in attaining agricultural sustainability. Hence, involvement of farming community in decision-making, implementation and training farmers would help in achieving agricultural and livestock development goals.

40

Role of Agri-Clinic and Agribusiness Centers for Agri-Preneurship Development

Pankaj Kumar
Department of Veterinary and Animal Husbandry Extension Education
Bihar Veterinary College, BASU, Patna

Saroj Kumar
Department of Veterinary and Animal Husbandry Extension Education
Bihar Veterinary College, BASU, Patna

Puspendra Kumar Singh
Department of Department of Veterinary and Animal Husbandry Extension Education, Bihar Veterinary College, BASU, Patna

---

Introduction

Agriculture and allied sectors contributing significantly to rural employment generation. It also contributes almost 18% of GVA (Gross Value Added) in Indian Economy at current prices (Economic Survey of India 2016-17). It remains sustaining livelihood security with nutritional security and help in social transformation of the country. Second half of 20th century witnessed the change of traditional and subsistence Indian agriculture into a commercial activity. Green revolution of sixties paved the way for entry of agribusiness companies selling seeds, fertilizers, pesticides and farm machineries. Agriculture today faces many challenges which include globalization and market liberalization, food price crises, natural resource depletion, climate change, rapid urbanization, changing production and consumption patterns, demographic changes etc. Market driven agriculture production is need of the hour since marketing has become a challenge for small farmers. Agri-preneurship development can be key in this scenario.

Conceptual development of Agri-preneurship

Agri-Preneurship refers to entrepreneurship in agriculture. Entrepreneurship is viewed to have the ability to generate and build a vision from practically nothing. It is a dynamic process, which contributes to creation of incremental wealth and building of an improved life style. Entrepreneurship like technology "is a meta economic event, something that profoundly influences and indeed shapes the economy without itself being a part of it" (Drucker, 1984: 13). J.B. Say (1767-1832) had for instance said "the entrepreneur shifts economic resources out of an area of lower and into an area of higher productivity and yield". Joseph Schumpeter (1883-1950)-the only one among the major modern economists, who had examined entrepreneurship in some depth and postulated thereon, had described an entrepreneur as an innovator playing the role of a dynamic businessman adding material growth to economic development." As Adam Smith wrote in his *Theory of Moral Sentiments* the urge of an entrepreneur to make profit and accumulate capital "first prompted men to cultivate the ground, to build houses, to found cities and commonwealths and to invent all the sciences and arts which ennoble and embellish human life." Entrepreneurship has traditionally been defined as the process of designing, launching and running a new business, which typically begins as a small business, such as a start-up company, offering a product, process or service for sale (Yetisen et al. 2015).Entrepreneurship is a concept that encompasses transforming an idea or vision into a "new business or new venture creation, or the expansion of an existing business, by an individual, a team of individuals, or an established business" (Reynolds et al. 1999). Entrepreneurs are usually creative, take opportunities and accept risks, and can quickly change business strategies to adapt to changing environments. They are often innovators (Kahan, 2012). While usually being innovative and creative, farmers often lack experiences, access to services, people, or markets, and skills to have realistic chances to succeed as entrepreneurs (Wongtschowski et al. 2013). As per Butler (2006), an entrepreneur is a complex combination of Personality, Attitude, Skills and Motivation like interacting factors.

Agri-clinic and Agribusiness Centre

Each year, nearly 17000 agri. Graduates pass out from different State Agricultural Universities and other recognized Universities. Out of these, nearly half get employed/goes for higher education and rests remain unemployed. Therefore, Ministry of Agriculture, Govt of India felt the need for utilization of this unemployed but trained manpower for providing privatized extension services to farming community. as well as providing them employment opportunities. In this backdrop, an innovative scheme called Agri-clinic and Agribusiness Centre (AC & ABC) was launched by Govt. of India in collaboration with National Bank for Agricultural and Rural Development (NABARD) on 9th April, 2002.

The overall responsibility of implementation of this scheme was given to National Institute of Agricultural Extension Management (MANAGE), Hyderabad. The scheme is aimed at development of Agri-preneurs through training, establishing agricultural ventures.

Agri-clinic: The ventures which provide expert services and advice to farmers on cropping practices, technology dissemination, crop protection from pests & diseases, market trends and prices of various crops in the markets and also clinical services for animal health etc. are called Agri-clinic. Effective services of Agri-clinic would ultimately enhance the productivity of crops/animals.

Agribusiness Centres: These are the commercial ventures to provide input supply, farm equipment's on hire and other services. The major aim is to provide employment to trained agriculture graduates.

In order to enhance viability of the ventures, Agriculture Graduates may also take up in agriculture and allied areas along with the Agri-clinics/Agribusiness Centres under the AC & ABC Scheme.

Objectives of AC & ABC Scheme

- To supplement efforts of public extension by necessarily providing extension and other services to the farmers on payment basis or free of cost as per business model of agri-preneur, local needs and affordability of target group of farmers.
- To support agricultural development; and
- To create gainful self-employment opportunities to unemployed agricultural graduates, agricultural diploma holders, intermediate in agriculture and biological science graduates with PG in agri-related courses.

AC & ABC Model and Stakeholders involved in implementation

The scheme is operated by different entities that perform their individual task to operate the scheme in a successful manner. Below is the diagrammatical explanation of the roles and responsibilities of each entity in the flow of the scheme.

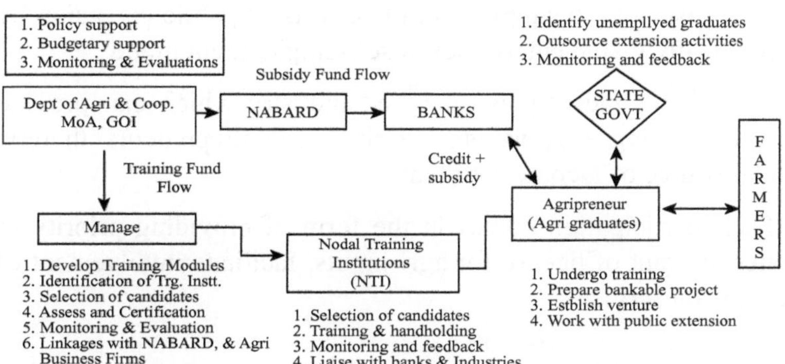

Fig.: AC & ABC Model with all stakeholders and their functions

DOAC & FW: Dept. of Agriculture Cooperation and Farmers Welfare, Govt of India provides the fund for this scheme through its extension division.

MANAGE: National Institute of Agricultural Extension Management, Hyderabad is the monitoring and overall implementing agency of this scheme. It is responsible for reviewing the performance of the nodal institutes; decide upon the training content, methodology and duration. Be a part of the selection committee for choosing the eligible candidates and set criteria for selection of nodal institutes.

Nodal Training Institutes (NTIs): These are institutes selected by MANAGE for conducting the training programmes for selected agriculture graduates and assist them in preparing bankable project. Once the project is over, it assist them in sanctioning of loan and successfully setting up of the ventures. There are a total of 140 NTIs identified by MANAGE which includes SAUs, State Govt. Institutes, NGOs, Agribusiness company, Institutes of Cooperative Management and Krishi Vigyan Kendras.

Banks: Banks could be nationalized/ commercial/cooperative and regional rural banks who would be the financing institution in the scheme. They are responsible for processing loan proposals and provide loans on approved proposals to the trained agriculture graduates. In addition to providing loan to the agri-preneur, they are also responsible for implementing announced policy on providing credit to such proposals.

NABARD: National Bank for Agricultural and Rural Development is the nodal institute for banks who is responsible for monitoring credit support to Agri clinics through the above mentioned banks. It is also responsible for extending refinance support to the banks under the scheme.

Agripreneurs: Agri-preneurs are the ultimate beneficiary of the scheme. They are agriculture graduates, post graduates and even doctorates who undertake training under this scheme and provide specialized extension and other services on fee-for-service basis and to supplement the efforts of public extension by providing economically viable enterprises in self-employment mode.

Input Industries: Input industry is an allied industry which can provide dealership, input stocking support etc. to the agri-entrepreneurs thereby creating a regular source of income for them.

State Govt: Their participation comes in the form of providing priority to trained graduates in grant of license for agri-inputs; facilitate involvement of ACABCs in extension services.

Progress of the AC & ABC Scheme

The scheme is operational in India since 1st April, 2002. A lot of agriculture graduates have been trained and many of them started their business ventures. This has been a journey of nearly 17 years. Therefore, we need to look on the salient achievements of the scheme since its beginning. A total of 72,784 Agriculture graduates have been trained by different Nodal Training Institutes from 1st April, 2002 till 29th October, 2020. Out of these, 30,567 candidates established their business ventures in different areas of agriculture and allied sectors like animal husbandry, dairy, poultry, goatery, fisheries etc. There were 32 activities related to agriculture and allied fields identified under this scheme for establishing business ventures by the trained agriculture graduates. Activities like AC& ABC, dairy, vermin-composting and crop production are amongst the most popular projects. The Agri-Clinics and Agri-Clinics and Agribusiness Centers together contributed 43.7% of total number of ventures established. The popularity of the Agri-clinics projects is mainly because of low investment and low risk.

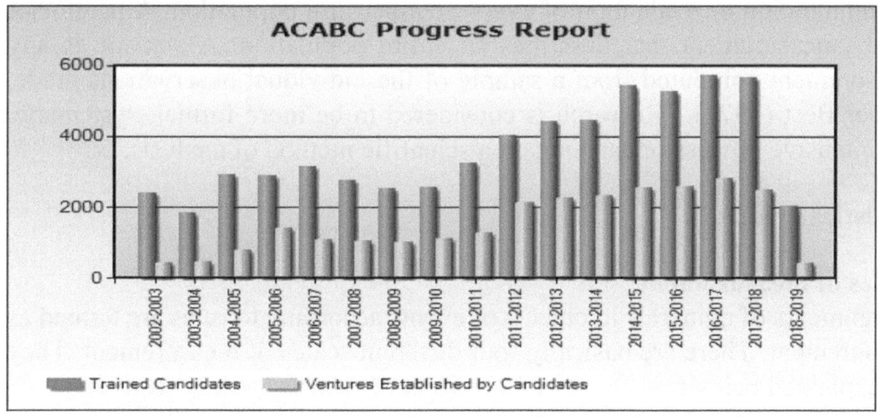

Source: http://www.agriclinics.net

Conclusion

This scheme is very good in terms of concepts and intention. If implemented properly, it can create a lot of employment opportunities to trained individuals. But Banks need to be sensitized, since many projects could not be started due to lack of finance from bank. One agri venture provides employment to many more people. Therefore, there is a need for pushing this scheme in North eastern states areas where there are many glitches. This scheme is a good option for development of entrepreneurs in agriculture and allied sector.

41

Application of Statistics in Social Science

Sukanta Biswas and Subhransu Mohan Nanda

Department of Veterinary & Animal Husbandry Extension Education
Faculty of Veterinary & Animal Sciences, WBUAFS, Kolkata, West Bengal

Introduction

A population is the set of all objects we wish to study. A sample is part of the population we study to learn about the population. A census may be defined as an enumeration or evaluation of every member of a population. A parameter is any measurement that describes an entire population. A statistic is any measurement computed from a sample of the individual observations made. As per Best (1977), "Research is considered to be more formal, systematic, and intensive process of carrying on a scientific method of analysis."

Statistical Methods

Scales of measurement

Assignments of numerals to objects or events according to rules are termed as measurement. There are basically four different scales of measurement. They are explained below:

a. Nominal scale

- In this scale, the numbers are assigned to objects or events which can be placed into mutually exclusive and exhaustive events.
- Eg: Male can be assigned with 1 and Female can be assigned with 2.

b. Ordinal scale

- In ordinal level of measurement, numbers are assigned to objects or events, which can be placed into mutually exclusive categories and be ordered into a greater or less than scale.
- The numbers assigned can be categorized as greater than or lesser than in order to indicate a relationship.

- Eg: The satisfaction level of poultry development programme by the respondents can be assigned 1 as most satisfied to least popular as 5.

c. Interval scale

- In this scale of measurement, numbers are assigned to objects or events which can be categorized, ordered and assumed to have an equal distance between scale values.
- The zero point is set arbitrarily.
- Eg: In a thermometer, 0 is set arbitrarily. The measurement is done with the interval scale.

d. Ratio scale

- As per Sproull, 1988, in ratio level of measurement, numbers are assigned to objects or events which can be categorized, ordered, assumed to have equal intervals between scale points and have a real zero point.
- Mathematical applications like multiplication, division can be used with this scale nut not with other scales mentioned earlier. Eg: 25:15 is equal to 5:3

Variables

They may be defined as attributes of any object, events, things or beings that vary and can be measured.

The different types of variables include

a. Dependent and Independent variables

- Dependent variables are said to be the effect of the independent variables. They may be defined as the phenomenon or characteristic hypothesized to be the outcome, effect, consequence or output of some input variables. This is represented by Y.
- Independent variables are presumed to cause of the dependent variables and is selected, manipulated or measured prior to measuring the outcome or dependent variable. They are represented by X_1, X_2, etc.
- Example: In a study conducted by Nanda *et al*, 2022 on Job satisfaction of veterinarians in relation with various socio-personal variables in Odisha and West Bengal, the following variables were taken into consideration:

Dependent variable

- Y: Job satisfaction of Veterinarians

Independent variables

- X_1: Age of the respondents

- X_2: Qualification of the respondent veterinarians
- X_3: Specialization of the respondents
- X_4: Nature of job
- X_5: Location of posting
- X_6: Job experience (in years)
- X_7: Distance of workplace from home

b. Qualitative attributes and quantitative variables

- Qualitative attributes are the attributes that cannot be manipulated after the research has started and they consist of categories that cannot be ordered in magnitude. Eg: Religion of the respondents
- Quantitative variables are the variables that can be ordered in magnitude and
- Composed of categories. They may be in greater or smaller amounts. Eg: Age, income of the respondents.

c. Continuous and Discrete variables

- They are the sub categories of the quantitative variables.
- Continuous variables are the variables that can be measured in exact degree of fineness or exactness.
- Discrete variables are the variables that can be determined by counting.

Sampling

The different types of sampling methods are explained below:

a. Probability Sampling

- In this type of sampling, the size of the parent population or universe from which the
- Sample is to be drawn must be known to the investigator.
- Each element has equal chance of being included in the sample.
- The different types of probability sampling methods are as follows:
- Simple random sampling:
  - Each of the elements has equal and independent chance of being selected.
  - The selection of a simple random sample is done by using the following methods:
- **Lottery system:** In this method, the name of each item is written in a slip of paper and all the papers are shuffled and selections of the items are done randomly.

- **Tables of random numbers**: random numbers are numbers that are computer generated according to a scheme whereby each digit is equally likely to be any of the integers 0,1,2...9 and does not depend on the other digits generated. The numbers are chosen independently, so any digit chosen has no influence on any other selection.
  - Eg: In research conducted by Nanda *et al*, 2020 entitled "Information needs of field veterinarians of coastal Odisha on dairy husbandry activities",120 number of field veterinarians were chosen randomly, 20 from each district. The study was conducted in 6 coastal districts namely Ganjam, Puri, Jagatsinghpur, Kendrapara, Bhadrak and Balasore.
- **Stratified random sampling:** In this case, the population is first divided into different groups and sampling is done from the individual groups.
- Proportionate stratified random: In this method, the researcher randomly draws the individuals in a similar proportion from each stratum of the population. Eg:
- **Disproportionate stratified random sampling:** In this case, the samples drawn from each stratum are not necessarily distributed according to their proportion in the population from where they have been randomly selected.
- **Cluster sampling:** This is that form of probability sampling where sampling units are groups of elements or clusters. Eg: Suppose there are 1000 farmers in a district. The sample needs to be 10% of the population. A particular block contains 100 farmers that make 10% of the total population. All the farmers of the blocks are selected as sample. This type of sampling is called as cluster sampling.

b. Non-probability sampling

In this form of sampling, the samples are chosen deliberately without random. Some of the important techniques of non-probability sampling methods are explained below.

- Quota sampling
- The entities are selected to be included in the sample until the same proportion of selected characteristics as per the population is reached.

Purposive sampling

- This is otherwise known as judgment sampling.
- In this case, the researcher has the liberty to choose the samples from a specified population based on the requirement of the study.

Systematic sampling

- In this case, every nth element is selected from the population or a list of elements.
- Eg: Every 7th roll number is selected from a total of 70 students in a class.
- Snowball sampling
- This is done in case of sociometry analysis.
- This method is used to find out the local leaders, opinion leaders and the lay leaders.
- Double sampling
- This form of sampling method is followed when the sampling is done two times.
- Eg: A questionnaire was sent to 1000 people. 400 filled responses were received after a stipulated period. From the 400 received responses, 100 are chosen and identified as the sample for the study.

Statistical Tests

The basic tests used in statistics include the use of 2 types of tests, i.e.

a. Parametric

Parametric statistics is a branch of statistics which assumes that sample data comes from a population that can be adequately modeled by a probability distribution that has a fixed set of parameters. Conversely a non-parametric model differs precisely in that the parameter set (or feature set in machine learning) is not fixed and can increase, or even decrease, if new relevant information is collected.

According to Seigel 1956, parametric tests are conducted under the following conditions.

1. The population from which the samples have been drawn should be normally distributed. This is known by the term "assumption of normality".
2. The variables must have been measured in interval or ratio scale.
3. The observations must be independent. The inclusion or exclusion of any case in the sample should not unduly affect the results of the study.
4. These populations must have the same variance or, in special cases, must have a known ratio of variance. This is called as homoscedasticity.

In cases where these conditions do not satisfy, it is always advisable to make use of non-parametric tests.

Different Types of Parametric Tests are Explained Below

Student's t-test

An Irish statistician, William Sealy Gossett in 1908 developed statistical method for testing the significance between the means of two different samples of same size. It was named as t-test. Since, Gossett used to write under pseudonym "student", t-test was named student's t-test by William Seeley. This test is also known as t-distribution or t-ratio. This test is applied to small samples only.

They are broadly divided into 2 types namely one sample t-test and two sample t-test

One sample t-test

This form of t-test is applied where the sample parameters are compared to population parameters. The size of the population must be small and is compared with the population.

$$t_c = \frac{|\overline{X} - \mu|}{s/\sqrt{n}} = \frac{|\overline{X} - \mu|}{SE}$$

$\overline{X}$ =Sample mean, μ = Population mean

S = standard deviation, n = number of observations

SE = Standard error

If $t_c < t_{tab}$ with n-1 degrees of freedom at chosen level of significance, H_0 is accepted. This means that there is no significant difference between sample mean and population mean.

Two sample t-test

This form of test is applied when we have 2 different samples and we compare between the parameters of these two samples. It is further divided into three categories.

a. Fischer's test

This form of test is applied when the variance of one sample equals with the variance of the other sample. Generally, when the samples are from the same breed or group, we consider that the variances are equal.

$$t_c = \frac{|\overline{X_1} - \overline{X_2}|}{\sqrt{s_c^2\left(\frac{1}{n_1} - \frac{1}{n_2}\right)}}$$

$$S_c^2 = \frac{(n_1 - 1)S_1^2 + (n_2 - 1)S_2^2}{n_1 + n_2 - 2}, S_c^2 = \text{combined variance}$$

b. Cochran's test

This test is used when the variance of one sample is not equal to the variance of the other sample. Samples from different breeds or different groups are said to have different variances.

$$t_c = \frac{\left|\overline{X}_1 - \overline{X}_2\right|}{\sqrt{\frac{s_1^2}{n_1} + \frac{s_2^2}{n_2}}}$$

$$t_{\text{tab}} = \frac{w_1 t_1 + w_2 t_2}{w_1 + w_2}, w_1 = \frac{s_1^2}{n_1} \text{ and } w_2 = \frac{s_2^2}{n_2}$$

t_1 is the tabulated value at $(n_1 - 1)$df

t_2 is the tabulated value at $(n_2 - 1)$df

c. Paired t-test

This form of the test is used when both the samples are of the same population. Different treatments are applied in the same population at different time intervals.

$$t_c = \frac{\left|\overline{d}\right|}{s_d / \sqrt{n}}, \overline{d} = \frac{\sum d_i}{n}, s_d^2 = \frac{1}{n-1}\left[\sum d_i^2 - \frac{\left(\sum d_i\right)^2}{n}\right]$$

F-test

- When more than 2 treatments are under study, t0 test has to be performed for every pair of treatments. But for simultaneous comparison of any number of treatments, it is done through ANOVA technique.
- **Treatment:** It is a set of conditions imposed on experimental unit. Here, the treatments are known as objects of comparison.
- **Experimental unit:** It refers to the unit to which a single treatment is applied in one repetition of the experiment.

Z-test

The z-test is another test under parametric statistics which is applied normally distributed. It is used to compare two means the sample mean and the perceived population mean. It is also used to compare the two samples' means taken from the same population. This test is applied when the samples are equal to or greater than 30. The z-test can be applied in two ways: the One-Sample Mean Test and the Two-Sample Mean Test. This is an extension of t-test.

$$z = \frac{\overline{x_1} - \overline{x_2}}{\sqrt{\frac{s_1^2}{n_1} + \frac{s_2^2}{n_2}}}$$

b. Non-Parametric Tests

- These are the tests that are performed in case of qualitative data.

Chi-square test

- It is used to know whether the given sample is in agreement with renowned theory.
- Different types of chi square tests are explained below:
- To test whether a particular population has a specific variance or not.

$H_0 : \sigma^2 = \sigma_0^2$

$H_1 : \sigma^2 \neq \sigma_0^2$

σ^2=Population variance

σ_0^2= Sample variance

$$\chi_{cal}^2 = \frac{(n-1)s^2}{\sigma^2}$$

n = number of observations

s^2 = sample variance

σ^2 = population variance

(n-1) degrees of freedom at level pf significance

If χ_{cal}^2 is less than χ_{tab}^2, null hypothesis is accepted else rejected.

Goodness of fit

In this form of chi square test, we check whether the observed frequency is equal to expected frequency.

If population is divided into k different groups and we want to test the frequency of these k different groups according to some specified law.

$$\chi_c^2 = \frac{\left(O_{ij} - E_{ij}\right)^2}{E_{ij}}$$

(k-1) degrees of freedom at level pf significance

If χ^2_{cal} is less than χ^2_{tab}, null hypothesis is accepted else rejected.

Correlation

- According to Croxton and Cowden, correlation is the degree of association or strength of relationship between two quantitatively measured or continuous variables. Different methods for determination of correlation are explained below:
- Karl Pearson's correlation coefficient (r) by co-variance method
  - It is a mathematical method for measuring the tendency of linear relationship between two variables.
  - This was introduced by Karl Pearson.
  - This measure of correlation is also known as Personian Correlation coefficient.
  - The correlation coefficient is a number between -1 and +1 whose sign is the same as the slope of the line and whose magnitude is related to the degree of linear association between two variables.
  - The value or r can be calculated by using the formula

$$r_{(x,y)} = \frac{\sum(x-\bar{x})(y-\bar{y})}{\sqrt{\sum(x-\bar{x})^2 . \sum(y-\bar{y})^2}}$$

- Correlation coefficient by Spearman's rank method
  - This method is used for qualitative variables such as efficiency, intelligence, honesty etc.
  - These variables can't be measured quantitatively, but can be arranged serially.
  - Correlation coefficient between any two of such qualitative variables cannot be calculated by Pearson's method.
  - The correlation coefficient between 2 variables in n no. of individuals can be calculated by the following formula

$$r = 1 - \frac{6\sum D^2}{n(n^2-1)}, \; r = \text{Spearman's rank correlation coefficient.}$$

  D represents the difference between the pair of same individuals in two corresponding rank characteristics.

  n = no of pairs of observations.

- In this method, different expressions of an attribute are arranged serially in order of preference.

- Such an ordered arrangement is called **ranking** and the ordinal number indicating the position of a given attribute in the ranking is called **rank**.
- Computation of Rank Correlation Coefficient by Spearman's method
  - The value of rank correlation coefficient (R) ranges between +1 and -1.
  - It can be calculated in three different situations.
  - When actual ranks are given

Rank in 1st series	Rank in 2nd series	Difference between ranks	Square of rank difference
R_1	R_2	R_1-R_2=D	D^2

$$r = 1 - \frac{6\sum D^2}{n\left(n^2 - 1\right)}$$

- When actual ranks are not given

a. In such cases, actual data is converted into ranks.

b. It means ranks are assigned by arranging the data in ascending order or in descending order.

c. In descending order, the highest value is given rank 1, and is ascending order the lowest value is ranked 1.

- When ranks are equal
- When two or more items in one series of data may have equal values, a common rank is given to all the items having same value.
- The common rank is the average of the ranks which these items would have occupied in the series, had they differed slightly from each other.
- Suppose, two items are ranked equal at fifth rank because of having equal value. Had they differed slightly, they would have been ranked as 5th and 6th.

  Their common rank will be $\frac{5+6}{2} = 5.5$.
- The formula for calculation of rank correlation coefficient in a series where two items have same value becomes:

$$r = 1 - \frac{6\left[\sum D^2 + \frac{1}{12}\left(m^3 - m\right) + \frac{1}{12}\left(m^3 - m\right)\right]}{n\left(n^2 - 1\right)}$$

- Kendal Tau correlation coefficient
  - This is a non-parametric measure of relationships between columns of ranked data. Tau correlation coefficient returns a value of 0 to 1, where 0 is no relationship and 1 is the perfect relationship.

- The different versions of the Tau are explained below:
- Tau-A and Tau-B are used for tables with equal columns and rows.
- Tau-C can be used for tables with unequal number of rows and columns.
  - Kendall's Tau = (C–D/C+D), where C is the number if concordant pairs and D is the number of discordant pairs.

Regression analysis

As per Panse and Sukhtatme, 1967, regression equation may be defined as the underlying relation between *y* and *x* in a bi-variate population and is said to represent the regression of the variate *y* on the variant *x*.

If *y* is the dependent variable and *x* is the independent variable, the linear regression equation can be written as $y = a + bx$

Multiple regression analysis is done to know the extent to which the independent variables, separately or jointly could predict or contribute towards the dependent variable. It basically measures the combined relation between a dependent and a series of independent variables.

Factor analysis

This analysis is employed by the researcher in order to establish commonness among a set of observed variables. The variables are grouped into factors by using this technique. The factors newly grouped, often termed as latent variables.

Principal Component analysis

This is the most widely used method of factor analysis. The first component extracted explains the maximum amount of total variance in the observed variables. The first component many be correlated with many variables. The second component will have two important characteristics. First, it explains a maximum amount of variance in the data set that was not accounted by the first component. Secondly, it will be uncorrelated with the first component.

Path analysis

This is a type of statistical analysis undertaken to obtain a clear picture of the direct and indirect effects of the independent variables on dependent variables. Singh and Chaudhary (1977), defined path coefficient as the ratio of the standard deviation of the effect due to a given cause to the total standard deviation of the effect.

Conclusion

Statistics plays an important role in the social science. Presently, many software are available for analyzing the research data. The most common among them include MS-Excel, IBM-SPSS, SAS, JASP, WOMBAT, HARVEY and Mat Lab. This software has helped in making the analysis in an easier manner.

42

Hunger-Poverty-Silence New Age Extension Strategy to Break The Lethal Combination

Sankar Kumar Acharya

Agricultural Extension, Bidhan Chandra Krishi Viswavidyalaya, Mohanpur West Bengal-741252

History of human civilization initiated with the struggle against hunger, it flourishes with the fight against poverty and turns oblivious with absence of voices being raised against these two bio-social lethal. If hunger is a pain, poverty is an agony, then, keeping silent against this carcinoma of civilization is no doubt a crime. Is it that poor people are put to an insurmountable silence by the ruthless hegemonies of political economy, or, they are silent, that's why they remain poor? Silence has been the lethal enzyme in transforming poverty into hunger, and, offers to a socio- chemical bond, poverty-hunger-silence; the bond that remains non-breakable as on date. Economists lament for poverty, nutritionists regret hunger, but the issues of silence and its cohesion to both hunger and poverty has seldom been scholastically delved into or dealt with. We can hope, a desperation of wishful thinking as it may be, shall drench the researchers who think and feel to explore a missing link between hunger and poverty, the silence or the social anemia of voices.

Hunger is the sauce of life that drives us to the golden harvest; it's the fire either, that destroys socio-ecological balances to invite ever increasing entropy. The UNO in its recent press release express concerns that more millions will die not due to COVID pandemic only, it is because of hunger and poverty. The humongous up surging of joblessness, economic disaster and social disorder due to this pandemic, the poor, hungry and voiceless people are going to die, a repetition of social Titanic episode can be as worst as an analogy

In India only close to 10 million migrant workers have become re-migrant for the worse destiny, a close to five million have lost their job or extremely vulnerable to a sudden joblessness due to economic apocalypse as reflected in a appalling -23 per cent growth revealed by the ministry of finance, India. The need of the hour is to elicit the factual data on the damaged and vulnerability status with an immediate restart of economical repairing and social healing process. We have no choice but to make people, those who are reeling under dire marginalization, free from fear psychosis by restoration of both economy and morals

Silence is the moth lethal inputs that make poor the poorer, deprived with a stubborn silence and the hungry with an unacceptable negotiation with social hegemony and extortion inflicted on the poor by the mighty richer community. So, a comprehensive research offers an inevitability of a study that would delineate and decipher the lethality of a venomous combination amongst and between hunger- poverty-silence, the trio that causes deadening consequences of deprived people and the civilization at length.

Even with the swashbuckling claim on growth and prosperity on the present civilization, the other side of this prosperity is so brick and disastrous that has no match for the past centuries even. Out of around 7 billion population of the world, 1.5 billion are hungry. They don't have adequate access to food, if it is there, the quality doesn't stand anywhere near to fulfill their calorie requirement. In India, 350 million people are living below the poverty line and of them, 200 million people have become victim to moderate to extreme hunger indexes. 42 per cent of the new born babies are under weight. 60 per cent of the children are suffering from moderate to high level of anaemia experiencing stunted growth

Beyond the curtain of hunger, there is another problem that is chronic hunger. Based on hunger index we the nation is occupying 100th position in the world (IFPRI Report, 2017). The scenario of chronic hunger is even worse and astoundingly it is worse than African nations as well.

Quoting back of Gunner Myrdal, a German analyst (Wrote 'Asian Drama'), the reasons for sluggish growth of Indian Agriculture is her Agricultural work force, who themselves are suffering from malnutrition, hunger and social impoverishment.

Indian agriculture is the largest but unorganized economic sector of the world. The farm entrepreneurs are suffering from both the vagaries of nature and market. The decelerating agricultural economy has thrown the growers into a vicious cycle of hunger, poverty and silence. Hunger here has been denoted by the level of food, calorie and nutrition intake by human bodies within the framework of minimum requirement set by World Health Organization (WHO) .Poverty here has been measured in terms of per capita income per month from a unit of holding, which is 121 million in India(NSSO data, 2014-2015).

The **silence** here is measured in terms of inability and impermeability to communicate with others or availing communication from others as to their need for survival and growth. The unique character of studying silence 'uninformed Diaspora' in India is that for farmers huge pile of information are there, but only a minuscule proportion is being accessed by the farmers. The voice for Minimum Support Price, crop insurance, health and nutrition, security and sustainability, is either plan fully unheard or they are refrained from uttering their voices to defend their stakes. The silent killer is the lethargy of uninformed life, when an individual is restrained either from accessing information or uttering opinion.

So, these three lethality are both technically and operationally combined together. Simply enough, it is to withstand the corollary that states Indian farmers are poor and that is why they are hungry; they are both poor and hungry because they are silent.

Some empirical experience

Artificial neural network helps us to interpret and estimate the nonlinear pathway of selected input variables on the output variables. Three distinct layers are over here, one is input layer the second is hidden layer wherein the errors are minimized through activation and the output layers or the dependent variables. For the graphical presentation of the first neural network we can find that communication variables(x11) and energy consumption variable(x12) have routed the distinct and dominant impact on the output variable hunger (y1). It has passed through the two hidden layers for the rationalization vis a vis the reduction of error. So we can predict hunger with least of errors from these two input variables, communication variables and energy consumption. Pattern as one of the important predictor for the level of hunger of the respondents

Now we are switching over to the second output variable poverty. Through the same way we can found that the management orientation X6 variable, stress perception on voice X9 variable and homestead land X10 variable have contributed in a decisive manner on the output variable poverty. Interestingly all these variables have been passed through three hidden layers for the management of their errors vis a vis estimation of their effect on the output variables

Now we are moving to words wherein all these output variables have been considered together and at the same time all the input variables have been taken care of. Here we can find that five hidden layers are there and through which all these input variables have generated their impact on the consequent variables those are hunger, poverty, voice and cognitive differential. We take one case for example that is X8. Here we can find that the X8 variable that is stress perception on poverty has passed through two hidden layers, one is hidden layer 1: 2 and the other is hidden layer 1:5 and after rooted through these two hidden layers as well as being reduced in terms of error these variable X8 has impacted on the output variable Y2 that is poverty. So we can see that whenever the respondents are under serious stress they are morose and don't show the interest to interact with others. Then they undergo a kind of withdrawal syndrome and then they lack the information about the projects simply because of there lethargy to access the same. So these variables if we see that to be taken care of to characterize the variable poverty. In another case we can find that the variable X11 that is communication variable after being passed through the hidden layer 1:1 and 1:5, they have been characterized the output variable Y4 that is cognitive differential. So, it is interesting to note that the communication variables are the main reason why the respondents have developed their different levels of cognitive differentials on the awareness of different government programmes. These four neural network paradigms have been successful in isolating the dominant variables, determining the number of hidden layers and ultimately how they have characterize the respective and corresponding output variables

Hunger poverty and voice are interrelated to each other and performing isochronously in the domain of entitlement and empowerment of the target respondents in the study.

When four consequent variables (hunger, poverty, voice and cognitive differential) have been estimated and elucidated in terms of 21 exogenous variables, it has generated unique and significant interaction and interrelation having huge strategic implications.

Hunger can well be estimated in case of farming respondents by Cropping intensity (x11), Livestock count (x12), Total crop yield (x15), poverty can be estimated by Cropping intensity (x11), Cost of cultivation (x16), Communication variables (x18), voice can well be estimated by Economic motivation (x4), Stress perception on poverty (x8), Livestock yield (x13) and cognitive differential can well be estimated through Stress perception on hunger (x7), Stress perception on voice (x9), Cropping intensity (x11), Livestock yield (13).

ANN for identifying dominant variables on hunger, poverty and voice

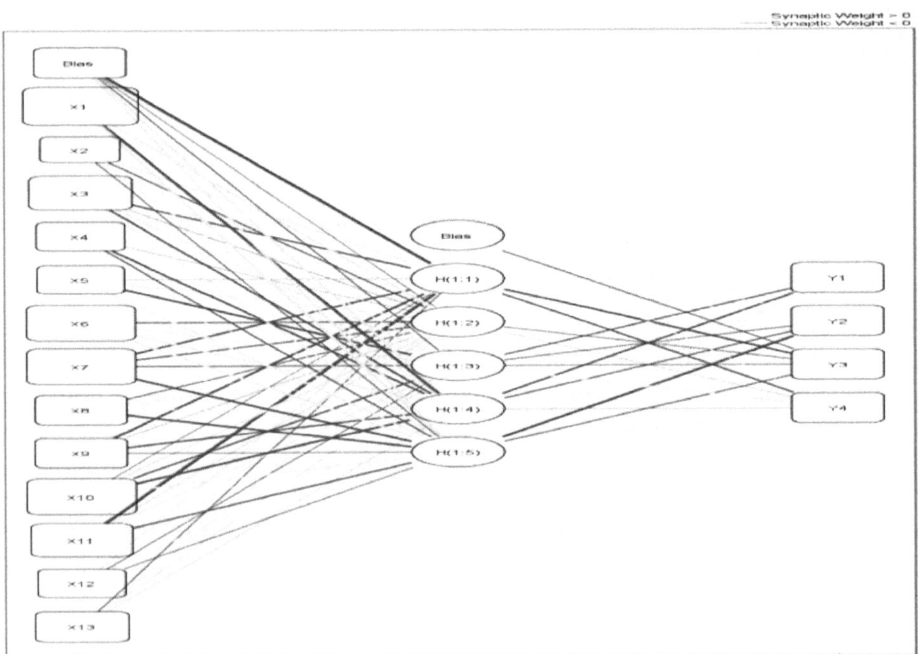

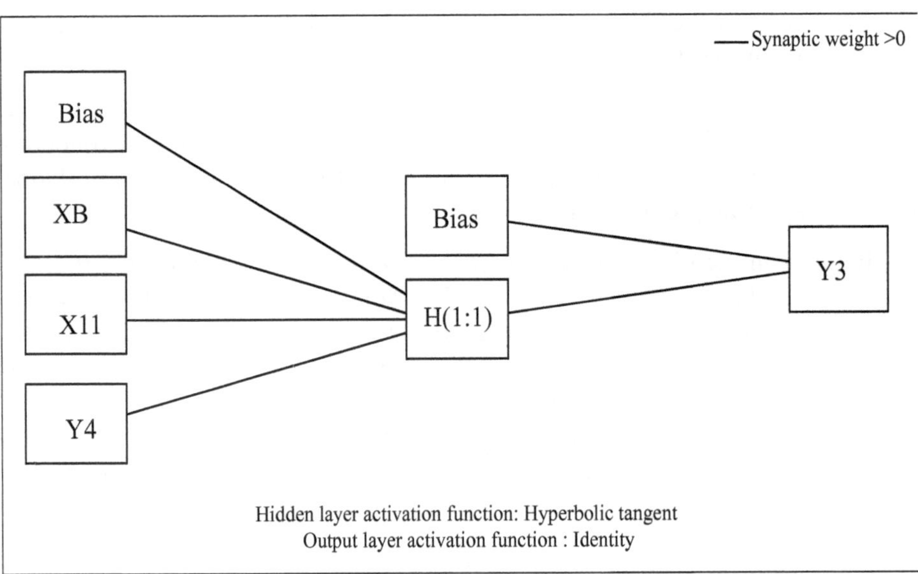

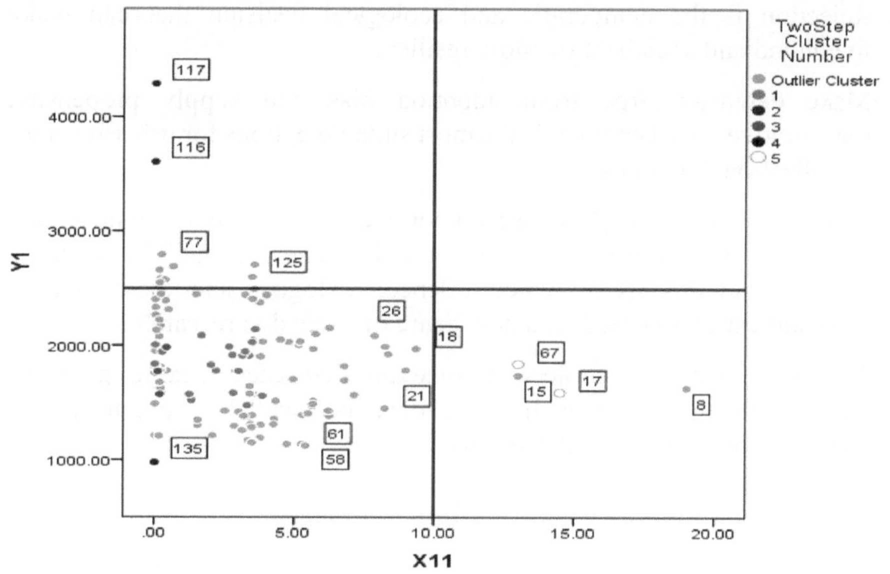

Diagnosing and detecting hunger and voice correlates in different quartiles

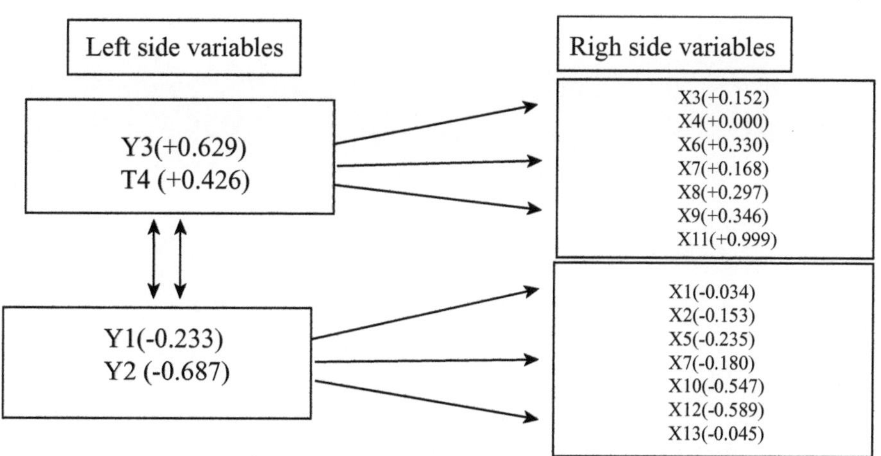

CCA to identify congenital movement of hunger-poverty, voice-cognitive differential amongst respondents

Strategy

1. Making poor rising voices can increase access to resource, technology and power.
2. Dialogues are the most critical inputs beyond money or fertilizer

3. Rejection is the democratic and ecological decision that can make livelihood and socialization more resilient.
4. Make extension free from adoption bias and supply propensity, regenerative social ecology is the most suitable options for ushering auto-socialization dynamics.
5. Voice, as endorsed by UN, of the poor and from the poor, are miserably missing from extension research in India. There should be an array of empirical models on voice, silence, dialogues and cross cultural communication to breed on a new genre of extension research.
6. Making development projects a voice and dialogues of target poor can successfully eliminate can eliminate social, political and economic *dalals* from the core of the social ecology.

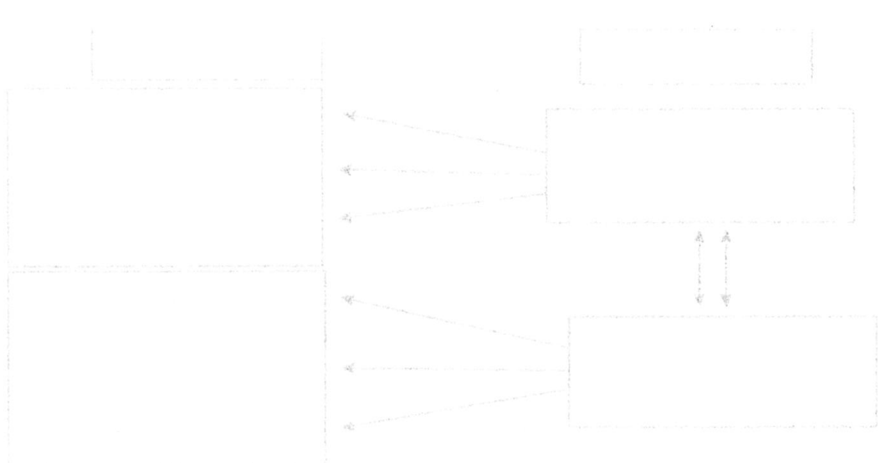

43

Upliftment of Socio-Economic Status of Rural People Through Diversified Aqua Farming Systems in India

Ashis Kumar Panigrahi

University of Burdwan, Burdwan, West Bengal

Introduction

Rural development focuses on development of rural man, woman and all things. Rural development influences the growth of economy in rural areas. Rural development mainly depends on agriculture. This agriculture reduces hunger in rural areas and increases food security. Bondad-Reantaso *et al.*, (2009) showed for rural development aquaculture act as a indicator. Brummett and Williams (2000) showed rural development of aquaculture in Africa.

Role of poverty alleviation by aquaculture

(a) Aquaculture creates employment in rural area

(b) Aquaculture gives nutrition to infants and women

(c) Vale of aquaculture is comparatively high.

(d) Rural people may income by selling the fish seed.

(e) Landless people can cage culture, mollusks culture in very short place.

Poverty alleviation & rural upliftment through various Integrated farming system:

Duck cum fish farming:

In duck cum fish farming, manure that enters into pond helps photosynthetic organism's growth. According to Ayyappan et al (1998) this fish farming is very common in China and Russia. For higher economic efficiency duck cum fish farming plays a crucial role in rural area. Revenue of duck cum fish framings are eggs, meat, fish. Rural people also eat duck meat when required.

Main benefits of duck cum fish farming are

(a) Culture pond supply good environment for duck.

(b) When the duck move into culture pond, it reduces duck feed.

(c) Dropping of ducks increases nutrient in pond

(d) When duck swim in pond it act as bio aerators

(e) Not required any extra land for this farming

(f) High survivability of ducks due to good environment

Paddy cum fish culture

In this method farmers produced rice with simultaneous production of fishes. As it is very easy process, farmers in rural area is highly benefited by paddy cum fish farming. India has many lakes, reservoir that helps farmers for the production of rice crop. Shingare *et al.,* (2020) showed, production of *Cyprinus carpio* per hector was 146.342 kg in Konkan region. Baruah *et al.,*(1999) showed , by rice cum fish farming 400- 450 kg per hector fish is produced whereas 2100 – 2300 kg per hector of rice is produced in Assam. Advantages of paddy cum fish culture are,

(a) No extra or supplementary food is required.

(b) By paddy cum fish culture harvesting was done within 90 days (Shingare et al. 2020)

(c) No additional training is required as rural people are well adapted for paddy culture.

(d) Fish excreta increases soil fertility.

Poultry cum fish farming

Research showed, in India 13000 tons of poultry dropping contains about 350 mt ton of proteins. This manure is used in rural area for agriculture. Poultry manure helps in plankton development. Fish used this poultry manure as food. This poultry manure have large amount of N, P. Beside this rural people rearing this poultry and sell this poultry egg, meat, etc.

Goat cum fish farming

Goat cum fish farming involves maximum production with very minimum cost. It also helps in resources utilization in aquaculture. Goat excreta include organic fertilizer. In goat excreta phosphorus have 1.78%, carbon have 60%.

Beside this goat urine have phosphorus and nitrogen. It is used as fish food. This system is very useful in rural area.

Cattle cum fish farming

Cattle dung directly enters into fish pond. This cattle dung act as manure in aquaculture in rural areas. In this type, cowsheds build near the fish pond as cow dung helps to develop plankton in pond. Here rural people benefit because only 5 cows can give about 4000 lit milk as well as 2000 kg fish per year.

Rabbit cum fish farming

Rabbit excreta contain high nitrogen and helps sustained growth of plankton. Beside rabbit mean is popular in some rural areas. In rabbit cum fish farming only 200 rabbit is require for 1 ha of aquaculture pond.

Pig cum fish farming

Pig excreta drained directly in fish pond as pig house are near the culture pond. Pig excreta have 70% digestible food and act as good fertilizer in culture pond. Culture of pig is very cheap process because pig eats rice bran, vegetables, etc. This pig food is very much available in rural areas and rural peoples are benefited by pig meats as well as fish also.

Ornamental fishery

Ornamental fishery is very common in rural areas due to low investment. People of rural area engaged in this fish culture. Ornamental fishery is a business in rural women. (Sinha et al. 2019) showed average income of self-help group from ornamental fishery is about 4500/ month.

Role of aquaculture in rural development

1. Fish increases brain development and stable metabolic processes.
2. Aquaculture provides food demand in Asia, Europe, etc.
3. Aquaculture helps to generate large number of employment in rural area.
4. Urban waste is recycling by aqua farming.
5. Rural infrastructure is developed by connecting roads.
6. Aquaculture encourages community efforts in rural areas.
7. In rural areas women are mostly engaging.

Year wise fish seed production in India (Directorate of fisheries, State govt/ UT's)

Year	Production (lakhs fry)
2014-15	393487
2015-16	354350
2016-17	357439
2017-18	444207
2018-19	481974
2019-20	521706

Gender involve in duck cum fish farming in Purulia –I block (Majhi 2016)

Village	Male	Female	Total
Shibdih	5	0	5
Ramnagar	5	0	5
Fatepur	5	0	5
Ralibera	5	0	5

Gender activity profile of ornamental fish culture (Sinha et al., 2019)

Activities	Women Involvement
Selection of breeders	Yes
Breeding	Yes
Nursing	Yes
Rearing	Yes
Feeding	Yes
Water quality check	No
Premises cleaning	Ye
Packing	Yes
Retail marketing	No
Whole sale marketing	Yes
Export	Yes

Supply of fish from other state (Ton) (Hand Book of Fisheries statistics, 2014, Govt of WB)

Name of the state	2011-12	2013-14
Andhra Pradesh	99818	76865
Orissa	57039	48966
Madhya Pradesh	7129	9080
Bihar	8912	6053

Risks of aquaculture production: Some risk factors in aquaculture production are as follows

1. Workers may injure during their work.
2. Fisherman workers suffer many diseases.
3. Snake biting
4 .Some chemicals that used in aquaculture may create health hazard.
5. Fungal infection
6. Pathogenic infection.

Conclusion

In integrated farming there is a huge efficiency of resources utilization. Manure of animal is used as fertilizer in pond. Rashid et al (2015) showed in slyest district 76.67 % people are highly benefited by farming of fish. Rural people rear poultry, duck. This poultry, duck gives high profit for rural areas. Beside this poultry, duck dropping used fish as food. Those farmers have very small land this faming helps as a source of income. So, income of rural people dependent on the different types of aqua farming.

References: Books, Journals Thesis & Other Resources

The Manuscript is a Multi-authorship composition, as contributed by 43 Nos. of nationally acclaimed, resource persons from Extension Education discipline in various national level Extension and research institutes, State Veterinary & Agriculture (SVU/SAU) Universities, ICAR-KrishiVgyan Kendras from Pan India. The Content of the resource document is not the original contribution of the resource persons, but innovative in perspective of knowledge, and skill development of the faculties/researchers/Extension education professionals in conceptualizing advance extension and communication strategies for sustainable livelihood generation through Animal Husbandry & allied farming system of for holistic development of the Country. As, the compilation is the collection of resource materials from various books, journals, thesis along with other online and offline resources, so there may found up to 95% percent Similarity index, from which the resources of the manuscripts are taken to make the documents an reflective and thought provoking. The Chief Editor, Editor & all authors of this compilation are duly acknowledged the contribution of all content provider to develop the resource documents and they are not demanding the contribution in the manuscript as their own and original one. The Editors & authors have developed this material only for better knowledge sharing among the intended reader/stakeholder unintentionally and unethically.*To avoid issue of plagiarism or any conflict of interest, whatever help taken from various cited books/thesis/journals/student papers along with other offline or online resources referred are cited as follows:*

References

A User's Guide to Measuring Local Governance UNDP 2022, https://www.undp.org /publications/ users-guide-measuring-local-governance-0accessed on January 25, 2022.

A. Lalitha, Suresh Chandra Babu. "Evaluation of Agricultural Technology Management Agency for dairy development", Elsevier BV, 201 9.

A.K. Singh, R. Roy Burman. "Agricultural extension reforms and institutional innovations for inclusive outreach in India", Elsevier BV, 2019.

Acharya R M. 1982. Sheep and Goat Breeds of India. FAO Animal Production and Health Paper 30, FAO of United Nations, Rome Italy.

Acharya, R. M., Misra, R.K. and Patil, V. K. (1982).Breeding Strategy for Goats in India.Indian Council of Agricultural Research, New Delhi, 111pp.

Adam, K.A. (2009). Some Ghanaian Traditional Practices of Forest Management and Biodiversity Conservation.In J.A. Parrotta, A. Oteng-Yeboah &, J. Cobbinah (Eds). Traditional Forest-Related Knowledge and Sustainable Forest Management in Africa. IUFRO World Series Volume 23. pp 121-122. Austria: IUFRO Headquarters, Vienna.

Aditya and Jirli Basavaprabhu (2010), ICT mediated agricultural extension: a survey of leading models and best practices, Journal of Progressive Agriculture, Vol.1, No.1. Pp: 74 83 (ISSN:2229-4244).

Aditya and JirliBasavaprabhu (2011), A study on social computing aspects on the students of Banaras Hindu University Journal of Global Communication, Vol.4, No.2. Pp: 148-161 (Print ISSN: 0974-0600, Online ISSN:0976-2442).

Aditya, A. K. Thakur and BasavaprabhuJirli (2014) Awareness about Social Computing among students.Asian Journal of Extension Education Vol 32 (1) Pp: 21-23 (ISSN: 0971 3115).

Aditya, BasavaprabhuJirli and A.K. Thakur (2014) Values Associated with the Students Using Social Media Tools. Journal of Community Mobilization and Sustainable DevelopmentVol 9 No. 1 Pp: 93-96, January-June 2014 (ISSN:2230-9047).

Aditya, Birendra Kumar, K. Abhinav and BasavaprabhuJirli (2014) Technology enabled learning in South Asia: A Review. Journal of Global Communication. Vol 7 No. 2 (July to December) Pp:128-134.

Agrawal, A. (1995). Dismantling the divide between indigenous and scientific knowledge. Development and Change.Vol. 26, No 3, 413-439.

Ahmed, M.M. (1994). Indigenous knowledge for sustainable development in the Sudan. Khartoum, Sudan: Khartoum University Press.

Ajay Kumar, Lesile L. Prince, Seiko Jose. "Sustainable wool production in India", Elsevier BV, 201 7.

Ajoy Mandal, M. Karunakaran, P.K. Rout, R. Roy. "Conservation of threatened goat breeds in India", Animal Genetic Resources/ Ressourcesgénétiques animales/ Recursos genéticosanimales, 201 4.

Anjana Anjana, Siran Mukerji, Purnendu Tripathi. "Prospects of Agriculture as a Lifelong Livelihood Option for Young Indian Rural Population", International Journal of Social Ecology and Sustainable Development, 2022.

Annual Report.2008 & 2010. Central Sheep & Wool Research Institute, Avikanagar.

Ashkanasy N S and Daus C S (2005), "Rumors of the Death of Emotional Intelligence in Organizational Behaviour are Vastly Exaggerated", Journal of Organizational Behaviour, Vol. 26, pp. 441-452.

Atteh, O.D. (1989). Indigenous local knowledge as key to local-level development:possibilities,constraints and planning issues in the context of Africa. Seminar onreviving local self-reliance: challenges for rural/regional development in Eastern andSouthern Africa.

B. Sudhakar Rao. "Rural Infrastructure: A Critical Issue for Farm Productivity in Asia", Asia-Pacific Journal of Rural Development, 2019.

BAHS,2014.http://dahd.nic.in/dahd/WriteReadData/Final%20BAHS%202014%2011.03.2015.pdf.

Balaji, N and Chakravarthi, P (2010). Ethnoveterinary practices in India- a review. Veterinary World, Vol. 3(12) pp 549-551.

Banhotra, A. and Gupta, J. 2016. Mapping of indigenous technical knowledge (ITK) on animal healthcare and validation of ITK's used for treatment of pneumonia in dairy animals. Indian Journal of Traditional Knowledge, 15 (2): 297-303.

Barau, D.A. and Olukosi, J.O. (2011) Logical Framework Analysis (LFA): An Essential Tool for Designing Agricultural Project Evaluation. Nigerian Journal of Basic and Applied Science.19(2): 260-268.

Benjamin J, Bessant J, Watts R; Making Groups Work: Rethinking Practices, Allen and Unwin, St. Leonards. 1997.

Bhatia, S. and Arora, R. 2005.Biodiversity and Conservation of Indian Sheep Genetic Resources - An Overview-Asian-Aust. J. Anim. Sci. 2005. 18(10): 1387-1402.

Bierenia L., Hill J; Virtual Mentoring and Human Resources Development. Advances in Developing Human Resources, 2009; 7 (4): 556 -568.

Birner Regina and Anderson Jock R (2007). How to Make Agricultural Extension Demand-Driven? The Case of India's Agricultural Extension Policy IFPRI Discussion Paper 00729.

Bizimana Nseknye 1997 Scientific evidence of efficacy of medicinal plants for animal treatment, Ethno veterinary Medicine: Alternatives for Livestock Development, Proceedings of an International Conference held in Pune, 4-6 Nov, 2: Abstracts, pp.11-12.

Boswell, W.R. and Boudreau, J.W. (2002) Separating the Developmental and Evaluative Performance Appraisal Uses. Journal of Business and Psychology.16: 391–412 https://doi. org /10.1023/ A:1012872907525.

Brackett M A, Rivers S E and Salovey P (2011), "Emotional Intelligence: Implications for Personal, Social, Academic and Workplace Success",Social & Personal Psychology Compass, Vol.5, No.1, pp. 88-103.

Brautigam, Deborah. 1991. "Governance: A Review." World Bank, Policy and Review Department, Washington, D.C.

Buresh, R.S., Cooper, P.S.M. (1999). The Science and Practise of Short-Term Improved Fallows: Symposium Synthesis and Recommendations. Agroforestry Syst., 47: 345-356.

Buzan, T.(1993) The Mind Map Book, 6 September 1993, ISBN 0-563-36373-8.

Capacity Building: file:///G:/CB_1/Capacity%20building%20-%20Wikipedia.html.Approach to training extension personnel.icarzcu3.gov.in › pdf › Technical › 8.pdf.

Cavalcanti C, Economic thinking, traditional economical knowledge and ethno economics, Curr. Socio, 50 (2002), 39-45.

Centre for Good Governance (2017). Handbook on Problem Solving Skills .

Chambers, R. 1987. Rural dev. Putting the last first.Longman Scientific and Technical,Essex. Pp 191-218.

Chander, M. and Prakashkumar, R. (2013). Investment in livestock extension activities by State Departments of Animal Husbandry (SDAH) in India: An appraisal. Indian Journal of Animal sciences, 83(2):185-189.

Chikaire J.U., Ani A.O., Atoma C.N., and Tijjani A.R; Capacity Building: Key to Agricultural Extension Survival. Scholars Journal of Agriculture and Veterinary Sciences, 2015; 2(1A):13-21.

Cohen, R.D.H., Sykes, C.D., Wheaton, E.E. and Stevens, J.P., 2002."Evaluation of the effects of Climate Change on Forage and Livestock Production and Assessment of Adaptation Strategies on the Canadian Prairies".University of Saskatchewan, Saskatoon.

Couillard, J., Garon, S. and Riznic, J. (2009) The Logical Framework Approach-Millennium. Project Management Journal.40(4):31-44. doi:10.1002/pmj.20117.

Coutts J, Roberts K, Frost F, Coutts A;Role of Extension in Building Capacity-What Works, and Why. 2005. Available at www.fao.org./sd/exdirect/Exan0015.htm.

Cruz R. V., et al. 2007 Asia. Climate change 2007: impacts, adaptation and vulnerability. In Contribution of Working Group II to the Fourth Assessment Report of the Intergovernmental Panel on Climate Change (eds Parry M. L., Canziani O. F., Palutikof J. P., van der Linden P. J., Hanson C. E.), pp. 469–506. Cambridge, UK: Cambridge University Press.

Curzi, Y., Fabbri, T., Scapolan, A. and Boscolo, S. (2019) Performance Appraisal and Innovative Behaviour in the Digital Era. Frontiers in Psychology. 10:1659. doi: 10.3389/fpsyg.2019.01659.

DAHD 2013.http://www.dahd.nic.in/dahd/bahs-2013.aspx.

Das, A., Raju, R. and Patnaik, N. M. (2020). Present Scenario and Role of Livestock Sector in Rural Economy of India: A Review. Int. J.Livest. Res, 10:23-30.

De Amitendu, H.P.S. Arya, B. Tudu and A. Goswami, 2004.Indigenous Technical Knowledge in Animal Husbandry.Livestock Research for Rural Development 16(8).

De Villiers K Anne 1996 Quantifying indigenous knowledge: A rapid method for assessing crop performance without field trials. Agricultural Research and Extension Network, Agren, July 1996.

de_Richter, Renaud K., Tingzhen Ming, Sylvain Caillol, and Wei Liu. "Fighting global warming by GHG removal: Destroying CFCs and HCFCs in solar-wind power plant hybrids producing renewable energy with no-intermittency", International Journal of Greenhouse Gas Control, 201 6.

Department of Agricultural Research and Education-DARE (2019). DARE gazette notification 2019. Ministry of Agriculture and Farmers' Welfare, Govt. of India, Retrieved from http://www.nbagr.res.in/Gazette.pdf.

Department of Animal Husbandry, Dairying and Fisheries-DADF (2019). DADF annual report 2018-19. Ministry of Agriculture & Farmers Welfare, Government of India, Retrieved from http://dadf.gov.in/sites/default/filess/Annual%20Report.pdf.

Deshmukh RR, Rathod VN and Pardeshi VN (2011). Ethno-veterinary medicine from Jalna.

Devaki, K and Mathialagan, P. 2015. Animal husbandry traditional knowledge in Kancheepuram district.International Journal of Science, Environment and Technology, 4(5):1289 – 1295.

Devendra, C and Burns, M. (1983), Goat production in the Tropics (Second Edition), Commonw, Agric. Bur., Fernham, Buckinghamshire, U.K, 183 pp.

Devendra, C. (1991), Goat production: An International perspective. Proceedings of the International Goat production Symposium. Tallahassee. Florida.

Dewalt, B.R. (1994). "Using indigenous knowledge to improve agriculture and natural Resource management."Human Organization 53 (2).pp.123-131.

Dey, M.M.& H.K. Upadhyaya. 1996. Yield Loss Due to Drought, Cold &Submergence Tolerance. District of Maharashtra state. Indian Journal of Traditional Knowledge,10(2):344-348.

Dourmad, J., Rigolot, C., and Hayo van der Werf, 2008.Emission of Greenhouse Gas: Developing management and animal farming systems to assist mitigation. Livestock and Global Change conference proceeding. May 2008, Tunisia.

Emery, A.R. (1996). The Participation of Indigenous Peoples & Their Knowledge inEnvironmental Assessment &Dev. Planning (draft). Centre for Traditional Knowledge: Ottawa, Canada.

Epstein, H. (1974). Vanishing livestock breeds in Africa and Asia. In: Proc. Ist World Congr. Genet.Appl. Livest. Prod. Editorial Garsi, Madrid 11:31-35.

Ethno-veterinary Medicine, Springer Science and Business Media LLC, 2020.

Extension and advisory services: at the frontline of the response to COVID-1 9 to ensure food security, Food and Agriculture Organization of the United Nations (FAO), 2020.

FAO, 2001.Production yearbook.FAO, Production year book (1998-2000).

FAO, 2009.Enabling agriculture to contribute to climate change mitigation. FAO, Rome.

FAO. (2007).In: Gender and Food Security : Women hold the key to food security. Published by Food and Agriculture Organization of the United Nations, Rome.

Flood, R.L (1995) Solving Problem Solving: A Potent Force for Effective Management. New York, Ny: Wiley.

FourParadigmsofAgriculturalExtension. RetrievedOctober8,2014, fromMy AgriculturalInformation Bank: http://agriinfo. in/default.aspx?page=topic&superid=7&topicid=1441.

Fulzule, R.M. and Meena, B.L. (1995). Training Needs of Tribal Women. Indian J. Dairy. Sc. 48: 551-553.

Fulzule, R.M. and Meena, B.L. (1995). Training Needs of Tribal Women. Indian J. Dairy. Sc. 48: 551-553.

G.R. Gowane, L.L.L. Prince, F.B. Lopes, C. Paswan, R.C. Sharma. "Genetic and phenotypic parameter estimates of live weight and daily gain traits in Malpura sheep using Bayesian approach", Small Ruminant Research, 2015.

Gardner, H. (1983). Frames of Mind. New York: Basic Book Inc.

Gerber, P. J., H. Steinfeld, B. Henderson, A. Mottet, C. Opio, J. Dijkman, A. Falcucci, and G. Tempio. 2013.Tackling climate change through livestock: a global assessment of emissions and mitigation opportunities. Rome: FAO. http://www.fao.org/3/a-i3437e.pdfGoogle Scholar.

Getachew Bekele Fereja. "The Impacts of Climate Change On Livestock Production and Productivities In Developing Countries: A Review", International Journal Of Research Granthaalayah, 201 6.

Ghatawal Jitendra Pal and BasavaprabhuJirli (2016) New Media activism among young learners, Journal of Global Communication. Vol 9 (special issue) Pp: 355-366.

Ghatawal Jitendra Pal and BasavaprabhuJirli (2018) Communication And Psychological Profile Of Central Office Employees Of Banaras Hindu University, International Journal of Agriculture Sciences (ISSN: 0975-3710 & E-ISSN: 0975-9107), Volume 10, Issue 12, 2018, pp.-6459-6461.

Ghatawal Jitendra Pal, JirliBasavaprabhu and Singh Awadhesh Kumar (2016) Recognition and Utility of NewMedia for Students.International Journal of Agriculture Sciences, Vol.8, No. 53, 2016, pp.-2761-2764 (ISSN: 0975-3710&E-ISSN: 09759107).

Girard B. (Ed), (1992), A Passion for Radio: Radio waves and community, Montreal: Black Rose Books. Library of Congress, electronic edition published in 2001 by Bruce Girard & Comunica – www.communica.org/passion retrieved on 27.01.2022).

GOI, (2016a), National Intellectual Property Rights Policy. Department of Industrial Policy and promotion.Ministry of Commerce and Industry, Government oflndia.

Goleman D (1995), "Emotional Intelligence", Bantam Books, New York.

Gopal R. Gowane, Arun Kumar, Chanda Nimbkar. "Challenges and opportunities to livestock breeding programmes in India", Journal of Animal Breeding and Genetics, 2019.

Harvir Singh Kasana, Krishna Dev Kumar. "Chapter 9 Project Management", Springer Science and Business Media LLC, 2004.

Hilderbrand ME; Capacity for Poverty Reduction: Reflection on Evaluations of System Efforts: IN Capacity Building for Poverty Eradication Analysis of, and Lessons from Evaluations of UN System Support to Countries; Efforts. United Nations, New York. 2008.

Hopkin-Thompson PA; Colleagues Helping Colleagues: Mentoring and Coaching. NASSP Bulletin, 2000; 85 (617): 28 – 36.

Hord SM; Professional learning communities: Communities of continuous inquiry and improvement. 1997.

Horton D; Evaluating capacity development: experiences from research and development organizations around the world. IDRC. 2003.

Horton D; Planning, Implementing and Evaluating Capacity Development. 2002. Available at www.portals.wI.wwr.bnl/files/ppne/capacity-development-isnar.pdg.

http://www.climate.org/topics/agriculture.html.

https://www.managementstudyguide.com/importance_of_motivation.htm.;https://www.linkedin.com.;https://www.courses.lumenlearning.com.https://www.mindtools.com.

Huitt, W.G. (2005)Current Trends in Psychology, Valdosta State University .

ICAR, (2006), ICAR Guidelines for Intellectual Property Management and Technology Transfer/ Commercialization.Indian Council of Agricultural Research, NewDelhi.

ICAR, (2014a), ICAR Rules and Guidelines for Professional Service Functions.Indian Council of Agricultural Research, New Delhi.

ICAR, (2014b), ICAR Guidelines for Internal Evaluation and Forwarding Research Papers to Scientific Journals and Data Management in ICAR Institutes. Indian Council of Agricultural Research, New Delhi.

ICAR, (2014c).National Agricultural Innovation Foundation.XII Plan EFC document approved.

IFAD, 2009.Comprehensive Report on IFAD's Response to Climate Change through Support to Adaptation and Related Actions.

IFPRI 2010. International Food Policy Research Institute- 2010 Annual Report.

IIRR (International Institute of Rural Reconstruction), (1996). Recording & Using IK- A Manual. IIRR: Silang, Philippines. IUCN/UNEP/WWF 1991 Summary - Caring for the Earth: A Strategy for Sustainable Living. Gland, Switzerland: IUCN/UNEP/WWF. Khartoum, Sudan: Khartoum University Press.

Indian Patent Office, Guidelines for processing of patent applications related to traditional knowledge and biological materials. Available at http://www.ipindia.nic.in /iponew/ TK_Guidelines_18 December 2012.pdf. Accessed on 06.03.2013.

Information resources on the internet. In: International Conference on Ethnoveterinary practices, 4th to 6th January 2010, Thanjavur, India.

IPCC (Inter-Governmental Panel on Climate Change). 2001. Third Assessment Report of the Intergovernmental Panel on Climate Change: The Scientific Basis (Working Group-I). Cambridge University Press, United Kingdom and NewYork, NY, USA, 881 pp.

IPCC . 2013. Summary for policymakers. In: Stocker, T.F., Qin, D., Plattner, G.K., Tignor, M., Allen, S.K., Boschung, J., Nauels, A., Xia, Y., Bex, V., Midgley, P.M., editors. Climate change 2013: the physical science basis. Contribution of Working Group I to the Fifth Assessment Report of the Intergovernmental Panel on Climate Change. Cambridge (UK)/ New York (NY): Cambridge University Press; p. 1535. Available from https://www.ipcc.ch/pdf/assessment-report/ar5/wg1/WGIAR5_SPM_brochure_en.pdfGoogle Scholar.

IPCC(Inter-Governmental Panel on Climate Change). 2007. Fourth Assessment Report of the Inter-governmental Panel on Climate Change: The Impacts, adaptation and vulnerability (Working Group III). Cambridge University Press, United Kingdom and New York, NY, USA.

J M Erskine. "Rural development: Putting theory into practice",Development Southern Africa, 1 985 jcreview.com.

Janis, I.L. (1982) Groupthink: psychological studies of policy decisions and fiascoes. Boston: Houghton Mifflin. ISBN 978-0-395-31704-4.

Jebáček, Ivo, and Marek Horák. "Measuring of a Nose Landing Gear Load during Take-Off and Landing", Applied Mechanics and Materials, 201 6.

Jennifer Mencl, Andrew J. Wefald, Kyle W. van Ittersum. "Transformational leader attributes: interpersonal skills, engagement & well being", Leadership & Organization Development Journal, 201 6.

Jessica A. Manzone, Julia Nyberg. "Chapter 4 Instruction-Expanded Virtual Education Model", IGI Global, 2021.

Jirli Basavaprabhu, Srivastava Susheel Kumar & Singh RSP (2006) A Study on attitude of UG students towards distance education in agriculture.JR. of Open Schooling Vol VI, No. 1 (Jan-June2006)pp.56-71.

JirliBasavaprabhu (2019) Paradigm shift in role of Extension Educationists in the light of e Mediated extension services Presented Lead paper in ISEE National Seminar on Socio Digital approaches for transforming Indian agriculture, November 20-22, 2019, CCS Haryana Agril University, Haryana.

JouniKuha, John H. Goldthorpe. "Path analysis for discrete variables: the role of education in social mobility", Journal of the Royal Statistical Society: Series A (Statistics in Society), 201 0.

Judge, T. A. and Ferris, G. R. (1993).Social Context of Performance Evaluation Decisions. The Academy of Management Journal. 36(1): 80–105. https://doi.org/10.2307/256513.

Judge, T.A., Ferris, G.R., 1993.Social Context of performance evaluation decisions. Academy of Management Journal 36 (1), 80–105.

Kalpana Sastry,R and Srivastava A. (2013). Emerging Intellectual Property Regimes and Traditional Knowledge Systems in Indian Agriculture. In: Indigenous traditional Knowledge for Promotion of Sustainable Agriculture, edited by V S Babu, K Suman Chandra & S M Ilyas (NIRD, Hyderabad, India), 2013,pp.145-160.

Kasana, Harvir Singh, and Krishna Dev Kumar. "Project Management", Introductory Operations Research, 2004.

Kinati, W. and Mulema, A. A. (2018). Gender issues in livestock production in Ethiopia. ILRI, Nairobi, Kenya.

Kogut B, Zander U; Knowledge of the firm, combinative capabilities, and the replication of technology. Organization science, 1992; 3(3):383-397.

Kothari Ashish (2015). —The seeds of revolution‖, India Together, October 30, 2015.

Kramer C Y 1957 Extn. of multiple range tests to group correlated means. Biometrics, 13: 13-18.

Kuhn, T.S. 1962. The structure of scientific revolutions.International Encyclopedia of United Science. USA.

Kujur Grace, M.N. Jha, B.N. Chaudhary, D.C. Kabdal, V.S. Deepkumar, R.C. Singh, P.A Deshmukh (2009), Media Support to Agriculture Extension: success stories of All India Radio, Prasarbharati, New Delhi.

Kumar, V and Sinha, K, (2015.) Status and Challenges of IPR in Agricultural Innovation inIndia". Journal of Intellectual Property Rights. Vol. 20, pp. 288-296.

L. Dash, S. Das, S. Mohanty, F. H. Rahman, S. K. Sahoo and S. N. Mishra (2020). Platform Based Housing System Improved Health and Reduced Mortality Percentage of Goats in FloodProne Area of Coastal Odisha. Advances in Research, 2020, 21(8): 10-17.

Larson, C. E., LaFasto, F. M. J. (1989). Teamwork: What must go right, what can go wrong. Newberry Park, CA: Sage.

Leichtman, H.M(1996) Helping Work Environments Work. Washington, D.C.: Cwla Press.

Lopes P N, Cote S and Salovey P (2006a), "An Ability Model of Emotional Intelligence: Implications for Assessment and Training. In Durskat V F, Sala & Mount G (Eds.) Linking Emotional Intelligence and Performance at Work, pp. 53-80, Lawrence Erlbaum Associates, Mahwah, NJ.

Lopes P N, Grewal D, Kadis J, Gall M and Salovey P (2006b), "Evidence that Emotional Intelligence is Related to Job Performance and Affect and Attitude at Work, Psicothema, Vol. 18, pp. 132-138.

Lu L, Cooper C L, Kao S F and. Zhou Y (2003), "Work Stress, Control Beliefs and Well-Being in Greater China: An Exploration of Sub-Cultural Differences between the PRC and Taiwan", Journal of Managerial Psychology, Vol. 18, No. 6, pp. 479-510.

M Utomo, L Pieter. "Strengthening Indonesian Farmers' Resilience Capacity of Disasters and Climate Change Through Development of Decision Support System: Challenges Lie Ahead", IOP Conference Series: Earth and Environmental Science, 2022.

Machiadikwe N Benjamin, Agbareevo Nwogu and Nmenna Victoria (2016). Level of Extension Agents Motivation and Effectiveness in Abia State, Nigeria: International Journal of Scientific and technology Research, Vol. 5 (04), April 2022.,

Macy, B. A., & Izumi, H. (1993). Organizational change, design and work innovation: A meta-analysis of 131 North American field experiments, 1961-1991. In W. Pasmore& R. Woodman (Eds.), Research in organizational change and development (pp. 235-313). Greenwich, CT: JAI.

Madhu, Pattanashetti and D.A. Nithya, (2012), —Awareness and preference of Krishi community radio programmes‖ Karnataka Journal of Agricultural Sciences, Vol. 25, No. 4, University of Agricultural Sciences, Dharwad, Karnataka.

MaharaGirijesh Singh, BasavaprabhuJirli and Ashok Rai (2013) m-Learning: An educational approach for Change in Hills of Uttarakhand. Journal of Global Communication.Vol 6 No. 2. Pp: 144-150.

MahekhkaAnuja (2007-08). Dissertation submitted to Mudra Institute of Communication, Ahmedabad.

Malathi Subramanian. "Chapter 1 6 Rural E Governance through the "Panchayati Raj" Institutions in India", IGI Global, 201 2.

Malik, K.K., &Pavarala, V. (2007). Other Voices: The struggle for community radio in India. Thousand Oaks, CA: Sage Publications.

Mandal Pankaj Kumar, Kirti and BasavaprabhuJirli (2016) Role of Information and Communication Technologies in Rural Development Journal of Global Communication. Vol 9 (special issue) Pp:129-133.

Martins A, Ramalho N and Morin E (2010), "A Comprehensive Meta-Analysis of the Relationship between Emotional Intelligence & Health", JR. of Personality & Individual Differences, Vol. 49, pp. 554-564.

Mathauda SS, Mavi HS, Bhangoo BS, Dhaliwal BK (2000). Impact of projected climate change on rice production in Punjab (India),Tropical Ecology 41(1): 95-98.

Mathur J.C and Neurath Paul (1959), —An Indian Experiment in Farm Radio Forums‖, UNESCO, Paris.

Mati BM; Capacity Development for Smallholder Irrigation in Kenya. International Crops Research Institute for Semi-Arid Tropics, Kenya, Nairobi. 2008.

May, Markham, Warr, Sue. "EBOOK: Teaching Creative Arts & Media 1 4+", EBOOK: Teaching Creative Arts & Media 1 4+, 201 1.

Mayer J D and Salovey P (1997), "What is Emotional Intelligence?" In: Salovey P and Sluyter D (Eds.). Emotional Development and Emotional Intelligence: Educational Implications. Basic Books, New York, pp. 3-31.

Mayer, R.E (1992) Thinking, Problem Solving, Cognition.2nd Ed. New York, Ny: W.H. Freeman.

Meena, R.L., B. Jirli, M. Kanwat and Meena, N.K. (2018).Mobile Applications for Agriculture and Allied Sector.Int.J.Curr.Microbiol.App.Sci.7(02), Pp: 2317-2326.

Milkovich, G. T. and Boudreau, J. W. (1997), Human Resource Mgmt, The McGraw-Hill companies Inc. U.S.A.

Millar J, Photakoun V, Connell J; Scaling Out Impacts: A Study of Three Methods for Introducing Forage Technologies to Villages in Lao PDR. Australian Center for I[nt]ernational Agricultural research,Australia. 2005.

Mishra D.C. (1990). New Directions In Extension Training. Dir. of Extension, Min. of Agriculture. New Delhi.

Mohammad Faysal Sarker , 2016, The Impact of Motivation on the Performance of Employees, Munich, GRIN Verlag, https://www.grin.com/document/376007.

Mohammad, A. and Singh, K. (2010) Management in Extension. Published by Director, National Dairy Research Institute, Karnal. Haryana.

N. B.Narasimha Prasad, E. Abdul Hameed. "Groundwater Management Strategies for Lakshadweep Island—A Case Study", ISH Journal of Hydraulic Engineering, 201 0.

Nafees Meah, Sheetal Sharma. "Chapter 1 9-1 Climate-Resilient Agricultural Development in the Global South", Springer Science and Business Media LLC, 2021.

Nagel, U. J. 1997. Chapter 2 – Alternative approaches to organizing extension: In: Improving Agricultural extension: A referenceManual. Swason B.E., R.PBentz a n d A.J. ofranko(eds). FAO.

Nasrullah, Amir(Dickson, K). "Critical analysis of micro enterprise policy development in developing countries: A case of Bangladesh", Brunel University Brunel Business School PhD Theses, 201 2.

NAVS 2015. Ethno-veterinary Medicine: A Concept for Sustainable Livestock Production.

NBA, (2008).The Biological Diversity Act 2002. At: http://nbaindia.org/content/25/19/1/act.html[Accessed on May 20,2016].

Nguyen, V.N. (2004). FAO programme on hybrid rice development &and use for food security and livelihood improvement. Paper presented at the Concluding Workshop of IRRI-ADB funded project 'Sustaining Food Security in Asia through Dev. of Hybrid Rice Technology', IRRI, Los Baños, Philippines,7–9, Dec. 2004.

Nikunj Rajyaguru, Shubhendu Vyas, Kunjan Vyas. "9 Internet of things platform for smart farming", Walter de Gruyter GmbH, 2021.

NITI Aayog, (2016).National Institution for Transforming India.At: http://niti.gov.in /content/self-employment-talent-utilization. [Accessed as on May26,2016].

Njuki, J. and Sanginga, P.C. (2013). In: Women, livestock ownership and markets: Bridging the gender gap in eastern and southern Africa. New York, USA: Earthscan USA/International Development Research Centre, Canada. Page 1-7.

Nongtdu G., Bordoloi R., Saravanan R., Singh R., & Singh N.U. (2012). Training Needs of Agricultural Extension Personnel in Meghalaya, Indian Journal of Hill Farming 25(1):1-8. kiran.nic.in › pdf › IJHF › Vol25_1 › Training_Needs.

Noor Wani, A Hakeem, Rahat Wani, Junaid Rishu. "Information and Communication Technology in Agriculture: A Kashmir Perspective", Asian Journal of Agricultural Extension, Economics & Sociology, 201 7.

Northouse, G. (2007). Leadership Theory and Practice.(3rd ed.) Thousand Oaks, CA: Sage Publications, Inc.

Office of Controller General of Patents Designs and Trade Marks.(2016). http://www.ipindia.nic.in/IPActs_Rules/IPActs_Rules.htm. [Accessed on June15,2016].

P. Biswas, B. Mahato, D. C. Mahato, F. H. Rahmanand Chinanshuk Ghosh (2020). Effect of Vermi-compost and Biochar on Growth andYield of Carrot in Red Lateritic Soils of Purulia District of West Bengal. International Journal of Plant & Soil Science, 2020, 32(8): 15-20.

Policy Paper No. 3. National Academy of Veterinary Sciences (India), New Delhi.

Ponnusamy. K, Gupa. J and Nagarajan, R (2009) Indigenous technical knowledge (ITK) in dairy .

PPV&FR Authority.(2016) Protection of Plant Varieties & Farmers' Rights Act, 2001.http://www. plantauthority.gov.in/gazette.htm. [Accessed on June15,2016].

Prajwalita Pathak, Vivek Kumar Nayak, Rebeka Sinha, Bilal Ahmad Ganaie. "Review on small ruminant conservation status and prospects in India", Tropical Animal Health and Production, 2020.

Punsalmaa B., 2006. Climate Change Vulnerability and Adaptation in the Livestock Sector of Mongolia. AIAAC, project No. AS06. Washington, USA.

R Nisha, R Arunachalam. "A study on awareness and adoption of the rational ITKs in Tea crop among the Hilly Tribes", Asian Journal of Agricultural Extension, Economics & Sociology, 2018.

R. Thangadurai, Srikant Sharma, Dushyant Bali, B.P. Rana, Vivek Mahajan, IndranilSamanta, SarbaniHazra. "Prevalence of Ocular Disorders in an Indian Population of Horses", Journal of Equine Veterinary Science, 201 0.

R.E. Evenson, R.W. Herdt, and M.Hossain, (eds.), Rice Research in Asia: Progress and Priorities. UK:International Rice Research Institute in Collaboration with CAB International; 1996.

Rai Ashok and BasavaprabhuJirli (2013) Information Technologies for e-Readiness.Journal of Communication Studies.Vol 31 No. December 2013 Pp: 28-33 (ISSN: 0970-554).

Rai Ashok, BasavaprabhuJirli and Abhishek Singh (2016) e-Readiness 4D: An Analysis Journal of Global Communication. Vol 9 No.1 Pp: 22-31.

Rai Ashok, BasavaprabhuJirli and Abhishek Singh (2018) e-Readiness: Its Relational Perspectives with Profile of Extension Functionaries. Journal of Global Communication.Vol. 11, No. 1, January-June 2018:65-75.

Rangnekar, D.V. 1998. Random thoughts on Ethno veterinary Practices and their Validation in relation to Livestock Development in India. ICAR short course entitled "Techniques for scientific validation and Evaluation of Ethno veterinary practices" pp. 24-27.

Rao, S.V.N., and Jain, D.K., 1993. Screening of technologies, Proceedings of the All India Dairy Husbandry Officers' Workshop held at NDRI, Karnal from 2nd-3rd Dec, 1993, p.40-46.

Rathinasabapathy, G, Rajasundaram, R.C and Punniamurthy. N, Ethnoveterinary medicine .

Ravikumar, R.K., D. Thakur, H. Choudhary, V. Kumar, A. S. Kinhekar, T. Garg, K. Ponnusamy, G.R. Bhojne, V.M. Shetty and V. Kumar, 2017. Social engineering of societal knowledge in livestock science: Can we be more empathetic? Veterinary World, 10(1): 86-91.

Ray, G. L. and Mondal, S. (2014) Research Methods in Social Sciences & Extension Education. Kalyani Publishers.

Reddy, M. N., and Swanson, B.E. (2006).Strategy for up-scaling the ATMA model inIndia. In Proceedings of the Association for International Agricultural and Extension Education (AIAEE) 22nd Annual Conference, Clearwater Beach,Florida, U.S.A.

Reforming and strengthening public agricultural extension and advisory service systems in smallholder farming", Food and Agriculture Organization of the United Nations (FAO), 2021

Richard Graham Nelson, Amir Azaron, SaminAref. "The use of a GERT based method to model concurrent product development processes", European Journal of Operational Research, 201 6 ride2rich.com.

Rohit Joshi, Atulya Narayan. "Performance Measurement Model for Agriculture Extension Services for Sustainable Livelihood of the Farmers: Evidences from India", Theoretical Economics Letters, 201 9 rtikolkata.cag.gov.in.

Rotberg, Robert (July 2014). "Good Governance Means Performance and Results". Governance.

S P Mukherjee, Bikas K Sinha, Asis Kumar Chattopadhyay. "Statistical Methods in Social Science Research", Springer Science and Business Media LLC, 201 8.

S. Bhatia, R. Arora. "Biodiversity and Conservation of Indian Sheep Genetic Resources - An Overview -", Asian Australasian Journal of Animal Sciences, 2005.

S. Pradhan, F. H. Rahman, S. Sethy, G. Pradhan and J. Sen (2020).Evaluation of Short Duration Drought Tolerant RiceVarieties in Drought Prone Areas of SubarnapurDistrict of Odisha. International Journal of Plant & Soil Science, 2020, 32(8): 21-26.

S. Sarkar, G. Das, F. H. Rahman, S. Biswas, S. Sarkar, S. Saha and B. Roy (2020). A Study on Use of Black Polythene Mulch as a Climate Smart Technology on Performance ofWinter Cucumber and Resource ConservationInTeraiAgro-climatic Zone of West Bengal. Current Journal of Applied Science and Technology, 2020, 39(12): 100-106.

Salas, E., Diazgranados, D., Klein, C., Burke, C. S., Stagl, K. C., Goodwin, G. F., &Halpin, S. M. (2009). Does Team Training Improve Team Performance? A Meta-Analysis. Human Factors: The Journal of the Human Factors and Ergonomics Society, 50(6), 903-933. doi: 10.1518/001872008X375009.

Salovey P and Grewal D (2005), "The Science of Emotional Intelligence", American Psychological Society, Vol. 14, pp. 281-285.

Salovey P and Mayer J D (1990), "Emotional Intelligence", Imagination, Cognition and Personality, Vol. 9, pp. 185-211.

Samir Yerpude, Tarun Kumar Singhal. "Enhancing New Product Development Effectiveness With Internet of Things Origin Real Time Data", Journal of Cases on Information Technology, 201 8.

Samuel, M.P., Sastry, Kalpana. R., Venkattakumar, R, (2014),"Status and prospects of IP regime in India: Implication forAgril. Education". Journal of IPR, Vol. 19, pp. 189- 201.

Sanborn, L. O., and Huszczo, G. E. (2007) "Encyclopedia of Industrial and Organizational Psychology." Thousand Oaks, CA: SAGE Publications, pp. 788-790. Web. 10 Nov. 2014. <http://dx.doi.org/10.4135/9781412952651>.

Sartorius, R.H. (1991) The logical framework approach to project design and management. Evaluation Practice. 12(2): 139-147 .

Sedigheh Nader Abadi, Hadi Aghassi, Emad Roghanian. "A multi-attribute GA for piecewise linear Time-Cost Trade-off Scheduling optimization", 201 1 World Congress on Information and Communication Technologies, 201 1.

Shawn Harmon, Graham Dutfield& Patricia Barclay (2010). Knowledge management & contextualization of IPR in innovation systems, SCRIPTed, 7 (1) (2010)32.-43.

Sheena Carlisle, Martin Kunc, Eleri Jones, Scott Tiffin. "Supporting innovation for tourism development through multi-stakeholder approaches: Experiences from Africa", Tourism Management, 201 3.

Shubeena, S., A. Hai, S.A. Hamdani and A.H. Akand, 2018. Indigenous Technical Knowledge (ITKs) Used by Farmers of Central Kashmir to Increase Production and Reproduction in Livestock. International Journal of Livestock Research, 8(8), 294-302.

Shubhransu Nayak, Satyaranjan Behera, Prasad Kumar Dash. "Potential of Microbia Diversity of Coastal Sand Dunes: Need for Exploration in Odisha Coast of India", The Scientific World Journal, 201 9.

Sidahmed, A. 2008.Livestock & Climate Change:Coping& Risk Management Strategies for a Sustainable Future. In Livestock & Global Climate Change conference proceeding, May 2008, Tunisia.

Simon,H.A.(1972) Human Problem Solving. Prentice Hall, Englewood Cliffs, NJ, (1972). "the most important book on the scientific study of human thinking in the 20th century".

Singh Akanchha and BasavaprabhuJirli (2018) Changing Perception and Awareness towards ICT along with Changing Roles of Stakeholders in Agriculture.Research Journal of Agril. Sciences Vol9(6):Pp.1412-1416, November-December (2018)(ISSN:0976-1675).

Singh, K.M., Meena, M.S., Swanson, B.E., Reddy, M.N. and Bahal,R.(2014) In-depth Study of the PluralisticAgricultural Extension System in India, MPRA Paper No. 59461, posted 26. October 2014 01:07 UTC, http://mpra.ub.uni-muenchen.de/59461.

Slote, M. (1983) Goods and virtues. Oxford: Clarendon Press.

Snedecor G W and Cochran W G 1994 Statistical Methods, 8th ed. Affiliated East-West Press, New Delhi.

Soam, S.K. (2009) Project Logical Framework. Published in Resource material-1 of Foundation Course for Agricultural Research Service. NAARM , Rajendranagar, Hyderabad.

Sonavale, K. P., Shaikh, M. R., Kadam, M. M. and Pokharkar, V. G. (2020). Livestock sector in India: a critical analysis. Asian J. Agri. Ext. Eco.Socio., 38(1):51-62.

Stella C. Nduka, Adetoun A. Oyelude. "Goge Africa: Preserving Indigenous Knowledge Innovatively through Mass Media Technology", Preservation, Digital Technology & Culture, 201 9.

Stephen P, Brien N, Triraganon R; Capacity Building for CBNRM in Asia: A Regional Review. 2006. Available at www.elcoftc.org/site/fundmm/dois/CABS/idrc-review.pdf.

Sternberg, R. J. (1994) Thinking and Problem Solving. 2nd Ed. San Diego, Ca: Academic Press.

Sulaiman, R.V. and Hall A.J. (2002) An innovation system perspective on the restructuring of agricultural extension- evidence from India, Outlook on Agriculture 30(4);235-243.

Sulaiman, R.V. and Hall A.J. (2004) Towards Extension Plus: opportunities & Challenges (Policy Brief). National Centre for Agriculture Economics & Policy research, ICAR, New Delhi.

Sulaiman, R.V. and Hall A.J. (2017).The Emergence of Extension Plus: Future for Extension-Beyond TOT. Agriculture and Rural Development Discussion Paper 8; Extension Reform for Rural Development. https://www.researchgate.net/publication/316736871.

Sulaiman, R.V., Hall, A.J. and Suresh, N. (2004) Emerging trends in private extension provision: a case of MSSL in India, Ag Ren Network Paper (forthcoming), Overseas Development Institute, UK.

Sunita Raina. "Chapter-6:Agricultural Extension Agents and Challenges for Sustainable Development", Springer Science and Business Media LLC, 2020.

Swanson B E (2006) The changing role of agricultural extension in a global economy. Journal of International Agricultural and Extension Education, 13(3):5-17.

Swanson R.A.(1984). Forecasting the economic bebefits of training, Performance and Institutional Journal.24(7): 10-11.

Swason, B.E. 2010.Changing extension paradigms within a rapidly changing global Economy. Rural Dev. News. "Advances in Construction Management", Springer Science and Business Media LLC, 2022

T. R. Sahoo, P. Mishra, F. H. Rahman, N. M. Mohapatra and S. N. Mishra (2020).The Response of Green Manuring of Sesbaniaaculeateon growth and Yield of Rice in Flood ProneArea of Coastal Odisha.Current Journal of Applied Science and Technology, 2020, 39(11): 13-1.

Tabing, L (2005), —How to Do Community Radio: A premier for community radio operators, UNESCO, New Delhi.

Thakur, D. and Chandra, M. (2006). Gender Based Differential access to information among livestock owners and its compact on household milk production. Indian J. Dairy. Sc. 59(6):401-404. https://www.unescap.org/sites/default/files/good-governance.pdf retrieved on 22/01/2022 at 14:32 hrs.

Thakur, D. and Chandra, M. (2006). Gender Based Differential access to information among livestock owners and its compact on household milk production. Indian J. Dairy. Sc.59(6):401-404.

The IMF and Good Governance, IMF. https://www.imf.org/en/About/Factsheets/The-IMF-and-Good-Governance Retrieved on January 26,2022.

The Sundarbans: A Disaster-Prone Eco Region, Springer Science and Business Media LLC, 201 9.

Thornton P., Herrero M., Freeman A., Mwai O., Rege E., Jones P., and McDermott J., 2008. "Vulnerability, Climate Change & Livestock – Research Opportunities & Challenges for Poverty Alleviation". ILRI, Kenya.

Understanding the links between agril. & health, International Food Policy Research Institute (IFPRI), 2006

United Nations. (1997). In: Report of the Economic and Social Council for 1997. A/52/3, Retrieved 18 September 1997 from www.un.org.

Usha Das, Souvik Ghosh. "Factors driving farmers' knowledge on climate change in a climatically vulnerable state of India", Natural Hazards, 2020.

V M Harivallabha, I Anithamahalakshmi, S. SenthamizhSelvi. "A model to improve the reliability of ICT in agriculture", 201 6 IEEE Technological Innovations in ICT for Agriculture and Rural Development (TIAR), 2016.

Velmurugan Ayyam, SwarnamPalanivel, SivaperumanChandrakasan. "Chapter 22 Aquaculture-Based Systems for Harmonious Development of Coastal Region", Springer Science and Business Media LLC, 201 9.

Verma, M.R., and Singh, Y.P., 1969. A plea for studies in Traditional Animal Husbandry. The Allahabad Farmer, 43(2): 93-98.

vikspedia.in. https://vikaspedia.in/agriculture/livestock/role-of-livestock-in-indian-economy (accessed on 12.02.2022).

WAAP book of the year - 2005, Wageningen Academic Publishers, 2005.

Warren,D.M. Using Indigenous Knowledge in Agricultural Development, World Bank Discussion Paper 127, Washington, 1991.

Wassmann, R., N.X. Hien, C.T. Hoanh, T.P. Tuong. 2004. Sea Level Rise affecting Vietnamese Mekong Delta: Water Elevation in Flood Season and Implications for Rice Production. Climatic Change 66 (1):89-107 .

World Bank (1997)"Knowledge and skills for information age, the first meeting of the Mediterranean Development forum" Mediterranean Development Forum, URL. http://www. worldbank. org/html/fpd/technet/mdf/objective.htm.

World Bank, 2007.Climate change adaptation in Africa: a microeconomic analysis of livestock choice. World Bank Policy Research Working Paper No. 4277, July 2007.

World Health Organization.(2003).In:Sexual health, human rights & the law. Geneva, ISBN 978-9241564984.

World Resources Institute. 2007. Earth Trends: Environmental Information. Available at http:// earthtrends.wri.org.

WTO,(2016).Overview: The TRIPS Agreement. At: https://www.wto.org/english /tratop_e/ trips_e/intel2_e.htm(Accessed on June15,2016).

Yakubu, DH, BZ Abubakar, TK Atala, and A Muhammed. "Use of Information and Communication Technologies among Extension Agents In Kano State, Nigeria", Journal of Agricultural Extension, 201 3.

ZhaoyuZhai, José Fernán Martínez, Victoria Beltran, Néstor Lucas Martínez. "Decision support systems for agriculture 4.0: Survey and challenges", Computers and Electronics in Agriculture, 2020.

Thesis/Dissertation Referred

Submitte to ABI College; American Intercontinental University Online; American Public University System; American University in the Emirates; Amity University; Arab Open University; Asia Pacific International College; Aspen University; Association of Business Executives; Ayrshire Regional College; Batangas State University; Bihar Agricultural University; Bridgepoint Education; Central Queensland University; Chandigarh University; Christ

University; Colorado Technical University Online; Coventry University; CSU, Long Beach; CVC Nigeria Consortium; Danford College; EDMC; Ekiti; Far Eastern University; Federal Polytechnic, Ilaro; Fiji National University; Flinders University; Florida Institute of Technology; Georgia Military College; Great Zimbabwe University; Griffith College Dublin; Higher Education Commission Pakistan; Hindustan College of Science Technology; Indian Institute of Management; Institute of Art Design and Technology; Institute of Rural Management; Institute of Tourism Studies; Intercollege; Jamia Milia Islamia University; Kabarak University; Kentucky Wesleyan College; Kingston University; Kozep-europaiEgyetem; Laureate Higher Education Group; Leeds Metropolitan University; London School of Science & Technology; Maastricht School of Management; Mancosa; Manukau Institute of Technology; Middle East Technical University; Myerscough College, Lancashire; National Law University New Delhi; National School of Business Management NSBM, Sri Lanka; North West University; Ohio University; Orissa University of Agriculture & Technology; Oxford Brookes University; Regenesys Business School; Republic of the Maldives; Republic Polytechnic; Runshaw College, Lancashire; S.P. Jain Institute of Management and Research, Mumbai; Saint Paul University; Savannah State University; School of Business and Management ITB; Segi University College; Sikkim Manipal University, Ghana; SIM Global Education; Sim University; Southern New Hampshire University - Continuing Education; St. Petersburg College; Strayer University; Symbiosis International University; Teachers' Colleges of Jamaica; The Robert Gordon University; The WB National University of Juridical Sciences; Trevecca Nazarene University; Universiti Putra Malaysia; UniversitiTeknologi MARA; University of Derby; University of Dubai; University of East London; University of Greenwich; University of Hong Kong; University of KwaZulu-Natal; University of Leeds; University of Luton; University of Northampton; University of Northumbria at Newcastle; University of Queensland; University of Rwanda; University of Science and Technology, Yemen; University of South Africa; University of South Australia; University Of Tasmania; University of Technology, Sydney; University of the Philippines Los Banos; University of the Sunshine Coast; University of the West Indies; Univ. of Wales central institutions; University of Wales, Lampeter; University of Westminster; University of Witwatersrand; University of Zimbabwe; Visayas State University; Westford School of Management; XLRI Jamshedpur.

Website Referred

www.aarohilife.org; www.aau.ac.in; www.abongobimedia.com; www. academycool.com; www.activeremedy.org; www.aesanetwork.org; www.

aesonnigeria.org; www.aged.tamu.edu; www.agriclinics.net; www.agrigoaexpert.res.in; www.agriinfo.in; www.agrilinks.org; www.agris.nic.in; www.aguijrssh.com; www.ajas.info; www.aleap.org; www.alleducationjournal.com; www.animalmedicalresearch.org; www.antiessays.com; www.apexjournal.org; www.ardaf.org; www.assamagribusiness.nic.in; www.atarikolkata.org; www.authorstream.com; www.baif.org.in; www.basicknowledge101.com; www.betuco.be; www.biotecharticles.com; www.breathehr.com; www.britishecologicalsociety.org; www.care.org; www.cgg.gov.in; www.champa.kku.ac.th; www.chsd-theresacollege.net; www.cigr.org; www.citeman.com; www.clairenewton.co.za; www.companysarthi.com; www.conference.bonfring.org; www.coursehero.com; www.cred.be; www.crispindia.org; www.cropandweed.com; www.cmoe.com; www.c-rural.eu; www.csu.edu.au; www.daff.gov.za; www.devalt.org; www.dodl.klyuniv.ac.in; www.downtoearth.org.in; www.dphu.org; www.drishtiias.com; www.du.ac.in; www.eapk.org.ua; www.ecronicon.com; www.egyankosh.ac.in; www.elgaronline.com; www.employeepedia.com; www.entomoljournal.com; www.eolss.net; www.ethnovetweb.com; www.exinfm.com; www.extncon201 7.org; www.fao.org; www.frontiersin.org; www.gadfcs.org; www.geeksforgeeks.org; www.gjoee.org; www.globalacademicgroup.com; www.goodsensemaking.com; www.grin.com; www.gwp.org; www.harti.gov.lk; www.hillagric.ac.in; www.icfa.org.in; www.icrisat.org; www.iedunote.com; www.iedunote.com; www.ifad.org; www.ifpri.org; www.iicd.org; www.iimahd.ernet.in; www.ijmra.us; www.ijpab. com; www.ijstr.org; www.ilearncana.com; www.ilo.org; www.iloencyclopaedia.org; www. impactafya.com; www.indeed.com; www.indiagri.in; www.indiainfoline.com; www.indiastudychannel.com; www.inseeworld.com; www.internationalpolicybrief.org; www.iosrjournals.org; www.ipms-ethiopia.org; www.iqpcevents.com; www.ircwash.org; www.i-scholar.in; www.i-scholar.in; www.joe.org; www.kre publishers.com; www.krishisanskriti.org; www.krishisewa.com; www.lankaweb.com; www.lcsc.edu; www.lifeeducare.com; www.lkouniv.ac.in; www.local2030.org; www.lrrd.org; www.manage.gov.in; www.managementcentre.co.uk; www.managementskillscourses.com; www.mdpi.com; www.moef.nic.in; www.naarm.ernet.in; www.nature.com; www.navsindia.org; www.nbpgr.ernet.in; www.ncap.res.in; www.ncbi.nlm.nih.gov; www.ncirl.ie; www.nicra.iari.res.in; www.nicra-icar.in; www.nwlink.com; www.oer.unn.edu.ng; www.oerafrica.org; www.onlinegtu.com; www.organic-center.org; www.panchayat.gov.in; www.phyto journal.com; www.pops.int; www.printsasia.co.jp; www.projectenergize.org.nz; www.projecttopics.org; www.psychologytoday.com; Www.readbag.com; www.regioniiiems.com;

www.researcherslinks.com; www.researchgate.net; www.researchjournal.in; www.rural21.com; www. sac.org.bd; www.salto-youth.net; www.savjetodavna.hr; www.saylor.org; www.scielo.br; www.scopemed .org; www.scribd.com; www.searo.who.int; www.shirinzarqatherapist.com; www.simplilearn.com; www.slideshare.net; www.studymode.com; www.successtonicsblog.com; www.sundarini.organic; www.syngentafoundation.org; www.thehindubusinessline.com; www.thepharmajournal.com; www.toppers4u.com; www.toppr.com; www.udsspace.uds.edu.gh; www.ukessays.com; www.un.org; www.unescap.org; www.united.ac.in;

www.universityofcalicut.info; www.uou.ac.in; www.Valamis.com; www.vernetztes-denken.de; www.vet erinarypaper.com; www.vikaspedia.in; www.walshmedicalmedia.com; www.wassan.org; www.wethepeople.co.in; ww.worldbank.org; www.worldwidejournals.com; www.agric.gov.ab.ca; www.wds.world bank .org;

Other Online Resources

Academic.oup.com; aciar.gov.au; aesonnigeria.org; africicted.za.org; ageconsearch.umn.edu; ag-extension.blogspot.com; agricoop.gov.in; agriinventionjournal.com; agriodisha.nic.in; agritech.tnau.ac.in; agropedia.iitk.ac.in; answers.yahoo.com; arca-eg.org; archive.org; ariscom.in; asti.cgiar.org; ataribengaluru.icar.gov.in; atarik.res.in; ataripune.icar.gov.in; baadalsg.inflibnet.ac.in; baou.edu.in; benthamopen.com; biosciencediscovery.com; blog.ipleaders.in; blog.peerwith.com; blog.vantagecircle.com; bmsit.ac.in; boris.unibe.ch; brainly.in; bspublications.net; buildinformi.blogspot.com; businessdocbox.com; byjus.com; carbonmarketwatch.org; careersdocbox.com; ccari.res.in; ccsniam.gov.in; cdn.cseindia.org; cgspace.cgiar.org; change-management-toolbook.com; cirb.icar.gov.in; cirdap. org; Climate; coek.info; comms.southsudanngoforum.org; community.powerbi.com; compendium.gfras.org; conference.ifla.org; content.yudu.com; core.ac.uk; corporatefinanceinstitute.com; csankitasingla.blogspot.com; cseindia.org; csnm.kku.ac.th; cssri.org; cyberleninka.org; d.researchbib.com; dac.gov.in; damaacademia.com; de.scribd.com; departments.agri.huji.ac.il; digitalcollections.sit.edu; digitalcommons.unl.edu; discuss.itacumens.com; doaj.org; docplayer.net; docslide.us; documents.mx; documents.worldbank.org; dokumen.pub; drrajivdesaimd.com; dspace.gipe.ac.in; dspace.stir.ac.uk; dspace.uii.ac.id; dspace.unijos.edu.ng; eagri.org; earthref.org; ebin.pub; ebooks.lpude.in; eclipse.mu.ac.in; edo.csdpnigeria.org; edu.greenecosystem.in; egyankosh.ac.in; ejmcm.com; employment news.gov.in; en.wikipedia.org; enemsmicrosystresearchspot.blogspot.com; epdf.tips; eprawisdom.com; eprints.cmfri.org.in; eprints.lancs.ac.uk; epubs.icar.org.in; epw.in;

erl.ucc.edu.gh:8080; es.scribd.com; essence-journal.com; etd.aau.edu.et; ethnovetweb.com; files.eric.ed.gov; fliphtml5.Com; fr.scribd.com; fscluster. org; fsir.in; fud.edu.ng; globalforumras.org; govinfo.me; graphjam.memebase. com; greedhead.net; haryanakisanayog.org; hdl.handle.net; hdr.undp.org; heartlandmci.com; hillagric.ac.in; home.snu.edu; hrbdf.org; icar.naarm.ernet. in; icarrcer.in; icarzcu3.gov.in; ictupdate.cta.int; Id.scribd.com; idl-bnc.idrc.ca; igau.nic.in; iisjcm.org; ijarcs.info; ijas.iaurasht.ac.ir; ijcmas.com; ijellh.com; ijirset.com; ijitjournal.org; ijlr.org; ijmr.net.in; in.indeed.com; indianjournals. com; indiraisbs.ac.in; indusblog.com.pk; innovation.brac.net; inside.6q.io; ; ipindia.nic.in; ir.amu.ac.in; issuu.com; iuu.ac; jcreview.com; jendytamelab. wordpress.com; joe.org; journalcjast.com; journalijpss.com; journalofscience. org; journals.covenantuniversity.edu.ng; journals.pen2print.org; journals. sagepub.com; karriere-muster.1afirma.at; kipdf.com; Kiran.nic.in; krishi. icar.gov.in; krishikosh. egranth.ac.in; krishisanskriti.org; krishivistar.gov. in; ksmith2.teammetro.net; legalsutra.com; library.enaca.org; library.wur.nl; link.springer.com; lionsclubsindia.org; madhavuniversity.edu.in; madridge. org; mafiadoc.com; magazines.odisha.gov.in; managementstudyguide. com; medium.com; mindamas-journals .com; mirror.iasri.res.in; mpra. ub.unimuenchen.de; my mande.org; nbagr.icar.Gov.in; ngosindia.com; nhm. nic.in; nicra-icar.in; nopr.niscair.res.in; notesperdues.wordpress.com; notion press.com; odishaahvs.nic.in; opac.elte.hu; openknowledge.worldbank.org; orgprints.org; pathofupsc.blogspot.com; pdfcoffee.com; pdfs.semanticscholar. org; petererni.ch; planningcommission.gov.in; planningcommission.nic.in; powerpointpresentationon.blogspot.com; prakshal.com; praphansarn.com; pria.org; ps-survival.com; pt.scribd.com; pt.slideshare.net; purehost.bath. ac.uk; qi.nhsrcindia .org; raghukulcs.com; refubium.fu-berlin.de; reliefweb. int; repository.au-ibar.org; repository .sustech.edu; research.ijcaonline.org; rgvi.gtk.szie.hu; ride2rich.com; rtikolkata.cag.gov.in; sameti.org; saspjournals. com; scienceandnature.org; scindeks.ceon.rs; sdgasiapacific.net; seea.org.in; shag. com.ua; sharmasridhar1.blogspot.com; shodhganga.inflibnet.ac.in; silo. pub; siteresources.worldbank.org; skillville.in; slidelegend.com; slideplayer. com; snehamumbai.org; sodel.jnujaipur.ac.in; spvet.it; superioressaypapers. com; teca.fao.org; theeis.com; thereaderwiki.com; theses.lib.polyu.edu. hk; tind-customer-agecon.s3.amazonaws.com; tnau.ac.in; trendsresearch. org; ujcontent.uj.ac.za; uk.practicallaw.thomsonreuters.com; ukstudent. elevateeducation.com; unesdoc.unesco.org; unpan1.un.org; vdocuments.mx; vibdoc.com; vital.seals.ac.za:8080; wajeh.net; wbuafscl.ac.in; wizardsolution. yolasite.com; works.bepress.com; world-food.net; wps.prenhall.com.